MITOCHONDRIAL DNA - NEW INSIGHTS

Edited by **Hervé Seligmann**

Mitochondrial DNA - New Insights
http://dx.doi.org/10.5772/intechopen.72029
Edited by Hervé Seligmann
Assistant to the Editor(s): Ganesh Warthi

Contributors

Hovorun, Ol'Ha Oleksandrivna Brovarets', Jaime Villegas, Verónica Burzio, Lorena Lobos-Gonzalez, Claudio Villota, Mariela Araya, Francisca Guevara, Luis Burzio, Steinar Daae Johansen, Tor Erik Jørgensen, Eric Faure, Roxane-Marie Barthélémy, Liu Jianbin, Concepcion De-La-Rua, Montserrat Hervella, Edoardo Errichiello, Tiziana Venesio, Ganesh Warthi, Hervé Seligmann, Herve Seligmann, Genaro Gabriel Ortiz, Mario Mireles-Ramírez, Héctor González-Usigli, Miguel A Macías-Islas, Oscar Kurt Bitzer-Quintero, Erandis D Tórres-Sánchez, Angélica L. Lizeth Sánchez López., Luis Javier Ramírez-Jirano, Mónica Ríos-Silva, Blanca M Torres.Mendoza

First published in London, United Kingdom, 2018 by IntechOpen
IntechOpen is the global imprint of INTECHOPEN LIMITED, registered in England and Wales, registration number: 11086078, The Shard, 25th floor, 32 London Bridge Street
London, SE19SG – United Kingdom
Printed in Croatia

British Library Cataloguing-in-Publication Data
A catalogue record for this book is available from the British Library

Additional hard copies can be obtained from orders@intechopen.com

Mitochondrial DNA - New Insights, Edited by Hervé Seligmann
p. cm.
Print ISBN 978-1-78984-265-4
Online ISBN 978-1-78984-266-1

Meet the editor

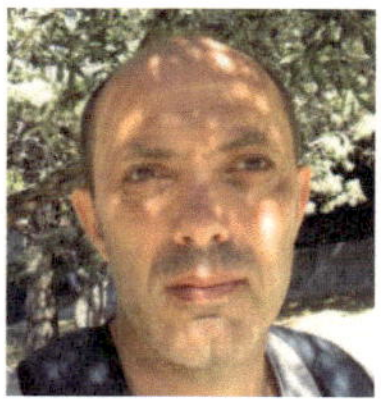

Hervé Seligmann's focus on mitochondrial DNA developed when searching for molecular mechanisms explaining developmental stability in lizards, a major topic during his PhD thesis at the Hebrew University of Jerusalem. During subsequent appointments at the University of Chicago, University of Oslo, again in Jerusalem and at Aix-Marseille University, he described >5 molecular processes affecting whole organism morphology and life history traits. This lead to the uncovering of several types of cryptic coding systems, which he describes for vertebrate mitochondria. These range from switches between alternative genetic codes (mainly stop codon translation), expanded codons, and several alternative transcriptions, based on systematic alterations of the template DNA (research ongoing).

Contents

Preface

The mitochondrial genome has always been the stepchild of modern molecular biology, perhaps because it is falsely considered as a quantitatively negligible curiosity. However, mitogenomes are probably at the crossroads of molecular biology and evolution. Mitogenomes, under constraints for size reduction, probably reflect the origin of life and its primordial coding systems by multiplying various types of sequence multifunctionalities. The evolution of mitochondrial genetic codes and the apparent use of different translation and transcription rules are notable examples. Notably, mitochondrial tRNAs differ from other tRNAs, putatively suggesting independent origins of mitochondrial tRNAs when translation evolved from transcription.

Recent phylogenetic analyses of mitochondrial proteomes also suggest that mitogenomes are an independent branch of the tree of life. Indeed, mitogenomes use an elusive non-complementary circular code that differs from the otherwise near universal self-complementary circular code used in most pro- and eukaryotes to regulate the ribosomal translation frame, as circular code motifs are conserved in tRNAs and rRNAs. This might reflect that mitogenomes are rare exceptions to Chargaff's rule that complementary nucleotides have approximately equal frequencies on any long enough single-stranded DNA or RNA sequence, evaded by single stranded genomes and organellar genomes, including mitogenomes. For mitogenomes, this is probably due to strand asymmetric replication that causes directional mutation gradients in nucleotide contents along the genome, according to distances from heavy and light strand replication (and transcription) origins.

Until additional independent evidence is found, we stick to the accepted view that mitochondria are ultrasymbiontic alphaproteobacteria. Nevertheless, the ancestral synteny observed between amoeban mitogenomes and genomes of their parasites, the giant viruses, could fit the view that mitochondria are an independent lineage, and/or that giant viruses developed from hypothetical, rare endospore-like structures formed by stressed mitochondria or their proteobacterial ancestor while switching cellular hosts. Indeed, giant viruses might be an independent, though controversial, fourth major lineage of life. Another point that mitochondria teach us in relation to the origins of life relates to the main axis of RNA evolution, from tRNA-like to rRNA-like. Several alignments and structural evidence suggest that tRNA accretions formed rRNAs, and in particular the ribosomal translational core. Mitochondrial ribosomes include, instead of a 5S rRNA subunit, a structural element consisting of an otherwise regular tRNA.

This short compilation of chapters on mitogenomes reflects the importance of mitogenomes to some extents in relation to molecular biology (chapters 1-4) as a tool in population genetics and reconstructing recent evolution (chapters 5-7), and also in the management of economically important populations, including humans (chapters 8-10).

Mitogenomes prepare more surprises such as this example perhaps even unexpected to some authors of chapters in this book: some eukaryota lack mitochondria. Mitochondria will continue to open our minds.

Hervé Seligmann
The Natural History Collections
The Hebrew University of Jerusalem
Jerusalem, Israel

Section 1

Molecular Biology

Chapter 1

True Mitochondrial tRNA Punctuation and Initiation Using Overlapping Stop and Start Codons at Specific and Conserved Positions

Eric Faure and Roxane Barthélémy

Additional information is available at the end of the chapter

http://dx.doi.org/10.5772/intechopen.75555

Abstract

In all the taxa and genomic systems, numerous *trn* genes (specifying tRNA) exhibit at specific conserved positions nucleotide triplets corresponding to stop codons (TAG/TAA). Similarly, relatively high frequencies of start codons (ATG/ATA) occur in fungi/metazoan mitochondrial-*trn* genes. The last nucleotide of these triplets is the first involved in the 5′-D- or 5′-T-stem, respectively. Their frequencies are tRNA species dependent. The products of these genes which bear one or two types of these codons are called ss-tRNAs (for stop/start). Metazoan mt-genomes are generally very compact, and many same strand overlapping sequences may simultaneously code for tRNAs and mRNAs. However, this study suggests that overlaps are not a direct mechanism to substantially reduce genome size. For protein-encoding genes, occulting possible overlaps, there are only alternative start codons and/or truncated stop codons, but the first putative in-frame standard initiation codon or complete stop codon is in the upstream or downstream overlapping ss-*trn* sequences, respectively. Even if, to date, experimental data are missing, stress signals might regulate producing extended or not proteins. Finally, possible implications of tRNA/mRNA hybrid molecules in the "RNA world" to "RNA/protein world" transition will be discussed.

Keywords: mitochondrion, tRNA origin, start codon, stop codon, overlap, origin of life, RNA world

1. Introduction

Transfer RNAs are key partners in the ribosome-translation machinery. Generally, they are composed of c.70–90 nucleotides (nts). Moreover, they are the most abundant nucleic acid species, constituting up to 10% of all cellular RNAs [1]. Therewith, the number of tRNA molecules is, e.g., about 2×10^5 in *Escherichia coli* and 3×10^6 in yeast cell [2]. Due to their anticodon, they read genetic information on mRNAs and deliver codon specified amino acids attached to their distal 3′-extremity for peptide bond synthesis on the ribosome. In this sense, tRNA is a key molecule which makes it possible to pass from a covalent bond between a RNA and an amino acid (fossil trace of the RNA world to the RNA/protein world transition) to peptide bonds (RNA/protein world). Genes specifying tRNAs (noted *trn*) are present in prokaryotic and nuclear genomes and in most of the DNAs of organelles (chloroplasts and mitochondria). Usually, tRNAs have a characteristic canonical cloverleaf secondary structure made up of the aminoacyl acceptor-stem and the D-arms (as it contains dihydrouridine), anticodon-arms, and T-arms (for the sequence TΨC where Ψ is pseudouridine), the hairpins, or "arms" consisting of a stem (helicoidal region in 3D) ending in a loop (**Figure 1**). The lengths of each arm, as well as the loop "diameter," vary from the tRNA type and from species to species. Furthermore, deduced *trn* sequences and even sequenced mature tRNAs exhibit reduced D-arms or T-arms or even lacking at least one of them, and in the extreme situation such as in *Enoplea* (nematodes) mitochondrial (mt)-*trn* genes are totally armless [3]. However, around 90% of the mt-tRNAs fold into the canonical cloverleaf structure [4]. In all the genetic systems, the tRNAs can carry a myriad of idiosyncratic posttranscriptional chemical modifications (e.g., http://modomics.genesilico.pl/; http://www.genesilico.pl/rnapathwaysdb/), and the total number of modified nts is nearly 120 [1]. Moreover, tRNAs become functional by postprocessing addition of the 3′-terminal CCA sequence. Modifications can also be necessary to ensure correct folding [4]. The tRNA folds into an L-shaped 3D structure in which two helical domains (acceptor/T and D/anticodon) are perpendicularly arranged. This particular juxtaposition of the two functional centers, the anticodon and the acceptor terminus, is essential for tRNA function. The

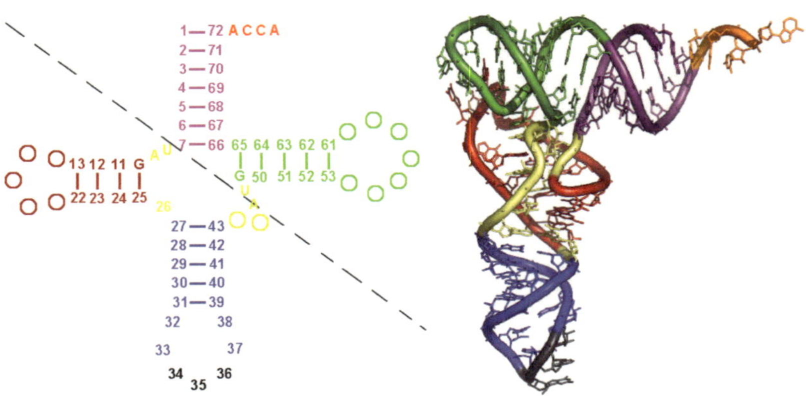

Figure 1. Typical cloverleaf secondary structure of a metazoan mt-ss-tRNA (left) with 3D image of an L-shaped tRNA (right). In 2D structure, the standard numbering was applied [5]. The first two nucleotides of the variable region and those of the D-loops and T-loops were represented by circles. The diagonal dashed line indicates the approximate separation between the "top half" and the "cherry-bob"/"bottom half". Nucleotide types were given for UAG10 and AUG49 triplets, the discriminator base (which is preferentially an A), and the CCA tail at the 3′-end. Short lines connect nucleotides forming Watson-Crick pairing within stems. Coloring: acceptor-stem in purple, D-arm in red, anticodon-arm in blue with the anticodon in black, T-arm in green, and CCA tail in orange. The yellow segments represented respectively in descending order of size, the variable region (connector 2), the connector 1 and the nt 26. 3D structure reproduced with the kind permission of Prof. N.R. Voss (Roosevelt University, Ill.) https://commons.wikimedia.org/wiki/File:3d_tRNA.png.

two domains are linked together by connector regions, one between the acceptor- and D-stems (connector 1) and the second between the anticodon- and T-stems (connector 2 which has a variable length from 0 to 21 nts and is also named variable region hereafter V-R) [5].

The ribosome allows the best possible spatial arrangement of the various partners and ensures catalysis, but the adaptor molecule which acts as a link between codes of mRNA and amino acids of polypeptides is the tRNA. In order to fill this major role, tRNAs have two distinct characteristics corresponding to two different genetic codes, the anticodon and the operational codes. The latter which is mainly embodied in the acceptor-stem allows to bind covalently and with high specificity an amino acid to a tRNA, a reaction catalyzed by a specific aminoacyl-tRNA synthetase (aaRS) [6]. The operational code might have actually predated the "classic" code associated with anticodons [7]. Moreover, the tRNAs exhibit diversity in uniqueness, all of them must be similar for entering the ribosome machinery; therefore, they generally look structurally homogeneous, especially in their secondary and tertiary structures even if "non-classical" tRNAs are known [3]. Moreover, cloverleaf structure and especially the tertiary interaction network governing the L-shaped tRNA architecture imply conserved and semiconserved bps and nts. On the other side, each type of tRNA structures must interact specifically with aaRSs and posttranscriptional modification enzymes, which implies that parts of their sequences and of their structures (as the V-R size) allow to distinguish them.

Reduced bacterial and most organelle genomes do not encode the full set of 32 tRNA species required to read all triplets of the standard genetic code according to the conventional wobble rules. Superwobbling where a single tRNA species contains modifications of the anticodon-loop, such as an hypermodified uridine at the wobble position 34 of the anticodon, reads all 4 nts at third codon position and has been suggested as a possible mechanism for how reduced tRNA sets may be functional [8]. Indeed, many metazoan mtDNAs have only a total of 22 tRNAs, apparently sufficient to recognize all codons (two tRNAs each for serine and leucine and one tRNA for each of the other 18 amino acids). However, superwobbling induces a reduced translational efficiency, which could explain why most organisms have adopted pairs of isoaccepting tRNAs over the superwobbling mechanism [9]. Moreover, e.g., in Cnidaria (sea anemones, corals, etc.) or Chaetognatha (marine invertebrates), current mtDNAs have lost several of their *trn* genes, and the absence of an apparently full set of mt-*trn* genes has also been mentioned [10]. Studies have investigated the fate of missing tRNAs and their corresponding aaRSs [11], and in many cases, the lost tRNAs are functionally replaced by imported nucleus-encoded tRNAs [10]. However, recent search strategies suggest that efficient reanalyzes detect several tRNA-like structures (TLS), which can be efficient tRNAs [12].

Compared to mitochondria found in other eukaryotic kingdoms, those of metazoa are massively reduced in their genetic structure [4]. Their mtDNA is a short, circular molecule that generally contains about 13 intronless, protein-coding genes, all of which are involved in aerobic respiration (also called oxidative phosphorylation) [13]. Moreover, the coding sequences of genes are usually separated by at most a few nts and long polycistronic precursor transcripts may be processed into mature mRNA and rRNA by precise cleavage of the 5′ and 3′-termini of the flanking tRNAs. This processing, which is known as the tRNA punctuation model [14], is mediated by RNase P and Z endonucleases, respectively [15]. However, this model is not always applicable, genes are not bound by *trn* genes or these latter may not be involved in the processing of precursor RNAs. Besides, in several taxa mt-mRNAs, rRNAs and even tRNAs may be oligoadenylated or polyadenylated [16]. This has numerous consequences with potentially dual and opposite roles: this promotes transcript stability or offers a target for initiating degradation. Overlapping genes on the same DNA strand occur throughout metazoa [17]. Therefore, the termination points of the protein-encoding genes could be difficult to infer as stop codons (generally UAA or UAG) may be absent. It is accepted that abbreviated stop codons (U or UA) are converted to UAA codons by polyadenylation after transcript cleavage, and this has been confirmed by analyzes of transcripts in some cases [18]. Sometimes, the initiation codon may also not have been detected. For several protein-encoding genes, the question of a possible overlapping with adjacent downstream or upstream *trn* genes is often raised [19]. Moreover, overlaps between adjacent mt-*trn* genes are frequent, but it is out of our topic [19, 20].

Incidentally, in 2004, searching for chaetognath mt-*trn* genes [21], it was observed that tRNAs bear nt triplets corresponding to stop or start codons at precise conserved positions, and this constitutes the original topic of this chapter.

2. Material and methods

Most of the research was done in two databases which include primary sequences and graphical representations of tRNA 2D structures, tRNAdb (http://trna.bioinf.uni-leipzig.de/DataOutput/) contained more than 12,000 *trn* genes from 579 species belonging to prokaryotes and eukaryotes, whereas in mitotRNAdb (http://mttrna.bioinf.uni-leipzig.de/mtDataOutput/), 30,525 metazoan mt-*trn* genes belonging to 1418 species were recorded [22]. Despite a bias for metazoa, these two databases provide powerful and fast search engines. Alignments were generated by Clustal W (www.ebi.ac.uk/clustalw/), whereas secondary structures were predicted by tRNAscan-SE (http://lowelab.ucsc.edu/tRNAscan-SE/) [23]. BLAST analyzes were conducted using the website: https://blast.ncbi.nlm.nih.gov/Blast.cgi.

3. Results and discussion

3.1. Frequencies of TAR10 and ATR49 triplets in various taxa

Visual observations of tRNA deduced 2D structures suggested that nt triplets which could correspond to stop or start codons seemed to be particularly represented at specific positions. The UAR (R for purine) triplets at position 8–10 in the standard numbering and therefore will be named UAR10, whereas the potential initiation codons whose last nt is at the position 49 will be called AUR49 (**Figure 1**). We chose to number the codons only according to their last nt because the nt 47 is frequently missing in the metazoan mt-tRNAs. Analyzes focus on DNA; hence, these are usually annotated TAR or ATR instead of UAR or AUR. All the tRNAs which bear one or both of these codons are named ss-tRNAs (ss for stop and start) or ss-*trn* for the corresponding genes. Using tRNAdb and mitotRNAdb databases, these triplets' frequencies were investigated in different taxa including nuclear and organelle genomes for eukaryotes (**Table 1**). Excluding taxa for which the number of *trn* genes is too low for statistical

	Nb	TAG	TAA	TAR	ATG	ATA	ATR	TAR+ ATR	TAR+ATR/ATR
Eubacteria	6383	62.2	0.63	62.8	1.61	0.20	1.82	0.58	31.9
Proteobacteria	2602	63.2	0.81	64.0	1.00	0.12	1.11	0.35	31.0
α-proteobacteria	613	67.7	0.16	67.9	0.65	0.16	0.81	0.65	80
Archaea	1081	49.2	0.93	50.1	0.00	0.09	0.09	0	0
Eukaryotes									
nuclear	2226	40.0	0.36	40.3	0.18	0.13	0.31	0.18	57.1
plastids	399	50.4	13.85	64.2	4.01	3.01	7.02	5.76	82.1
Viridiplantae*	160	59.4	7.50	66.9	3.16	1.25	4.38	3.75	85.7
Fungi*	299	32.8	8.36	41.1	4.01	13.04	17.06	11.71	68.6
*Porifera**	491	53.4	14.46	67.8	8.15	14.66	22.81	18.94	83.0
*Acoelomata**	418	45.7	9.09	54.8	17.22	7.18	24.40	13.16	53.93
*Pseudocoelomata**	277	70.0	11.55	81.6	1.08	1.08	2.17	1.44	66.7
*Protostomia**	4854	38.4	12.46	50.8	14.61	25.48	40.09	20.00	49.9
*Deuterostomia**	24398	49.6	2.25	51.8	18.89	7.99	26.89	14.46	53.8

Metazoan taxa are in italics. *Abbreviation*: Nb, number of *trn* genes. TAR + ATR for % of *trn* genes bearing the two types of triplet. * Mitochondria.

Table 1. Percentage of TAR10 and ATR49 triplets in various taxa independently of the V-R size.

analysis, TAR10 always occurs at high frequencies, whether in prokaryotic, nuclear, or organelle genomes. Values range from 41.1% for fungi to 81.6% for pseudocoelomates. In all the taxa and all tRNA species combined, the percentage of TAG10 triplets is always significantly higher than those of TAA10. The differences are very important in prokaryotic and nuclear genomes, since the percentage of TAA10 is always less than 1, while that of TAG10 is at least 40%. Within the organelle genomes, the difference is smaller but can vary by a factor of 2.5–22.

As the TAR10 triplet (principally TAG) is present in at least 40% of the *trn* genes for all taxa and genomic systems combined, it could have been present in *trn* genes of the Last Unicellular Common Ancestor (LUCA), which presumably lived some 3.5–3.8 billion years ago [24]. It is probably an ancestral character which was present in proto-*trn* sequences. As the percentage of TAA10 strongly increases in *trn* genes of organelles, one can ask whether this character was not already present in their bacterial ancestor. It is now assumed that despite their diversity, all mitochondria derive from an endosymbiotic α-proteobacterium which has been integrated into a host cell related to Asgard Archaea approximately 1.5–2 billion years ago [25]. However, the earliest fossils possessing features typical of fungi date to 2.4 billion years ago [26]. Moreover, the eukaryotic cells would be chimeras constituted of an archaebacterium and one or more Eubacteria [27]. In addition, all current models for the origin of eukaryotes suggest that the eukaryotic common ancestor had mitochondria. Therefore, as the level of TAA10 is very low in *trn* genes of α-proteobacteria, it could therefore be a derived trait that may be related to the increase in AT% in mtDNA and/or recognition constraints by mt-aaRSs and modification enzymes. Similarly, it is generally accepted that all chloroplasts and their derivatives are derived from a single cyanobacterial ancestor [28], and in current cyanobacteria, the respective percentage of TAG10 and TAA10 triplets are 62.5 and 3.6, respectively. The increase in the percentage of TAA10 characterizes organelles.

In all the taxa for all tRNA species combined, the ATR49 triplets are always present in smaller numbers than TAR10. Moreover, their numbers are negligible except in organelle genomes, mainly mitochondria. The low level of ATR49 triplets in Pseudocoelomata is due to the frequent absence of T-arm in their mt-tRNAs. In mitochondria, in some taxa, the frequency of ATG49 is higher than of ATA49, while in others, the opposite occurs. The variability is not surprising, given approximately 2 billion years of mtDNA evolution [29]. It must be noted that the nt G is overrepresented at the 5′-end of the 5′-acceptor- and D-stems, quite often at the 5′-end of the T-stem but rarely at the equivalent position of the anticodon-stem. In taxa where the percentage of ATA49 is higher than those of ATG49, G is most often not the nt majority at the 5′-end of the T-stem. Moreover, differences between the relative percentages of ATG49 and ATA49 could be due, at least in part, to variations in the AT% in organelle DNAs. The percentage of ATR49 is very low in α-proteobacteria and weaker in this last taxon compared to all Proteobacteria or Eubacteria, and it is also very weak in cyanobacteria, and so the significant rate of ATR49 triplets would seem to be a derived condition of organelle DNAs rather than a conserved primitive state lost in current prokaryotes. This trait probably appeared during the transition from endosymbiotic bacterium to permanent organelle that implied massive evolutionary changes including genome reduction, endosymbiotic and lateral gene transfers, and emergence of new genes and the retargeting of proteins [25]. The timing of the mt-endosymbiosis and of the proto-mitochondria to mitochondria transition is uncertain, but one might trace the origin of the ATR49 triplets between at least the first eukaryotic common ancestor (FECA) and the last eukaryotic common ancestor (LECA). A second event occurred, at least, in the mitochondria of the ancestors of Opisthokonta (i.e., Metazoa and Fungi), which would have led to a net increase in numbers of ATR49. ATR49 means that the last two nts of the V-R are AT. It turns out that this mainly concerns the mt-*trn* genes, whose V-R has only 4 nts, which are almost exclusively present in the Fungi/Metazoa clade.

There are large differences in the frequencies of the TAR10 and ATR49 triplets depending on the species of *trn* genes (**Table 2**) and taxa (data not shown), and the selective variations in some taxa suggest that the increase in frequency for some types of triplets would be much more recent than mentioned above; in addition, decreases are also observed. There are, however, very conservative trends such as the presence of ATR49 triplets in genes specifying tRNA-Ala. Analyzes on mt-*trn* genes of Deuterostomia for which a great number of sequences for each type are available (from 1085 to 1382) show that only the tRNA-Cys and tRNA-Glu species have intermediate TAR10 percentages (**Table 2**). In all other tRNA species, the values are extreme, 9 and 10 tRNA species with values ranging from 0.4 to 9.8% or greater than 82.4%, respectively (**Table 2**). In contrast, half of the tRNA species have low ATR49 percentages (≤ to 10.8), and for only four types percentages are ≥77.8. There would also be a tendency suggesting that tRNA species with very high or very low percentages of TAR10 most often have low ATR49 (the tRNA species with the 7 highest and the 8 lowest TAR10 percentages exhibit 10 out of 11 of the lower percentages for ATR49).

3.2. Examples of putative implications of TAR10 and ATR49 as stop and start codons

In order to investigate possible implications of TAR10 and ATR49 triplets in translation, analyzes were performed in GenBank using as keywords: "TAA stop codon is completed by the addition of 3' A residues to the mRNA", "alternative start codon" or "start codon not determined" and mitochondrion (or mitochondrial DNA) complete genome. Then, it was researched whether upstream (for start codon) or downstream (for stop codon) of the protein-encoding gene was a *trn* gene. When a *trn* gene was found, TAR10 or ATR49 triplets were searched, and the same investigation

	Trp	Asp	Arg	His	Gly	Phe	Gln	Ala	Thr	Pro	Val
TAG	95.3	98.0	93.1	91.8	97.0	97.5	97.5	94.2	92.6	91.7	81.9
TAA	4.1	1.0	5.5	6.7	1.4	0.8	0.0	1.7	3.0	2.2	0.5
TAR	99.4	99.0	98.6	98.5	98.4	98.3	97.5	95.9	95.6	93.9	82.4
ATG	1.1	1.2	0.0	6.1	0.1	70.6	0.0	89.4	20.4	11.8	8.7
ATA	9.7	0.7	0.5	50.4	0.0	7.2	0.0	7.5	0.7	5.2	16.1
ATR	10.8	1.9	0.5	56.5	0.1	77.8	0.0	96.9	21.1	17.0	24.8
	Glu	Cys	Met	Leu1	Tyr	Leu2	Ser1	Lys	Ser2	Asn	Ile
TAG	16.6	17.0	0.7	8.1	7.1	5.9	0.1	2.4	1.2	1.1	0.4
TAA	8.8	0.6	9.1	0.3	0.1	0.0	3.0	0.2	0.3	0.2	0.0
TAR	25.4	17.6	9.8	8.4	7.2	5.9	3.1	2.6	1.5	1.3	0.4
ATG	2.0	17.7	95.6	0.1	9.8	0.2	0.0	8.1	42.7	1.9	32.5
ATA	2.2	3.1	0.3	1.1	14.4	3.2	0.0	0.1	0.5	0.6	52.0
ATR	4.2	20.8	95.9	1.2	24.2	3.4	0.0	8.2	43.2	2.5	84.5

The *trn* genes are represented by three-letter codes of amino acids. The tRNAs are ordered by decreasing TAR10 percentages. The percentage values ≥ to 77.8, between 17.0 to 56.5 and ≤ to 10.8 are underlined in yellow, blue, and green, respectively.

Table 2. Percentages of TAR10 and ATR49 by mt-***trn*** gene species in Deuterostomia.

was then made in conspecific mt-genomes. Using this strategy, these triplets have been only found in metazoan mtDNAs, in which overlapping mt-*trn* genes have long been known.

An example of putative uses of TAR10 triplets as stop codons is presented in **Table 3** for a subclass of parasitic flatworms (Platyhelminthes : Eucestoda). Their mt-genetic code has only UAG and UAA as stop codons, avoiding possible bias due to use of other types of termination codons. In 51 among 66 complete mt-genomes, the first in-frame potential stop codon of the *cox1* gene is in the downstream *trnT* gene (24 cases with TAG10 suggesting a 10 nt overlap between *cox1* and *trnT* genes). Authors considering that this long overlap would be impossible have proposed a number of alternative options favoring overlap avoidance (e.g., [30]). (1) *cox1* might use an earlier atypical stop codon. (2) The 3′-end of the *cox1* mRNA could have an abbreviated stop codon (U or UA instead of UAG10) upstream the *trnT* gene which is completed by polyadenylation. (3) If in the potential long transcript, the cleavage would occur just after G10, the *cox1* mRNA would end with the complete UAG10 as stop codon and the first 10 nts of the *trnT* gene would be added by an unknown editing process. (4) The *trnT* gene would be shorter in its 5′-end lacking the nts from 1 to 8 or 9, e.g., this has been proposed for the mt-*trnT* of Cyclophyllidea (*Echinococcus granulosus*, *Hymenolepis diminuta*, and *Taenia crassiceps*). If the full stop codon is used, then there is only a single nt (G10) overlap between *cox1* and *trnT*. Moreover, if the end of the *cox*1 gene is at the level of T9, the stop codon would complete by polyadenylation; whereas if the protein gene has a complete stop codon, the nt G10 would be added by edition. In the alternative structures, the D-arm is absent, whereas it is typical for this tRNA in digeneans (a class of Platyhelminthes) and in other phyla. However, mt-*trnT* genes issuing from Cyclophyllidea for which the first potential stop codon is at different positions (upstream or downstream the *trnT* gene, or in this last gene but upstream or downstream TAG10 or at this last position) exhibit

Order	Family	Species and accession numbers	TAR10	stop cod.
Bothrioce-phalidea	Bothriocephalidae	*Schyzocotyle nayarensis* (KX060589*)	TAG^{X}	
		Schyzocotyle acheilognathi (KX589243, KX060588, KX060587, KX060590-KX060595), *Senga ophiocephalina* (KX434430)	TAG	TAG§
Caryo-phyllidea	Capingentidae Lytocestidae	*Atractolytocestus huronensis* (KY486754*), *Breviscolex orientalis* (KY486752*), *Khawia sinensis* (KY486753*)	TAG^{X}	
	Caryophyllaeidae	*Caryophyllaeus brachycollis* (KT028770)	none	TAA$^{\&}$,
	Lytocestidae	*Khawia sinensis* (KR676560)	TAG	TAA$^{\&}$,
Cyclo-phyllidea	Anoplocephalidae	*Anoplocephala magna* (KU236385), *A. perfoliata* (KR054960)	TAG	TAG§
		Moniezia benedeni (KX121040), *M. expansa* (KX121041)	TAG	TAG$^{\mu}$
	Hymenolepididae	*Hymenolepis diminuta* (AF314223*), *H. nana* (KT951722), *P. c.* (KR611041*)	TAG^{X}	
		Drepanidotaenia lanceolata (KR817910)	none	TAG$^{\$}$
		Cloacotaenia megalops (KU641017*)	TAG	TAA$^{\&}$
	Paruterinidae	*Cladotaenia vulturi* (KU559932*)	TAG^{X}	
	Taeniidae	*Echinococcus granulosus* (AF297617, KJ559023), *Hydatigera parva* (NC_021141), *Taenia arctos* (NC_024590), *T. crassiceps* (AF216699), *T. solium* (AB086256), *Versteria mustelae* (NC_021143)	TAG^{X}	
		Hydatigera krepkogorski (NC_021142)	TAG	TAA$^{\$}$
		Echinococcus canadensis (AB208063, AB235847, AB235848), *E. equinus* (AF346403, NC_020374), *E. multilocularis* (AB018440*), *E. oligarthrus* (AB208545), *E. ortleppi* (AB235846), *E. shiquicus* (AB208064)	TAG	TAG$^{\$}$
		Echinococcus vogeli (AB208546*), *Taenia asiatica* (NC_004826), *T. crocutae* (NC_024591), *T. hydatigena* (FJ518620, GQ228819), *T. multiceps* (FJ495086, GQ228818), *T. pisiformis* (GU569096), *T. regis* (NC_024589), *T. saginata* (AY684274), *T. taeniaeformis* (JQ663994, FJ597547)	TAG	TAA$^{\&}$
		Echinococcus granulosus (KU601616)	TAG	TAA$^{\mu}$
Diphyllo-bothriidea	Diphyllobothriidae	*Diphyllobothrium latum* (AB269325, DQ985706), *D. nihonkaiense* (EF420138, AB268585), *Diplogonoporus balaenopterae* (NC_017613), *D. grandis* (NC_017615), *Spirometra erinaceieuropaei* (KU852381, AB374543)	TAG^{X}	
		Spirometra decipiens (KJ599679*)	TAG	TAA$^{\&}$
Proteoce.	Proteocephalidae	*Testudotaenia* sp. (KU761587)	TAG^{X}	

Species names are followed by their accession number(s). *: sequences for which the authors of these latter considered that there was an abbreviated stop codon and this latter was upstream the *trn* sequence. Symbols: ^{X} TAR10 was the first in-frame putative stop codon; §, $^{\$}$, $^{\&}$ and $^{\mu}$, the putative stop codon was upstream the *trn* gene (*tg*), in the *tg* but upstream or downstream TAR10 or nts 8–10, downstream the *tg*, respectively. *Abbreviations*: *P. c., Pseudanoplocephala crawfordi*; Proteoce., Proteocephalidea; stop cod., putative stop codon according to the authors of the sequences.

Table 3. Position of the first complete in-frame stop codon of the ***cox1*** gene versus the following ***trnT*** gene in Cestoda (Platyhelminthes).

similar secondary structures, including a D-arm. In addition, the high level of nt conservation in the 5′-end of the *trnT* genes of cestoda (i.e., G1, G2, T7, T8, A9, G10, T11, T12 and A14) suggests strongly that the 5′-acceptor-stem and the D-stem are under positive selection. All this implies that the hypothesis of D-armless tRNAs is, according to us, improbable.

Concerning the putative ATR49 start codon, in GenBank, the number of complete mt-genomes found using the keywords previously mentioned was relatively low; moreover, in some cases, the upstream gene encoded a protein, specified a rRNA and/or there was only one mention for a given taxon. A significant example within Deuterostomia (frogs) is presented in **Table 4**. In the superfamily Hyloidea, the ATA49 triplet is frequently the first potential complete start codon at the level of the gene pair encoding and specifying NAD1 and tRNA-Leu2, respectively. In two families (Bufonidae, Hylidae), for all the sequences (16 belonging to 14 different species), the first ATR triplet found in frame in the ORF of the *nd1* gene is ATA49. For four sequences belonging to three other frog families, the ATR49 triplet is missing from the *trnL2*

Family	Species and accession numbers	ATA49 triplet	Alternative start codon
Dendro.	*Anomaloglossus baeobatrachus* (NC_030054)	none	AAA[§]
Bufonidae	*Bufo gargarizans* (NC_008410*), *B. japonicus* (NC_009886*), *B. melanostictus* (NC_005794*), *B. stejnegeri* (NC_027686*), *B. tibetanus* (NC_020048*), *Bufotes raddei* (NC_028424*)	ATA[X]	
	Bufo gargarizans (KM587710, KU321581)	ATA[X]	TAA
Cerato.	*Telmatobius chusmisensis* (KT949346), *T. bolivianus* (NC_020002)	none	TTG
Heleo.	*Heleophryne regis* (NC_019998*)	none	GTG
Hylidae	*Dryophytes suweonensis* (NC_032380*), *Hyla annectans* (NC_025309*), *H. chinensis* (NC_006403*), *H. japonica* (NC_010232*), *H. suweonensis* (NC_034238*), *H. tsinlingensis* (KU601448*, NC_026524*), *H. ussuriensis* (NC_029410*)	ATA[X]	

[X]: ATA49 as the first putative in-frame start codon. *: "start codon not determined" according to the authors of the sequences. Alternative start codons are given by the authors of the sequences. [§]: alternative start codon in the *trn* gene. *Abbreviations*: Dendro, Dendrobatidae; Cerato., Ceratophryidae; Heleo., Heleophrynidae.

Table 4. Position of the first putative start codon of the *nad1* gene versus the upstream gene specifying tRNA-Leu2 in Hyloidea, a superfamily of frogs.

gene; moreover, an ATA triplet is integrally present in the V-R of the *trnL2* gene of *Heleophryne regis*, but it is not in frame with the following gene. For these last four cases, the authors of the sequences proposed alternative start codons. This seems obligatory, but this has not been experimentally verified. For several authors who have sequenced parts of mtDNAs of Hylidae, the *nd1* gene would start at ATA49 for about 140 sequences (e.g., Roelants and Bossuyt [31]).

In the two studied taxa, Blast analyzes of the NCBI ESTs and SRA (SequenceRead Archive) databases have been performed, but no result supports the proposed hypotheses: transcripts starting at an ATR49 or terminating at a TAR10 were not found. However, for each taxon, few mt-transcripts occur, and fully matured transcripts are even rarer.

3.3. Why mt-*ss-trn* genes with TAG10 and ATR49 triplets as putative stop and start codons only occur in Metazoa?

Foremost, biases in the search strategy cannot be excluded, but the important point to note is that mt-genomes of animals, fungi, protists, and plants differ drastically in all major characteristics including gene content and large size variation. Generally, metazoans have ultra-compact mtDNAs (from c.10,000 to c.50,000 bp); usually, nonfunctional sequences are rapidly eliminated, and there are short intergenic regions and frequent overlaps [13]. However, nonbilaterian mt-genomes have higher variation in size, gene content, shape, and genetic code [32]. The mtDNA size range is from 30,000 to 90,000 bp in fungi, and generally, intergenic regions are relatively long. A broader range of mtDNA size is found in higher plants (from 0.2×10^6 to about 11.3×10^6 bp [33]), and the largest known mt-genome in this lineage exceeds sizes of reduced bacterial and nuclear genomes [34]. The increased sizes of plant mtDNAs are mostly due to noncoding DNA sequences, large inserted nuclear regions, and many introns and not to a large increase in gene numbers. The nuclear-derived sequences amount to up nearly half of their size as in melon [35], and so presence of mt-*trn* genes with nuclear origin cannot be excluded. Although not directly correlated, intergenic distances are generally much higher in larger genomes, reducing the number of overlaps. In addition, the situation of plant mt-tRNAs is very complex. Indeed, they contain few "native" tRNAs expressed from true mt-*trn* genes. They possess "chloroplast-like" *trn* genes inserted into the mtDNA. They compensate the loss of mt-*trn* genes by importing several nucleus-encoded tRNAs [36]. In addition, most often in plants, the standard code applies to the reading of organelle genomes, even if ATA is frequently used as start codon. Metazoan mt-genomes are generally small, very constrained and exhibit several gene overlaps between *trn* and protein-encoding genes or between *trn* genes. Their tRNAs have sequence and structural peculiarities and tend to shortening [19]. Our exploration is not exhaustive, but this might explain the presence of putative stop or start codons specifically within mt-*ss-trn* genes of this taxon.

One may wonder why the hypotheses concerning the TAR10 and ATR49 triplets were not proposed before? At least, the presence of these characteristic triplets could have been observed by some authors but considered as having no connection with the translation of neighboring protein genes. Among the first sequenced and the most studied were mt-genomes of *Homo sapiens* (J01415) and *Mus musculus* (J01420). In these latter, no putative start or stop codon occurs at these positions within *trn* sequences adjacent to protein genes (data not shown).

3.4. Some known structures in the living world bearing a start or stop codon at least in part of a stem-loop structure

In the living world, many nucleic sequences with secondary structures playing a physiological role involving stop and/or start codons have been discovered. Some representative examples are briefly presented here. (1) The tropism switching of the bacteriophage BPP-1 is mediated by a phage-encoded diversity-generating retroelement, which introduces nt substitutions in a gene that specifies a host cell-binding protein (*Mtd*) [37]. The nt substitutions are introduced in a variable repeat located at the 3′-end of this gene. Two nts after this region, the UAG stop codon is present, and its last nt is situated at the 5′ beginning of the 5′-stem of a hairpin. Both the UAG codon and hairpin are required for phage tropism switching. (2) Programmed translational bypassing is a process, whereby ribosomes "ignore" a substantial interval of mRNA sequence. In a bacteriophage T4 gene, bypassing requires translational blockage at a "takeoff codon" immediately upstream of the UAG stop codon, and both codons are in the 5′-stem of a hairpin; moreover, this region is mobile [38]. (3) The operon *flgFG* of the bacterium *Campylobacter jejuni* can encode two genes (*flgF* and *flgG*). Its expression in *E. coli* produces a fusion protein probably due to ribosomal frameshifting (translational hopping) [39]. The putative hop region contains, among others, a hairpin beginning by the last nt of the UAA stop codon of the first mRNA. The AUG start codon of the second gene is in the loop of the following hairpin. (4) In Eubacteria, riboswitches are regulatory segments of DNA or mRNA that can bind a small molecule (the effector), which repress or activate their cognate genes at transcriptional and/or translational levels. In the riboflavin and *cob* operons, conformational changes can form a stem loop which sequesters the translational start site, consisting of the Shine-Dalgarno (SD) sequence plus start codon thus preventing gene translation [40]. (5) Bacterial transfer-messenger RNAs (tmRNAs) have dual TLS and mRNA-like properties. They rescue stalled ribosomes on mRNAs lacking proper translational stop signal; the tRNA-like structure acts first as an alanine-tRNA, and then the short mRNA reading frame is translated and the product is released [41]. This *trans*-translation terminates at the stop codon terminating the tmRNA reading frame. This stop can be in a little loop or totally or partially integrated in the stem of a hairpin-like structure. In eukaryotes, structurally reduced tmRNAs (no mRNA-like domain) rarely occur in chloroplasts [42] and in mt-genomes (in Jakobids, presumably close to the most ancient living eukaryotes with bacterial-like mt-genome) [41]. Moreover, tmRNA TLSs function even without any canonical initiation factors. These examples show that start or stop codons located in hairpin may have various functions, as we suggest for TAR10 and ATR49.

3.5. Multifunctionality of tRNAs

Ancient tRNAs probably had diverse functions in replication and proto-metabolism before protein translation [43] and modern tRNAs have also various functions in all the living organisms [1]. These functions include cell wall synthesis, protein N-terminal modification, nutritional stress management, porphyrin biosynthesis (heme and chlorophyll), lipid remodeling, and initiation of retrovirus reverse transcription. Accumulating experimental evidence suggests also that they have important regulatory roles in translation, viral infections, and tumor development (reviewed in [44]). Mt-tRNAs interfere with a cytochrome *c*-mediated apoptotic pathway and promote cell survival [45] and function as replication origins [46]. Moreover, nuclear-tRNA abundance and modifications are dynamically regulated, and tRNAs and their tRNA-derived RNA fragments (tRFs) are centrally involved in stress signaling and adaptive translation [47, 48]. This suggests that the choice of cleavage sites of mRNA transcripts with or not part of the neighboring ss-tRNA could be dynamic and also respond to environmental changes. Some of the noncanonical translation functions of tRNAs can also be driven or enhanced by their ability to adopt different complex three-dimensional structures, and these conformational changes can be linked to functional states [49]. Moreover, the tRNA multifunctionality has also been considered to be, at least in part, random due to the high amount of tRNA species within the cell [1]. In addition, the mt-*trn* genes represent natural pause sites for replication forks and could also prone double-strand breaks [50], and their role, as "punctuation signals," for processing of mtDNA polycistronic transcripts has already been mentioned.

Enormous numbers of tRFs in all domains of life were found in the last decade [44]. In the plant *Arabidopsis thaliana*, nucleus-, plastid-, and mt-encoded tRNAs can produce tRFs [36]. The tRFs are not randomly degraded tRNAs. Experiments showed several functions including regulation of tumor development and viral infections [44]. Degradations resulting from cleavages at TAR10 and ATR49 triplets could produce a conformation exhibiting two loops linked by a forked-stem structure, roughly resembling a pair of cherries, so called "cherry-bob" (**Figure 2**). Our hypothesis predicts this structure which however has never been observed [51].

3.6. Other putative roles of TAR10 and ATR49

Metazoan mt-genomes are believed optimized for rapid replication and transcription. Potentially, TAG10 and ATR49 make transcription/translation more complex but perhaps more efficient. Examples in the Section 3.2 (i.e., Eucestoda) suggest mt-overlaps appeared 100s millions of years (MY) ago, enabling co-evolution between protein-encoding genes and those specifying tRNA.

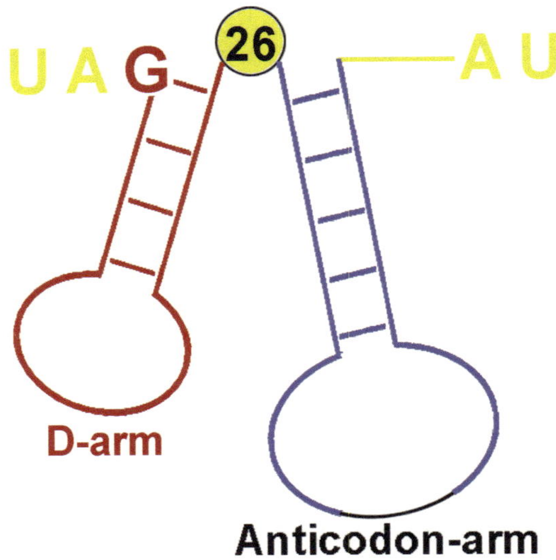

Figure 2. 2D "cherry-bob"/"bottom half" structure. AUG/UAG triplets are discussed in text. Colors as **Figure 1**.

Overlaps involve numerous constraints for genes including sequence bias. Constraints are probably less stringent for *trn* genes, which can evolve rapidly because relatively standard secondary structure coupled with a specific anticodon might suffice for tRNA function [52]. Incomplete cloverleaf structures may also be repaired post-transcriptionally [53].

Alternative processing might be possible for the production of either a supposed complete mRNA or a complete tRNA. In the first case, the synthesis of new complete mRNAs could be promoted by high mitosolic tRNA numbers. Moreover, amino acid starvation can regulate mt-tRNA levels [54]. However, if mt-tRNAs already present are not destroyed, translation would not immediately stop because mt-tRNA half-life which is lower than that of their cytosolic counterparts can nevertheless exceed 10 h [54]. Moreover, aberrant mt-tRNAs can be corrected by RNA editing during or after transcription, and this process appeared independently several times in a wide variety of eukaryotes [5]. As an extreme example, due to large overlaps between *trn* genes, up to 34 nts are added post-transcriptionally during the editing process to the mt-tRNA sequences encoded in an onychophora species, rebuilding the acceptor-stem, the T-arm, and in some extreme cases, the V-R and even a part of the anticodon-stem [55]. In that species, several edition types must be combined, including template-dependent editing [55]. This last example suggests that complete tRNA could be restored after a cleavage just upstream of ATR49. However, edition of parts of the 5′-end of tRNAs seems more problematic. Besides, mRNAs with upstream or downstream ss-tRNA can form a partially double strand region with a homologous ss-tRNA at the level of the acceptor-stem. This might induce mRNA degradation via antisense mechanisms. In bacteria, uncharged tRNAs cause antisense RNA inhibition [56], and small interfering cytosolic tRNA-derived RNAs exist [57]. Modifications (methylation, edition, etc.) of incomplete tRNAs generated after cleavages of polycistronic transcripts at TAR10 or ATR49 triplets would indicate regulatory functions.

Putative use of TAR10 or ATR49 triplets affects protein length. When in frame, this could generate a protein at least 3 or 9 amino acids longer, respectively. Extension length depends on positions of upstream stop codons completed by polyadenylation and/or on downstream (alternative) initiator codons. Not only complete proteins may be functional. Depending on cleavage positions in polycistronic transcripts, consequences may be neutral, disadvantageous, or favorable in specific contexts. In yeast, extended proteins can increase fitness under stress conditions [58]. In addition, in bacteria and in organelles, alternative initiation codons decrease efficiency [5], and it must be noted that ATR49 triplets are "canonical" start codons.

In other conditions, incomplete mRNAs could be favored. Mitosolic mRNA accumulations can be due to lack of translation because of tRNA paucity. Thus, high mRNA levels might indirectly promote cleavage of entire tRNA transcripts while reducing the synthesis of new functional mRNAs and favoring translation of those which are already present into proteins. Presence/absence of hairpins involving stop or start codons might regulate translation. This regulation could involve proteins that stabilize the hairpins or posttranscriptional modifications. Moreover, translational products of "incomplete" mRNAs might have housekeeping functions.

Regulation of alternative processing producing either complete tRNAs or complete mRNAs requires elucidation. Factors, probably proteins, need characterization. Note that metazoan mt-*atp8* and *atp6* genes overlap (mainly by 10 bp in vertebrates) and are transcribed as joint bicistronic transcript [59]. This proven overlap is inherent to mt-metabolism. Hence, similar overlaps assumed for TAR10 triplets are plausible.

Overlap conservation might reflect the need to produce bicistronic transcripts (5′-tRNA-mRNA-3′ or 5′-mRNA-tRNA-3′) or functional constraints at protein level (i.e., preserving specific amino acid patterns upstream or downstream the ORF). When overlap regions have conserved, amino acid sequences at the protein N- or C-terminal functional constraints at protein level for overlaps are probable [19]. In viruses, mutation rates are low in DNA regions coding for multiple protein products in separate reading frames (called overprinted genes) because point mutations compatible with functional products from all frames are rare. In these regions, the frame is said "close off." Partial overlap between protein-encoding genes and *ss-trn* genes would present similar situations explaining greater conservation of extremities of protein and tRNA sequences when the corresponding genes overlap. This lock almost only concerns the ss-tRNA's "top half," limiting changes in the region interacting with many processing enzymes. The *ss-trn* genes could also regulate translation upstream, bicistronic mRNA/ss-tRNA transcripts could be more stable, and likewise, ss-*trn* genes could also play roles in replication and transcription.

3.7. Methylation of *trn* genes and tRNAs and their possible roles in transcription and translation

Methylation is much rarer in mt- than nuclear-DNA [60]. However, these might occur at *trn* genes (particularly around TAR10 and ATR49) and might have deleterious consequences especially because differential mtDNA methylations are linked to aging and diseases (including diabetes and cancers) [60]. Methylation of nts of UAR10 and AUR49 is known as those of A9 and G10 which can be important for correct tRNA foldings [61]. We are unaware whether posttranscriptional modifications occur on bicistronic mt-transcripts containing complete or partial tRNAs. This would be worth investigating including possible consequences on maturation and translation.

3.8. Reassignments of codons and ss-tRNA

Several codon-amino acid reassignments are known, mainly from mitochondria [62, 63]. In 11 different mt-genetic codes, UGA stops code for tryptophan and AUA codes for methionine instead of isoleucine in 8 and 5 mt-genetic codes, respectively [63]. Both reassignments avoid potential errors along traditional wobble rules. Reassigning UGA-stop to UGA-Trp fits the "capture" hypothesis, and UGA codons mutate first to synonymous UAA codon in AT-rich mt-genomes. Then, UGA reappears occasionally by mutations, free for "capture" by an amino acid, like Trp [64]. AUA is frequently used as alternative initiation codon. Its reassignment to internal sense Met codon could also have evolved in AT-rich genomes. Moreover, the standard genetic code assigns six codons to arginine, whereas two would fit arginine's relatively low frequency in current proteins [65]. In 8 out of 11 mt-codes, different strategies reduce Arg codons to four, AGR reassignments to other amino acids (in six genetic codes), lack of two Arg codons (CGA and CGC yeast mt-code), and AGR as terminators in vertebrates. These AGR codons were believed mt-stop codons since early vertebrate evolution [66]. However, at least in humans, AGRs are not recognized terminators [67], suggesting that AGRs have no assignment. Hence, the vertebrate mt-genetic code could be the most optimized known genetic code (that of yeast was not retained because four Leu codons were reassigned to Thr). Characteristics of the nt triplets at the position 8–10 and ending at position 49 should be analyzed for each mt-genetic code.

3.9. Origin of the cloverleaf structure of tRNA and ss-tRNA

Various models could explain tRNA origins (see reviews [68–70]). The modern tRNA cloverleaf structure might result from direct duplication of primordial RNA hairpins (e.g., [68]). However, studies lend strong support to the "two halves" hypothesis [43], in which tRNAs consist of two coaxially stacked helices with presumed independent structural and functional domains. These correspond to the "top half" containing the acceptor-stem and the T-arm and the "bottom half" with the D-arm and anticodon-arm (**Figure 1**). The 2D representation of the latter corresponds to the "cherry-bob" structure (**Figure 2**). The "top half" of modern tRNA embeds the "operational code" in the identity elements of the acceptor-stem that interacts with the catalytic domain of specific aaRSs and is recognized by RNases P and Z and the CCA-adding enzyme (therefore mainly RNA end processing reactions) [70, 71]. This domain also interacts with translation elongation factor Tu and one rRNA subunit [71]. The importance of this domain in most macromolecular interactions involving tRNAs (including *in vitro* even when it is detached from the "bottom half") suggests that these half's specificities were established before the tRNA's "bottom half," presumably incorporated later [72]. Growing evidence for tRNA elements involved in both RNA and DNA replication with the 3′-end playing a determinant role has led to the idea that the "top half" initially evolved for replication in the RNA world before the advent of protein synthesis [73]. The supposed evolutionarily recent tRNA "bottom half" provides genetic code specificity. This suggests late implementation of the standard genetic code and late appearance of interactions between the tRNA "bottom half" and ribosomes [74]. Whether the "bottom half" derived from a loop or extra loop belonging to the "top half" or was an independent structural and functional domain that was subsequently incorporated into the "top half" remains unresolved [71]. Some authors suggest independent evolutionary origins [71, 72].

The study of ss-tRNAs suggests a model partially explaining canonical tRNA origins (**Figure 3**). The DNA region specifying the "bottom half" would be integrated in a sequence that can specify the "top half" but at the junction between the parts corresponding to the 3′-end of the 5′-acceptor stem and the 5′-end of the 5′-T-stem.

On the other hand, the "bottom half"/"cherry bob" structure could also be integrated at RNA level, either in the RNA world by intermolecular RNA-RNA recombination or template switches or later with retrotranscription events. Fujishima and Kanai [70] also proposed an equivalent model where a long hairpin corresponding to about the "top half" region merged with a viral RNA element corresponding to the "bottom half" to give the TLS found in modern viral genomes (who however possessed a pseudoknotted acceptor-stem). Besides, rare pre-tRNA molecules from the three domains of life exhibit an intron. The intron's origin is debated. The "introns-early" scenario assumes most of them were lost during evolution, and the opposite scenario theorizes that introns were inserted into some *trn* genes after their emergence [75]. To date, our hypothesis would rather favor the second scenario, even though it could be considered that the "cherry bob" structure could be an ancestral intron becoming unspliceable.

In tRNAs, the two first nts of both UAR10 and AUR49 belong to connector 1 and 2, respectively. They are thus at the junction between the top and bottom halves and are very close physically in the 3D structure (**Figure 1**). The belonging of some of the nts of the TAR10 and ATR49 triplets to either of the two parts is not discussed here because the theoretical model of **Figure 3** is applicable independently of "bottom half" extremities. However, as the V-R is important for aminoacylation [76], ATR49 triplets could rather integrally belong to the "top half." The tRNA L-shape is stabilized by various tertiary interactions of the V-R with the D-arm and between the D- and T-loops. Nucleotides of the connectors form contacts with the D-arm, and in some

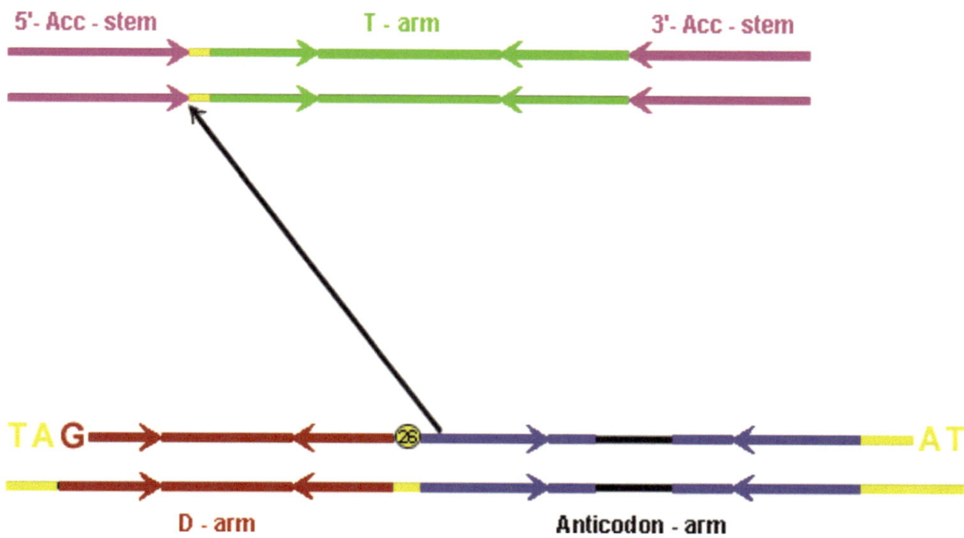

Figure 3. Proposed model for the origin of genes specifying tRNAs with canonical cloverleaf structure. It can be summarized by insertion (follow the arrow) of the region specifying the "bottom half" into those specifying the "top half". Here, the entire TAG10 triplet presumably belonged to the "bottom half" region as well as the first 2 nts of ATG49. Colors as **Figure 1**.

tRNAs, the G10 can establish potential tertiary interactions with a nt of the V-R upstream the putative start codon [77]. At least in cytosolic tRNAs, frequently U8 and sometimes U48 form noncanonical pairs. Moreover, generally, base pair 15–48 is more conserved in mt-tRNAs than 8–14, and this is probably due to the fundamental role played by the first in maintaining the tRNA L-shape [5]. UAR10 and AUR49 had to play first only a role in the L-shaped tertiary structure of tRNAs, and their implication as codons, if it exists, would be only a derived character. It was hypothesized that DNA punctuation evolved from 2D structures signaling polymerization initiation, termination, and/or processing to linear sequence motifs, which further evolved to translational signals [78]. In ss-tRNA, UAR10 triplet probably already plays a structural role in proto-tRNAs, whereas AUR49 would have appeared only during the evolution of organelle tRNAs and was related to L-shaped tertiary structures of organelle tRNAs and due to severe genome reduction and extreme base compositions. The opposite hypothesis would imply that the AUR49 triplet would have been a plesiomorphic character counter-selected in large genomes but kept in certain bacterial genomes up to mt-ancestors.

3.10. tRNAs at the origin of all the nucleic members of the RNA/protein world

Some authors have hypothesized that tRNAs may be the precursors of mRNAs, rRNAs (and therefore proto-ribosomes), and also of the first genomes. Several suggested similar origins for tRNA and rRNA [79]. Analyzes of sequences and secondary structures of ribosome suggested that the ribosomal peptidyl transferase center (PTC) which forms peptide bonds between adjacent amino acids originates from fused proto-tRNAs [80]. Strikingly, the ribosome is a ribozyme, since only RNA catalyzes peptide bond formation [81]. Otherwise, current eubacterial rRNAs themselves could encode several tRNAs [82] and chaetognath *16S rRNA* genes appear as tRNA nurseries [12] (or the opposite). Eubacterial 5S rRNAs contain TLSs similar to alanine and arginine tRNAs [82], exhibiting tRNA-like 2D structures [83]. Some suggest that rRNAs are fused tRNA molecules [80].

Molecular biology dogmatically assumes that "tRNA genes are of course entirely noncoding" [84]. But in 1981, Eigen and Winkler-Oswatitsch suggested that in the RNA world to the RNA/protein world transition, ancestral tRNAs were mRNAs [85]. Assuming that the first mRNAs had been recruited from proto-tRNAs, it follows that TLSs were inside viral and cellular mRNAs [86]. Self-recognition between tRNA-like mRNAs and canonical cloverleaf tRNAs could stabilize these molecules and produce proto-proteins [87]. The first proteins potentially emerged from junctions of ancestral tRNAs, and among the modern proteins, the only polymerase which matched with tRNAs translated like a mRNA was the RNA-dependent RNA polymerase [87]. Otherwise, eubacterial rRNAs could also encode several active sites of key proteins involved in the translation machinery [82]. Then, analyzes of sequences and secondary structures of ribosomes suggested that these derived from tRNAs also functioned as a protogenome [82]. The very parsimonious syncretic model "tRNA core hypothesis" assumes that some proto-tRNAs were classical tRNAs and also functioned as rRNAs and mRNAs, a self-recognition between these molecules allowed to obtain proto-proteins [88].

Assuming that the ATR49 triplets are a primitive character lost during the first genome expansions and that they could already act as an initiation codon seems too speculative, but RNA structures having characteristics of ss-tRNAs could have accumulated many advantages in

http://dx.doi.org/10.5772/intechopen.75555

the RNA/protein world. Structures with both start and stop codons partially in a stem-loop (as ss-tRNA), constituting basic signals for translation, could be a missing link of the RNA world hypothesis. Furthermore, in these proto-tRNAs, 3D structures could act as initiation and termination signals before the emergence of standard codons. Moreover, mRNAs in the form of ss-tRNA or a combination of several of these molecules would have been relatively stable. The cloverleaf structure could facilitate its entry into the PTC, and then interactions with other factors could allow a short region to be in linear form and thus could be read. Upstream and downstream of the linear region, the arrangement in hairpins protected the proto-mRNA from degradation during its reading, and as soon as a long enough region was read, it could take again its original 3D structure. Otherwise, circular proto-mRNAs derived from ss-tRNA-like molecules could not be excluded, although the hypothesis of circular tRNA-like ancestor ("proto-tRNA") was first proposed by Ohnishi in 1990 [89]. Furthermore, nuclear-encoded mt-tRNAs of Kinetoplastid protists are imported into the mitochondrion, and circularized mature tRNA molecules are produced probably by mt-endogenous RNA ligase activity (*in vivo* or during mt-isolation) [90]. Moreover, in red and green algae and possibly in one Archaea, the maturation of permuted *trn* genes, in which the sequences encoding the 5′-half and 3′-half of the specific tRNA are separated and inverted on the genome, needs the formation of a characteristic circular RNA intermediate which after cleavage at the acceptor-stem generates the typical cloverleaf structure with functional termini [91]. If in a ss-tRNA with a T-loop of 7 nts, the nt72 is ligated to the nt1; this creates a small ORF starting with a start codon (AUR49), which potentially codes for a peptide of 12 amino acids if UAR10 is used as stop codon. However, the circularization could be done elsewhere than at levels of nts 72 and 1. Thus, UAR10 would not be in frame, and therefore, this could allow the synthesis of smaller or longer peptides. To date, the formation of this type of structure and its translation remains hypothetical; however, experimental data shown that circular RNAs can be translated in prokaryotic and eukaryotic systems in the absence of any particular element for internal ribosome entry as SD sequence, poly-A tail, or cap structure [92]. Therefore, the evolutionary advantage of a circular proto-mRNA is also posited to be the simplicity of its replication mechanism and not be able to be degraded by the extremities that do not have one.

Besides, the fusion of tRNA-like mRNA and a classical tRNA could be at the origin of the ancestors of tmRNAs, and it can be mentioned just for guidance that the size of the tag peptide encoded by bacteria is of the same order of magnitude as those corresponding to putative translation of a ss-tRNA from the ATR49 triplet. Moreover, evolution of self-charging proto-tRNAs may also be selected [93], it has even been proposed that the activity of the juxtaposed 2′/3′-OHs of the tRNA A76 ribose qualifies tRNA as a ribozyme [94] and some RNAs (the early tRNA adaptor) must have had the ability to undergo 3′-aminoacylation. It has also been previously shown that many hairpin-structured RNAs bear ribozyme activity. These catalyze self-cleavage and ligation reactions [95]. In addition, it remains possible that circular ss-tRNAs with amino acid-anchored structure could be at the origins of tmRNAs. Indeed, two-piece bacterial tmRNAs (e.g., in α-proteobacteria) are encoded by a circularly permuted gene sequence implying that pre-tmRNA is processed, and that the two pieces are held together by noncovalent interactions. Moreover, in line with an α-proteobacterial origin of mitochondria, probable mt-encoded circular permuted *tmRNA* genes have been found in the oomycete (water mold) *Phytophthora sojae* and in the jakobid *Reclinomonas americana* [96]. A proto-*trnA* gene could be at the origin of modern tmRNAs [41]. Metazoan mt-*trnA* genes combine the highest levels of TAR10 and ATR49 triplets (>95% for each), but in the prokaryotic world, if the rate of TAG10 is always higher than 91%, only one ATR49 occurs in Eubacteria and none in Archaea.

4. Conclusions

Studies strongly suggest that the tRNA cloverleaf structure unfolded prior to the appearance of a fully functional ribosomal core, making it one of the most ancient RNAs of the RNA world [70, 97] or even the oldest [98]. Though the "RNA-world" hypothesis is well accepted, the successive events leading to the emergence of different partners playing a role in translation and the involvement of tRNAs in this evolution are highly controversial coveted field [99]. However, some hypotheses as the "tRNA core" [88] strongly suggest that tRNAs would be at the origin of the primitive genetic material and gave rise to mRNA and rRNA, as well as the conformational structure of the first proto-ribozymes. The base module being a pleiofunctional RNA that can adopt the cloverleaf structure is found today in various sequences without direct link with translation. One may conclude that "one should not change a winning secondary structure." In a precellular context, a molecule with ss-tRNA characteristics (small ORF associated with cloverleaf structure) would be advantageous. Putatively, ss-tRNA-like molecules cumulating both tRNA and mRNA functions would have been the first molecules on Earth to support nonrandom protein synthesis.

The antiquity of ss-tRNAs can be discussed, and it is very likely that the TAR10 (and especially TAG) triplets played very early a critical role in the tertiary folding of some tRNAs. Their implication in translation termination would be an exaptation where firstly, they were part of a structural signal. Origin of ATR49 triplets is less clear perhaps tracing to the first endosymbiosis. Hence it would be apomorphic (derived character). Analyzes by taxa and tRNA species suggest a nonhomogeneous evolution. At the beginning of the RNA/protein world, it has quickly become essential to start peptide synthesis at particular codons and one cannot exclude that ATR49 was an ancestral state which would have not been retained as intergenic spaces increased. Analyzes of known tRNAs of α-proteobacteria and cyanobacteria could suggest that in organelles, ATR49 triplets would have been selected with genome reduction. Organelle genomes may be under increased pressure for size reduction with resulting overlaps (see, [100]). However, several features strongly suggest that overlapping genes are not a direct mechanism to substantially reduce genome size. Gene overlaps allow mtDNA genome compaction while avoiding the loss of tRNA genes [53]. Nevertheless, overlaps may allow a more efficient control in the regulation of gene expression, the regulatory pathways are simplified, and the number of proteins (and genes) required decreases [100]. Among others, short antiparallel overlaps may be involved in antisense regulatory mechanisms. Consequently, genomes with compact sizes enable putatively less flexible but more efficient physiologies.

The selection of tRNAs had to be done mainly on two seemingly opposite criteria, stability and plasticity, making it a kind of Swiss army knife of the RNA world. This explains that beyond their central role in protein synthesis, tRNAs have many other crucial functions. To date, it can be hypothesized that ss-tRNAs might regulate gene expression, stress responses, and metabolic processes. Indeed, *in silico* analyzes allowed to speculate that several overlapping sequences may code simultaneously for mRNAs and tRNAs in most of the metazoan mt-genomes. These overlaps can have a variable (sometimes large) number of nts; however, when annotating their genomes, several authors voluntarily underestimated the number and the size of overlaps, speculating that there would be upstream abbreviated stop codons or downstream alternative start codons but most often without any direct demonstration so far. However, the high number of possible overlaps on the same strand in which the first in-frame complete stop codon or standard start codon are located at specific positions in the sequences of *trn* genes (TAR10 and ATR49, respectively) strongly suggest an exclusive relationship between obtaining tRNAs and translation of mRNAs and/or the development of repair system to keep the two genes functional due in some cases to co-evolution during several hundred MY. We can therefore speculate that ss-*trn* genes could allow true tRNA punctuation and initiation. Noted that ss-tRNAs seem to be hybrid molecules which would contain three essential coding or decoding informations in the form of nt triplets (i.e., anticodon and stop/start codons) which are all at least in part integrated into stem or loop; moreover, after the ATR49, nt triplets play the role of internal sense codons. To date, it is unclear what biochemical mechanism would allow to choose between different alternate cleavage sites, leading to the complete tRNA rather than to the mRNA or *vice versa*, but reduced/expanded proteins can be functional, and various processes including editing suggest this also for incomplete tRNAs. Hence, despite lacking experimental evidence, TAR10 and ATR49 triplets have probable roles, including regulation. Future analyzes of the processed bicistronic transcripts (tRNA/protein-encoding or the contrary) are required. Moreover, even if mt-*trn* genes are most often expressed at very low levels [53], only direct sequencing of tRNAs can validate transcription, epitranscriptomic maturation and can pinpoint nt modifications including post-transcriptionally edited positions. Purified native, or even synthetic, tRNAs should also be tested for their *in vitro* activity to confirm the functionality of aberrant transcripts. Similar experiments must be made on the flanking mRNAs and their products. If as we think, ss-tRNAs could play regulatory roles, initially experiments should compare stress and nonstress conditions.

Here, the bias for metazoan mtDNA does not allow for a complete picture of variation in the entire eukaryotic world, and protist mt-genomes should also be considered. Special attention should also be paid to noncanonical base pairings potentially formed by UAR10 and AUR49 nts, in perspective with tRNA structure and V-R length. Accounting for TAR10 and ATR49 triplet presences in the algorithms predicting tRNAs could improve mt-genome annotations, reducing numbers of false positives and negatives, and more accurately determine tRNA termini while accounting tRNA species, taxa, and genomic systems.

MtDNA plays a central role in apoptosis, aging, and cancer [13]. Moreover, mt-diseases are among the most common inherited metabolic and neurological disorders [101]. In addition, as new functions and new mechanisms of action of tRNAs are continuously discovered [1] and as ss-*trn* genes could affect the cellular dynamic during normal and stress conditions leading to pathologies, potential subtleties of action and regulation of these genes and products should be more thoroughly investigated.

Conflict of interest

The authors declare no potential commercial or financial conflicts of interest.

Author details

Eric Faure* and Roxane Barthélémy

*Address all correspondence to: eric.faure@univ-amu.fr

Aix Marseille University, CNRS, Centrale Marseille, I2M, Marseille, France

References

[1] Barciszewska MZ, Perrigue PM, Barciszewski J. tRNA-the golden standard in molecular biology. Molecular BioSystems. 2016;**12**:12-17. DOI: 10.1039/c5mb00557d

[2] Li S, Mason CE. The pivotal regulatory landscape of RNA modifications. Annual Review of Genomics and Human Genetics. 2014;**15**:127-150. DOI: 10.1146/annurev-genom-090413-025405

[3] Wende S, Platzer EG, Jühling F, Pütz J, Florentz C, Stadler PF, Mörl M. Biological evidence for the world's smallest tRNAs. Biochimie. 2014;**100**:151-158. DOI: 10.1016/j.biochi.2013.07.034

[4] Bernt M, Braband A, Schierwater B, Stadler PF. Genetic aspects of mitochondrial genome evolution. Molecular Phylogenetics and Evolution. 2013;**69**:328-338. DOI: 10.1016/j.ympev.2012.10.020

[5] Lang BF, Lavrov D, Beck N, Steinberg SV. Mitochondrial tRNA structure, identity and evolution of the genetic code. In: Bullerwell CE, editor. Organelle Genetics. Berlin: Heidelberg; 2012. pp. 431-474. DOI: 10.1007/978-3-642-22380-8_17

[6] Francklyn C, Perona JJ, Puetz J, Hou YM. Aminoacyl-tRNA synthetases: Versatile players in the changing theater of translation. RNA. 2002;**8**:1363-1372. DOI: 10.1017/S1355838202021180

[7] Schimmel P, Giege R, Moras D, Yokoyama S. An operational RNA code for amino acids and possible relation to genetic code. Proceedings of the National Academy of Sciences of the United States of America. 1993;**90**:8763-8768. DOI: 10.1073/pnas.90.19.8763

[8] Agris PF, Vendeix FA, Graham WD. tRNA's wobble decoding of the genome: 40 years of modification. Journal of Molecular Biology. 2007;**366**:1-13. DOI: 10.1016/j.jmb.2006.11.046

[9] Rogalski M, Karcher D, Bock R. Superwobbling facilitates translation with reduced tRNA sets. 1. Nature Structural & Molecular Biology. 2008;**15**:192-198. DOI: 10.1038/nsmb.1370

[10] Huot JL, Enkler L, Megel C, Karim L, Laporte D, Becker HD, Duchêne AM, Sissler M, Maréchal-Drouard L. Idiosyncrasies in decoding mitochondrial genomes. Biochimie. 2014;**100**:95-106. DOI: 10.1016/j.biochi.2014.01.004

[11] Haen K, Pett W, Lavrov D. Parallel loss of nuclear-encoded mitochondrial aminoacyl-tRNA synthetases and mtDNA-encoded tRNAs in Cnidaria. Molecular Biology and Evolution. 2010;**27**:2216-2219. DOI: 10.1093/molbev/msq112

[12] Barthélémy RM, Seligmann H. Cryptic tRNAs in chaetognath mitochondrial genomes. Computational Biology and Chemistry. 2016;**62**:119-132. DOI: 10.1016/j.compbiolchem.2016.04.007

[13] Ladoukakis ED, Zouros E. Evolution and inheritance of animal mitochondrial DNA: Rules and exceptions. Journal of Biological Research-Thessaloniki. 2017;**24**:2. DOI: 10.1186/s40709-017-0060-4

[14] Ojala D, Montoya J, Attardi G. tRNA punctuation model of RNA processing in human mitochondria. Nature. 1981;**290**:470-474. DOI: 10.1038/290470a0

[15] Levinger L, Mörl M, Florentz C. Mitochondrial tRNA 3′ end metabolism and human disease. Nucleic Acids Research. 2004;**32**:5430-5441. DOI: 10.1093/nar/gkh884

[16] Kyriakou E, Chatzoglou E, Zouros E, Rodakis GC. The rRNA and tRNA transcripts of maternally and paternally inherited mitochondrial DNAs of *Mytilus galloprovincialis* suggest presence of a "degradosome" in mussel mitochondria and necessitate the re-annotation of the l-rRNA/CR boundary. Gene. 2014;**540**:78-85. DOI: 10.1016/j.gene.2014.01.080

[17] Fiedler M, Rossmanith W, Wahle E, Rammelt C. Mitochondrial poly(A) polymerase is involved in tRNA repair. Nucleic Acids Research. 2015;**43**:9937-9949. DOI: 10.1093/nar/gkv891

[18] Wolstenholme DR. Animal mitochondrial DNA: Structure and evolution. International Review of Cytology. 1992;**141**:173-216. DOI: 10.1016/S0074-7696(08)62066-5

[19] Morrison D. How and where to Look for tRNAs in Metazoan Mitochondrial Genomes, and What you might Find when you Get there [Internet]. 2010. DOI: 10.1101/001875 Available from: http://arxiv.org/abs/1001.3813 [Accessed: 2018-01-25]

[20] Reichert A, Rothbauer U, Mörl M. Processing and editing of overlapping tRNAs in human mitochondria. The Journal of Biological Chemistry. 1998;**273**:31977-31984. DOI: 10.1074/jbc.273.48.31977

[21] Faure E, Casanova JP. Comparison of chaetognath mitochondrial genomes and phylogenetical implications. Mitochondrion. 2006;**6**:258-262. DOI: 10.1016/j.mito.2006.07.004

[22] Jühling F, Mörl M, Hartmann RK, Sprinzl M, Stadler PF, Pütz J. tRNAdb 2009: Compilation of tRNA sequences and tRNA genes. Nucleic Acids Research. 2009;**37**:D159-D162. DOI: 10.1093/nar/gkn772

[23] Lowe TM, Eddy SR. tRNAscan-SE: A program for improved detection of transfer RNA genes in genomic sequence. Nucleic Acids Research. 1997;**25**:955-964. DOI: 10.1093/nar/25.5.0955

[24] Dodd MS, Papineau D, Grenne T, Slack JF, Rittner M, Pirajno F, O'Neil J, Little CT. Evidence for early life in Earth's oldest hydrothermal vent precipitates. Nature. 2017;**543**:60-64. DOI: 10.1038/nature21377

[25] Roger AJ, Muñoz-Gómez SA, Kamikawa R. The origin and diversification of mitochondria. Current Biology. 2017;**27**:R1177-R1192. DOI: 10.1016/j.cub.2017.09.015

[26] Bengtson S, Rasmussen B, Ivarsson M, Muhling J, Broman C, Marone F, Stampanoni M, Bekker A. Fungus-like mycelial fossils in 2.4-billion-year-old vesicular basalt. Nature Ecology & Evolution. 2017;**1**:141. DOI: 10.1038/s41559-017-0141

[27] Margulis L, Dolan MF, Guerrero R. The chimeric eukaryote: Origin of the nucleus from the karyomastigont in amitochondriate protists. Proceedings of the National Academy of Sciences of the United States of America. 2000;**97**:6954-6959. DOI: 10.1073/pnas.97.13.6954

[28] Lewis LA. Hold the salt: Freshwater origin of primary plastids. Proceedings of the National Academy of Sciences of the United States of America. 2017;**114**:9759-9760. DOI: 10.1073/pnas.1712956114

[29] Lang BF, Gray MW, Burger G. Mitochondrial genome evolution and the origin of eukaryotes. Annual Review of Genetics. 1999;**33**:351-397. DOI: 10.1146/annurev.genet.33.1.351

[30] Le TH, Blair D, McManus DP. Mitochondrial genomes of parasitic flatworms. Trends in Parasitology. 2002;**18**:206-213. DOI: 10.1016/S1471-4922(02)02252-3

[31] Roelants K, Bossuyt F. Archaeobatrachian paraphyly and pangae and diversification of crown-group frogs. Systematic Biology. 2005;**54**:111-126. DOI: 10.1080/10635150590905894

[32] Lavrov DV, Pett W. Animal mitochondrial DNA as we do not know it: Mt-genome organization and evolution in Nonbilaterian lineages. Genome Biology and Evolution. 2016;**8**:2896-2913. DOI: 10.1093/gbe/evw195

[33] Gualberto JM, Mileshina D, Wallet C, Niazi AK, Weber-Lotfi F, Dietrich A. The plant mitochondrial genome: Dynamics and maintenance. Biochimie. 2014;**100**:107-120. DOI: 10.1016/j.biochi.2013.09.016

[34] Sloan DB, Alverson AJ, Chuckalovcak JP, Wu M, McCauley DE, Palmer JD, Taylor DR. Rapid evolution of enormous, multichromosomal genomes in flowering plant mitochondria with exceptionally high mutation rates. PLoS Biology. 2012;**10**:e1001241. DOI: 10.1371/journal.pbio.1001241

[35] Rodríguez-Moreno L, González VM, Benjak A, Martí MC, Puigdomènech P, Aranda MA, Garcia-Mas J. Determination of the melon chloroplast and mitochondrial genome sequences reveals that the largest reported mitochondrial genome in plants contains a significant amount of DNA having a nuclear origin. BMC Genomics. 2011;**12**:424. DOI: 10.1186/1471-2164-12-424

[36] Cognat V, Morelle G, Megel C, Lalande S, Molinier J, Vincent T, Small I, Duchêne AM, Maréchal-Drouard L. The nuclear and organellar tRNA-derived RNA fragment population in *Arabidopsis thaliana* is highly dynamic. Nucleic Acids Research. 2017;**45**:3460-3472. DOI: 10.1093/nar/gkw1122

[37] Guo H, Tse LV, Nieh AW, Czornyj E, Williams S, Oukil S, Liu VB, Miller JF. Target site recognition by a diversity-generating retroelement. PLoS Genetics. 2011;**7**:e1002414. DOI: 10.1371/journal.pgen.1002414

[38] Nosek J, Tomaska L, Burger G, Lang BF. Programmed translational bypassing elements in mitochondria: Structure, mobility, and evolutionary origin. Trends in Genetics. 2015;**31**: 187-194. DOI: 10.1016/j.tig.2015.02.010

[39] Loong Chan V, Louie H, Joe A. Expression of the flgFG operon of *Campylobacter jejuni* in *Escherichia coli* yields an extra fusion protein. Gene. 1998;**225**:131-141. DOI: 10.1016/S0378-1119(98)00516-2

[40] Nudler E, Mironov AS. The riboswitch control of bacterial metabolism. Trends in Biochemical Sciences. 2004;**29**:11-17. DOI: 10.1016/j.tibs.2003.11.004

[41] Macé K, Gillet R. Origins of tmRNA: The missing link in the birth of protein synthesis? Nucleic Acids Research. 2016;**44**:8041-8051. DOI: 10.1093/nar/gkw693

[42] Nan F, Feng J, Lv J, Liu Q, Fang K, Gong C, Xie S. Origin and evolutionary history of freshwater Rhodophyta: Further insights based on phylogenomic evidence. Scientific Reports. 2017;**7**:2934. DOI: 10.1038/s41598-017-03235-5

[43] Maizels N, Weiner AM. Phylogeny from function: Evidence from the molecular fossil record that tRNA originated in replication, not translation. Proceedings of the National Academy of Sciences of the United States of America. 1994;**91**:6729-6734. DOI: 10.1073/pnas.91.15.6729

[44] Xu WL, Yang Y, Wang YD, Qu LU, Zheng LL. Computational approaches to tRNA-derived small RNAs. Non-Coding RNA. 2017;**3**:2. DOI: 10.3390/ncrna3010002

[45] Hou YM, Yang X. Regulation of cell death by transfer RNA. Antioxidants & Redox Signaling. 2013;**19**:583-594. DOI: 10.1089/ars.2012.5171

[46] Seligmann H, Labra A. The relation between hairpin formation by mitochondrial WANCY tRNAs and the occurrence of the light strand replication origin in Lepidosauria. Gene. 2014;**542**:248-257. DOI: 10.1016/j.gene.2014.02.021

[47] Wang X, He C. Dynamic RNA modifications in posttranscriptional regulation. Molecular Cell. 2014;**56**:5-12. DOI: 10.1016/j.molcel.2014.09.001

[48] Schimmel P. The emerging complexity of the tRNA world: Mammalian tRNAs beyond protein synthesis. Nature Reviews. Molecular Cell Biology. 2017;**19**:45-58. DOI: 10.1038/nrm.2017.77

[49] Dethoff EA, Chugh J, Mustoe AM, Al-Hashimi HM. Functional complexity and regulation through RNA dynamics. Nature. 2012;**482**:322-330. DOI: 10.1038/nature10885

[50] Lenglez S, Hermand D, Decottignies A. Genome-wide mapping of nuclear mitochondrial DNA sequences links DNA replication origins to chromosomal double-strand break formation in *Schizosaccharomyces pombe*. Genome Research. 2010;**20**:1250-1261. DOI: 10.1101/gr.104513.109

[51] Raina M, Ibba M. tRNAs as regulators of biological processes. Frontiers in Genetics. 2014;**5**:171. DOI: 10.3389/fgene.2014.00171

[52] Yona AH, Bloom-Ackermann Z, Frumkin I, Hanson-Smith V, Charpak-Amikam Y, Feng Q, Boeke JD, Dahan O, Pilpel Y. tRNA genes rapidly change in evolution to meet novel translational demands. eLife. 2013;**2**:e01339. DOI: 10.7554/eLife.01339

[53] Doublet V, Helleu Q, Raimond R, Souty-Grosset C, Marcadé I. Inverted repeats and genome architecture conversions of terrestrial isopods mitochondrial DNA. Journal of Molecular Evolution. 2013;**77**:107-118. DOI: 10.1007/s00239-013-9587-7

[54] Schild C, Hahn D, Schaller A, Jackson CB, Rothen-Rutishauser B, Mirkovitch J, Nuoffer JM. Mitochondrial leucine tRNA level and PTCD1 are regulated in response to leucine starvation. Amino Acids. 2014;**46**:1775-1783. DOI: 10.1007/s00726-014-1730-2

[55] Segovia R, Pett W, Trewick S, Lavrov DV. Extensive and evolutionarily persistent mitochondrial tRNA editing in velvet worms (phylum Onychophora). Molecular Biology and Evolution. 2011;**28**:2873-2881. DOI: 10.1093/molbev/msr113

[56] Camps M. Modulation of ColE1-like plasmid replication for recombinant gene expression. Recent Patents on DNA & Gene Sequences. 2010;**4**:58-73. DOI: 10.2174/187221510790410822

[57] Honda S, Kawamura T, Loher P, Morichika K, Rigoutsos I, Kirino Y. The biogenesis pathway of tRNA-derived piRNAs in *Bombyx* germ cells. Nucleic Acids Research. 2017;**45**: 9108-9120. DOI: 10.1093/nar/gkx537

[58] Halfmann R, Jarosz DF, Jones SK, Chang A, Lancaster AK, Lindquist S. Prions are a common mechanism for phenotypic inheritance in wild yeasts. Nature. 2012;**482**:363-368. DOI: 10.1038/nature10875

[59] Stewart JB, Beckenbach AT. Characterization of mature mitochondrial transcripts in *Drosophila*, and the implications for the tRNA punctuation model in arthropods. Gene. 2009;**445**:49-57. DOI: 10.1016/j.gene.2009.06.006

[60] van der Wijst MG, van Tilburg AY, Ruiters MH, Rots MG. Experimental mitochondria-targeted DNA methylation identifies GpC methylation, not CpG methylation, as potential regulator of mitochondrial gene expression. Scientific Reports. 2017;**7**:177. DOI: 10.1038/s41598-017-00263-z

[61] Lorenz C, Lünse CE, Mörl M. tRNA modifications: Impact on structure and thermal adaptation. Biomolecules. 2017;**7**:2. DOI: 10.3390/biom7020035

[62] Seligmann H. Phylogeny of genetic codes and punctuation codes within genetic codes. Bio Systems. 2015;**129**:36-43. DOI: 10.1016/j.biosystems.2015.01.003

[63] NCBI. The Genetic Codes [Internet]. 2016. Available from: https://www.ncbi.nlm.nih.gov/Taxonomy/Utils/wprintgc.cgi#SG4 [Accessed: 2018-01-25]

[64] Osawa S, Jukes TH. Codon reassignment (codon capture) in evolution. Journal of Molecular Evolution. 1989;**28**:271-278. DOI: 10.1007/BF02103422

[65] Wallis M. On the frequency of arginine in proteins and its implications for molecular evolution. Biochemical and Biophysical Research Communications. 1974;**56**:711-716. DOI: 10.1016/0006-291X(74)90663-9

[66] Osawa S, Ohama T, Jukes TH, Watanabe K. Evolution of the mitochondrial genetic code. I. Origin of AGR serine and stop codons in metazoan mitochondria. Journal of Molecular Evolution. 1989;**29**:202-207. DOI: 10.1007/BF02100203

[67] Temperley R, Richter R, Dennerlein S, Lightowlers RN, Chrzanowska-Lightowlers ZM. Hungry codons promote frameshifting in human mitochondrial ribosomes. Science. 2010;**327**:301. DOI: 10.1126/science.1180674

[68] Di Giulio M. A comparison among the models proposed to explain the origin of the tRNA molecule: A synthesis. Journal of Molecular Evolution. 2009;**69**:1-9. DOI: 10.1007/s00239-009-9248-z

[69] Di Giulio M. The origin of the tRNA molecule: Independent data favor a specific model of its evolution. Biochimie. 2012;**94**:1464-1466. DOI: 10.1016/j.biochi.2012.01.014

[70] Fujishima K, Kanai A. tRNA gene diversity in the three domains of life. Frontiers in Genetics. 2014;**5**:142. DOI: 10.3389/fgene.2014.00142

[71] Maizels N, Weiner AM. The genomic tag hypothesis: What molecular fossils tell us about the evolution of tRNA. In: Gesteland RF, Cech TR, Atkins JF, editors. The RNA World. 2nd ed. Cold Spring Harbor Laboratory Press; 1999. pp. 79-112. DOI: 10.1101/087969589.37.79

[72] Sun FJ, Caetano-Anollés G. Evolutionary patterns in the sequence and structure of transfer RNA: A window into early translation and the genetic code. PLoS One. 2008;**3**:e2799. DOI: 10.1371/journal.pone.0002799

[73] Weiner AM, Maizels N. The genomic tag hypothesis: Modern viruses as molecular fossils of ancient strategies for genomic replication, and clues regarding the origin of protein synthesis. The Biological Bulletin. 1999;**196**:327-330. DOI: 10.2307/1542962

[74] Caetano-Anollés G, Wang M, Caetano-Anollés D. Structural phylogenomics retrodicts the origin of the genetic code and uncovers the evolutionary impact of protein flexibility. PLoS One. 2013;**8**:e72225. DOI: 10.1371/journal.pone.0072225

[75] Yoshihisa T. Handling tRNA introns, archaeal way and eukaryotic way. Frontiers in Genetics. 2014;**5**:213. DOI: 10.3389/fgene.2014.00213

[76] Larkin DC, Williams AM, Martinis SA, Fox GE. Identification of essential domains for *Escherichia coli* tRNA(leu) aminoacylation and amino acid editing using minimalist RNA molecules. Nucleic Acids Research. 2002;**30**:2103-2113. DOI: 10.1093/nar/30.10.2103

[77] Helm M, Brulé H, Friede D, Giegé R, Pütz D, Florentz C. Search for characteristic structural features of mammalian mitochondrial tRNAs. RNA. 2000;**6**:1356-1379. DOI: 10.1017/S1355838200001047

[78] El Houmami N, Seligmann H. Evolution of nucleotide punctuation marks: From structural to linear signals. Frontiers in Genetics. 2017;**8**:36. DOI: 10.3389/fgene.2017.00036

[79] Farias ST, Dos Santos Junior AP, Rêgo TG, José MV. Origin and evolution of RNA-dependent RNA polymerase. Frontiers in Genetics. 2017;**8**:125. DOI: 10.3389/fgene.2017.00125

[80] Farias ST, Rêgo TG, José MV. Origin and evolution of the Peptidyl Transferase Center from proto-tRNAs. FEBS Open Bio. 2014;**8**:175-178. DOI: 10.1016/j.fob.2014.01.010

[81] Noller HF. Evolution of protein synthesis from an RNA world. Cold Spring Harbor Perspectives in Biology. 2012;**4**:a003681. DOI: 10.1101/cshperspect.a003681

[82] Root-Bernstein MM, Root-Bernstein RS. The ribosome as a missing link in evolution. Journal of Theoretical Biology. 2015;**367**:130-158. DOI: 10.1016/j.jtbi.2016.02.030

[83] Mathews DH, Disney MD, Childs JL, Schroeder SJ, Zuker M, Turner DH. Incorporating chemical modification constraints into a dynamic programming algorithm for prediction of RNA secondary structure. Proceedings of the National Academy of Sciences of the United States of America. 2004;**101**:7287-7292. DOI: 10.1073/pnas.0401799101

[84] Bean A, Weiner A, Hughes A, Itskovits E, Friedman N, Rando O. Genome-wide histone modification patterns in Kluyveromyces Lactis reveal evolutionary adaptation of a heterochromatin-associated mark. bioRxiv 039776. DOI: 10.1101/039776

[85] Eigen M, Winkler-Oswatitsch R. Transfer-RNA, an early gene? Die Naturwissenschaften. 1981;**68**:282-292. DOI: 10.1007/BF01047470

[86] Ariza-Mateos A, Gómez J. Viral tRNA mimicry from a biocommunicative perspective. Frontiers in Microbiology. 2017;**8**:2395. DOI: 10.3389/fmicb.2017.02395

[87] Farias ST, Rêgo TG, José MV. A proposal of the proteome before the last universal common ancestor. International Journal of Astrobiology. 2016;**15**:27-31. DOI: 10.1017/S1473550415000464

[88] Farias ST, Rêgo TG, José MV. tRNA core hypothesis for the transition from the RNA world to the ribonucleoprotein world. Life (Basel). 2016b;**6**:15. DOI: 10.3390/life6020015

[89] Ohnishi K. Evolutionary meanings of the primary and secondary structures of the "UR-RNA", a primitive possibly self-replicating ribo-organism commonly ancestral to tRNAs, 5S-rRNA and virusoids. In: Gruber B, Yopp JH, editors. Symmetries in Science IV. Boston, MA: Springer; 1990. pp. 147-176. DOI: 10.1007/978-1-4613-0597-2_7

[90] Aphasizhev R, Karmarkar U, Simpson L. Are tRNAs imported into the mitochondria of kinetoplastid protozoa as 5′-extended precursors? Molecular and Biochemical Parasitology. 1998;**93**:73-80. DOI: 10.1016/S0166-6851(98)00022-X

[91] Soma A. Circularly permuted tRNA genes: Their expression and implications for their physiological relevance and development. Frontiers in Genetics. 2014;**5**:63. DOI: 10.3389/fgene.2014.00063

[92] Naoko ABE, Hiroshi ABE. Rolling circle translation of circular RNA. Seibutsu Butsuri. 2017;**57**:5-10. DOI: 10.2142/biophys.57.005

[93] Wolf YI, Koonin EV. On the origin of the translation system and the genetic code in the RNA world by means of natural selection, exaptation, and subfunctionalization. Biology Direct. 2007;**2**:198-223. DOI: 10.1186/1745-6150-2-14

[94] Safro M, Klipcan L. The mechanistic and evolutionary aspects of the 2′- and 3′-OH paradigm in biosynthetic machinery. Biology Direct. 2013;**8**:17. DOI: 10.1186/1745-6150-8-17

[95] Gwiazda S, Salomon K, Appel B, Muller S. RNA self-ligation: From oligonucleotides to full length ribozymes. Biochimie. 2012;**94**:1457-1463. DOI: 10.1016/j.biochi.2012.03.015

[96] Hafez M, Burger G, Steinberg SV, Lang BF. A second eukaryotic group with mitochondrion-encoded tmRNA: In silico identification and experimental confirmation. RNA Biology. 2013;**10**:1117-1124. DOI: 10.4161/rna.25376

[97] Harish A, Caetano-Anollés G. Ribosomal history reveals origins of modern protein synthesis. PLoS One. 2012;**7**:e32776. DOI: 10.1371/journal.pone.0032776

[98] Megel C, Morelle G, Lalande S, Duchêne AM, Small I, Maréchal-Drouard L. Surveillance and cleavage of eukaryotic tRNAs. International Journal of Molecular Sciences. 2015;**16**:1873-1893. DOI: 10.3390/ijms16011873

[99] Bhattacharyya S, Varshney U. Evolution of initiator tRNAs and selection of methionine as the initiating amino acid. RNA Biology. 2016;**13**:810-819. DOI: 10.1080/15476286.2016.1195943

[100] Johnson ZI, Chisholm SW. Properties of overlapping genes are conserved across microbial genomes. Genome Research. 2004;**14**:2268-2272. DOI: 10.1101/gr.2433104

[101] Sun H, Wang X, editors. Mitochondrial DNA and Diseases. Singapore: Springer; 2017. 230 p. DOI: 10.1007/978-981-10-6674-0

Chapter 2

Renaissance of the Tautomeric Hypothesis of the Spontaneous Point Mutations in DNA: New Ideas and Computational Approaches

Ol'ha O. Brovarets' and Dmytro M. Hovorun

Additional information is available at the end of the chapter

http://dx.doi.org/10.5772/intechopen.77366

Abstract

In this chapter, we formulate basic physico-chemical principles that define the micro-structural nature of the origin of the spontaneous incorporation and replication point errors—transitions and transversions—arising during DNA biosynthesis. At this point, we relied on the firstly discovered ability of the DNA base mispairs to tautomerize *via* the sequential intrapair proton transfer and highly stable, highly polar, zwitterionic transition states, accompanied by a significant shifting of the base mispairs toward DNA minor or major grooves. These tautomeric transitions are characterized by a change in geometry—from wobble to Watson-Crick and *vice versa*—of the purine·pyrimidine (A·T, G·C, G·T and A·C), purine·purine (A·A, A·G and G·G) and pyrimidine·pyrimidine (C·C, C·T and T·T) DNA base mispairs. Reported results allow us to explain, on one side, the origin of the mutagenic tautomers at the separation of the DNA strands before replication and, on the other side, how DNA base mispairs adapt to enzymatically competent size in the tight recognition pocket of the high-fidelity DNA polymerase.

Keywords: tautomeric hypothesis, spontaneous and induced point mutations in DNA, incorporation and replication point errors, mutagenic tautomerization, pairs of nucleotide bases, enzymatically competent conformation, DNA polymerase, DNA replication, hydrogen bond, van der Waals contact, quantum chemistry, Bader's quantum theory of atoms in molecules (QTAIM)

1. Introduction

High-fidelity DNA replication is a central issue in molecular biology [1]. During DNA replication, spontaneous point mutations [2–4] arise with frequencies $10^{-9} \div 10^{-11}$ [5–8] in functioning of living cells.

Nowadays, it is reliably known that the root cause of the origin of the spontaneous point mutations is the formation in the very tight, slightly deformable base pair recognition pocket of the high-fidelity DNA polymerase in its close state of the "wrong" DNA base pairs (i.e., mismatches) able to acquire in the process of thermal fluctuations the conformation of the correct Watson-Crick DNA base pair (i.e., enzymatically competent conformation), which guarantees their incorporation into the chemical structure of the synthesized DNA double helix [4].

In the literature, two approaches are currently presented, according to physico-chemical principles of the occurrence of the mispairs leading to spontaneous point mutations in DNA. One of them is the "tautomeric hypothesis" suggested by J. Watson and F. Crick [9], which consists in the spontaneous tautomeric transition of the DNA bases from canonical to mutagenic tautomeric forms leading to the formation of the adenine·cytosine (A·C*)/A*·C and guanine·thymine (G*·T)/G·T* (here and below, mutagenic tautomers are marked with asterisk) Watson-Crick-like mispairs with correct enzymatically competent conformation [10] containing mutagenic tautomers [11–13]. Despite great advances in experimental, in particular X-ray analysis [14, 15], NMR, in particular relaxation dispersion measurements [11–13, 16–18], and theoretical [19–21] investigations, there is no unique approach to the physico-chemical mechanisms enabling DNA bases in the canonical tautomeric form to acquire rare or mutagenic tautomeric form before the dissociation of the Watson-Crick nucleobase pairs into the monomers by the replication machinery in order to produce mispairs resulting in further misincorporations and as a result the spontaneous point mutations at the DNA replication. It is generally accepted in the literature that mutagenic tautomers of the DNA bases can arise *via* the double proton transfer (DPT) along intermolecular H-bonds in the Watson-Crick [22–25] and wobble [26] base pairs, and also in the protein-DNA complexes [27]. However, some authors also consider as the source of the origin of the spontaneous transitions the formation of the ionized DNA base pairs [28].

On contrary, according to second approach, other researchers believe that spontaneous point mutations arise due to the formation of the incorrect base pairs involving only DNA bases in the main, canonical tautomeric form—so-called wobble or shifted A·C and G·T base pairs [29, 30]. However, the mechanisms of their adaptation to the enzymatically competent sizes in the very tight, slightly deformable base pair recognition pocket of the high-fidelity DNA polymerase remain unclear [30, 31].

The common feature of these approaches is the absence of the general physico-chemical theory according the nature of these mispairs causing spontaneous point mutations, and the emergence of each of them is considered as a unique phenomenon. In the literature, there are no attempts or ideas aimed at combining these approaches into a unique, internally noncontradictory conception. Nevertheless, creation of such a microstructural theory is an interdisciplinary challenge with fundamental and applied consequences.

Thus, without clear understanding of basic mechanisms of the origin of spontaneous point mutations [32–34], it is difficult to develop a management strategy of genome instability and produce physico-chemical explanations of evolution [35, 36]; to design highly efficient mutagens—analogs of the nucleotide bases with targeted action for different purposes, in particular, for antiviral and anticancer therapy [37, 38]; to essentially increase precision of DNA-based nanodevices of biomolecular electronics as information carriers [39, 40]; to create synthetic macromolecular structures able to replicate with predetermined accuracy [41] and so on.

Here, we aim to reveal at the microstructural level the molecular grounds of intrinsic DNA mutability without involvement of external agents.

2. Computational methods

All geometric, energetic and vibrational calculations of the considered base mispairs and transition states (TSs) of their conversion have been performed by Gaussian'09 package [42] using B3LYP [43, 44] and MP2 [45] levels of quantum-mechanical (QM) theory combined with a wide variety of basis sets followed by the intrinsic reaction coordinate (IRC) calculations in the forward and reverse directions from each TS using Hessian-based predictor-corrector integration algorithm [46] in vacuum and in the continuum with $\varepsilon = 4$, which is characteristic for the active center of the DNA polymerase [47, 48]. Bader's quantum theory of Atoms in Molecules (QTAIM) was applied to analyze the electron density distribution [49]. Physico-chemical parameters have been estimated by the known formulas of physico-chemical kinetics [50].

3. Results and discussion

3.1. Classical mechanisms of DNA base tautomerization *via* DPT along two intermolecular H-bonds in H-bonded complexes

We established from the physico-chemical point of view that the generally accepted mechanism of the DPT along intermolecular H-bonds [22–29] cannot be the source of formation of mutagenic tautomers of DNA bases in the A·T(WC) and G·C(WC) Watson-Crick (so-called Löwdin's mechanism) [51–53] and G·T(w) wobble [54] base pairs, and also in the $m^1T{\cdot}CH_3COOH$, $m^9A{\cdot}CH_3COOH$, $m^1C{\cdot}CH_3COOH$ and $m^9G{\cdot}CH_3COOH$ complexes by the participation of DNA bases and side chains of the amino acids (m-methyl group) [55].

At this point, the A*·T* Löwdin's base pair is dynamically unstable and has a lifetime that is 6 orders of magnitude less than the characteristic time spent by DNA polymerase on the forced dissociation of the DNA base pairs into the bases (~10^{-9} s [32, 51, 52]). The short-lived G*·C* Löwdin's base pair escapes the DNA polymerase. The other final tautomerized complexes containing mutagenic tautomers of DNA bases are dynamically unstable: the value of the zero-point energy of the corresponding vibrational mode, in which frequency becomes imaginary at the transition state, is higher than the value of the reverse barrier (**Table 1**).

Tautomeric transition	ΔG^a	ΔE^b	$\Delta\Delta G_{TSy}{}^c$	$\Delta\Delta E_{TS}{}^d$	$\Delta\Delta G^e$	$\Delta\Delta E^f$	τ^g
MP2/aug-cc-pVTZ//MP2/6–311++G(d,p)							
A·T↔A*·T* [51–53]	11.95	12.26	10.29	12.40	−1.66	0.14	6.5×10^{-15}
G·C↔G*·C* [52]	9.22	8.22	9.69	13.28	0.47	5.06	1.6×10^{-13}
MP2/cc-pVQZ//MP2/6–311++G(d,p)							
G·T↔G*·T* [54]	11.78	12.12	9.47	12.58	−2.31	0.46	2.1×10^{-15}
MP2/6–311++G(3df,2pd)//M05/6–311++G(2df,pd)							
$m^1T \cdot CH_3COOH \leftrightarrow m^1T^* \cdot CH_3COOH$ [55]	5.63	6.48	7.24	10.45	1.60	3.97	1.9×10^{-12}
$m^9A \cdot CH_3COOH \leftrightarrow m^9A^* \cdot CH_3COOH$ [55]	8.21	7.23	6.68	8.52	−1.53	1.29	6.1×10^{-15}
$m^1C \cdot CH_3COOH \leftrightarrow m^1C^* \cdot CH_3COOH$ [55]	3.35	2.91	6.12	7.43	2.77	4.52	1.6×10^{-11}
$m^9G \cdot CH_3COOH \leftrightarrow m^9G^* \cdot CH_3COOH$ [55]	1.93	2.75	2.08	5.96	0.15	3.21	1.0×10^{-13}
MP2/cc-pVQZ//B3LYP/6–311++G(d,p)							
A·A*↔A*·A [65]	0.00	0.00	7.01	10.33	7.01	10.33	1.8×10^{-8}
A·G↔A*·G* [56]	10.07	9.58	9.63	11.46	−0.44	1.88	4.8×10^{-14}
G·G*↔G*·G [66]	0.00	0.00	5.51	8.33	5.51	8.33	8.2×10^{-10}
A·C*↔A*·C [57]	3.99	3.64	8.17	10.53	4.18	6.89	1.1×10^{-10}
G*·T↔G·T* [58]	1.22	1.19	2.63	5.61	2.63	5.61	8.1×10^{-13}
C·C*↔C*·C [64]	0.00	0.00	8.28	10.83	8.28	10.83	1.5×10^{-7}
C·T↔C*·T* [59]	9.15	8.99	9.55	11.38	0.40	2.39	2.1×10^{-13}
T·T*↔T*·T [63]	0.00	0.00	4.64	8.18	4.64	8.18	1.6×10^{-10}
$G \cdot G^*_{syn} \leftrightarrow G^* \cdot G^*_{syn}$ [60]	11.02	11.15	9.07	12.17	−1.96	1.02	4.1×10^{-15}
$A^* \cdot A_{syn} \leftrightarrow A \cdot A^*_{syn}$ [61]	13.98	14.71	14.15	16.43	0.16	1.72	1.1×10^{-13}
$A^* \cdot G^*_{syn} \leftrightarrow A \cdot G^*_{syn}$ [62]	1.89	2.20	2.42	4.60	0.52	2.40	2.2×10^{-13}

[a]The Gibbs free energy of the product relatively the reactant of the tautomerization reaction (T = 298.15 K).
[b]The electronic energy of the product relatively the reactant of the tautomerization reaction.
[c]The Gibbs free energy barrier for the forward reaction of tautomerization.
[d]The electronic energy barrier for the forward reaction of tautomerization.
[e]The Gibbs free energy barrier for the reverse reaction of tautomerization.
[f]The electronic energy barrier for the reverse reaction of tautomerization.
[g]The lifetime of the product of the tautomerization reaction.

Table 1. Energetic (kcal·mol^{-1}) and kinetic (in s) characteristics of the tautomeric transformations of the canonical Watson-Crick, wobble, model protein-DNA complexes, incorrect long, short and Watson-Crick-like mispairs of nucleotide bases *via* the DPT along the neighboring intermolecular H-bonds in vacuum.

3.2. Can mutagenic tautomers of the DNA bases be formed *via* the DPT in Watson-Crick-like mispairs?

Further, we investigated the physico-chemical mechanisms of the DNA bases tautomerization through the DPT along intermolecular H-bonds of incorrect DNA base pairs.

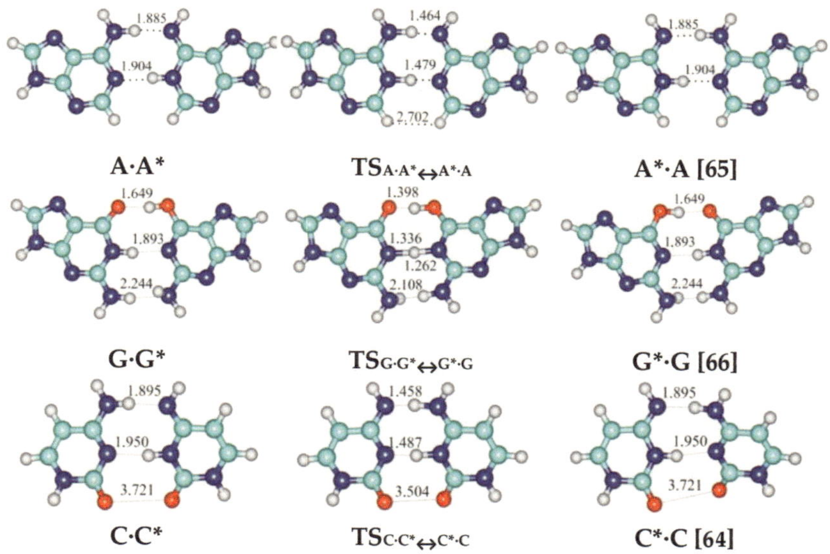

Figure 1. Geometrical structures of the three stationary structures (reagent, transition state and product) describing the progression of the tautomerization *via* DPT along intermolecular H-bonds in some mispairs (B3LYP/6–311++G(d,p) level of theory, ε = 1).

It was established that the A·G↔A*·G* [56], A·C*↔A*·C [57], G*·T↔G·T* [58], C·T↔C*·T* [59], $G{\cdot}G^*_{syn}$↔$G^*{\cdot}G^*_{syn}$ [60], $A^*{\cdot}A_{syn}$↔$A{\cdot}A^*_{syn}$ [61] and $A^*{\cdot}G^*_{syn}$↔$A{\cdot}G^*_{syn}$ [62] tautomerization processes occur without changing the tautomeric status of the initial DNA base pairs, since the terminal, tautomerized base pairs are dynamically unstable: low-frequency intermolecular vibrations cannot develop during their lifetime (**Figure 1**, **Table 1**). Hence, these transformations do not generate mutagenic tautomers.

During the tautomerization of the dynamically stable short T·T* [63] and C·C* [64] mispairs, as well as long A·A* [65] and G·G* [66] mispairs, mutagenic tautomers are distributed among the monomers with equal probability. This is important for understanding the consolidation of point mutations in subsequent rounds of DNA replication (**Figure 1**, **Table 1**). Short-lived, low-populated A*·C and G·T* mispairs are "providers" of the long-lived enzymatically competent A·C* [57] and G*·T base pairs [58], respectively, at the origin of the replication errors in DNA. Moreover, comparisons between calculated distances of intermolecular H-bonds with data from X-ray experiments [14, 15] show that incorrect A·C and G·T base pairs with Watson-Crick geometry occur in the A·C* and G*·T tautomeric forms in the active center of the high-fidelity DNA polymerase in its closed state.

Transition from vacuum to continuum with ε = 4, characteristics for the hydrophobic interfaces of the protein-DNA complexes, does not significantly influence the course of these tautomerization reactions and does not change the character of the obtained conclusions and generalizations.

Obtained data evidence that tautomeric hypothesis faces significant obstacles that could not be overcome without going beyond the classical framework that mutagenic tautomers of nucleotide bases are generated in the complexes by DPT protons along neighboring intermolecular H-bonds.

3.3. Novel mechanisms of the wobble (w)↔Watson-Crick (WC) tautomeric interconversions in the canonical and incorrect DNA base pairs as a key to understand origins of spontaneous transitions and transversions

For the first time, a novel theoretical approach to elucidate microstructural mechanisms of incorporation and replication point errors arising at the DNA replication was proposed. We show for the first time that pairs of nucleotide bases with Watson-Crick architecture of the H-bonding—classical, long, short, in which one or both bases are in the main or rare tautomeric forms, are in a slow tautomeric equilibrium with the corresponding wobble base pairs in comparison with the time, in which high-fidelity DNA polymerase spends on the incorporation of one nucleotide into the DNA double helix ($\sim 8.3 \times 10^{-4}$ s [67]). In fact, a novel pathway of the chemical reaction was discovered—tautomerization with significant changes of the geometry of the base pair—from Watson-Crick to wobble and *vice versa*.

We have discovered novel structural hypostases of the classical A·T(WC) and G·C(WC) Watson-Crick DNA base pairs arising due to their ability to switch into the wobble A*·T↑(w), $A{\cdot}T^*_{O2}$↑(w), A·T*↓(w) and G·C*↑(w), G*·C↓(w), G·C*↓(w), G*·C↑(w) H-bonded mismatches containing rare tautomers (**Figure 2**) [68]. Estimated populations of the tautomerized states of the A·T(WC) (6.1×10^{-9}–1.5×10^{-7}) and G·C(WC) (4.2×10^{-11}–1.4×10^{-9}) base pairs in the continuum with $\varepsilon = 4$ correspond to the interface of the protein-nucleic acid interactions. This evidences their involvement in nucleation of spontaneous point replication errors in DNA arising with frequencies $\sim 10^{-11}$–10^{-9} errors *per* replicated nucleotide.

We found for the first time the intrinsic ability of the purine·pyrimidine (A·C [69, 70] and G·T [69, 71]), purine·purine (A·A [72], G·G [72] and A·G [73]) and pyrimidine·pyrimidine (C·C [74], T·T [74] and C·T [73]) DNA base mispairs to perform wobble↔Watson-Crick tautomeric transitions *via* the sequential intrapair DPT and subsequent shifting of the bases relative to each other (**Figure 3**, **Table 2**). These nondissociative tautomerizations *via* the sequential PT are controlled by the highly stable ($\Delta E_{int} > 100$ kcal·mol^{-1}), highly polar and zwitterionic transition states of the type (protonated base)·(deprotonated base). These interconversions are accompanied by a significant rebuilding of the base mispairs with Watson-Crick architecture into the mismatches wobbled toward both DNA minor and major grooves and *vice versa*.

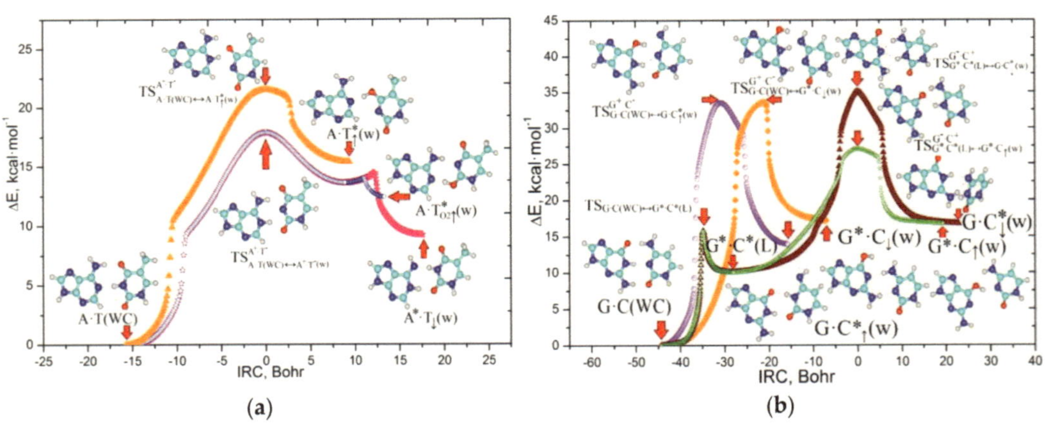

Figure 2. Energetic profiles of the mutagenic tautomerization *via* the wobbling of the (**a**) A·T(WC) and (**b**) G·C(WC) DNA base pairs to the H-bonded mismatches containing rare tautomers (B3LYP/6–311++G(d,p) level of theory, $\varepsilon = 1$) [68].

http://dx.doi.org/10.5772/intechopen.77366

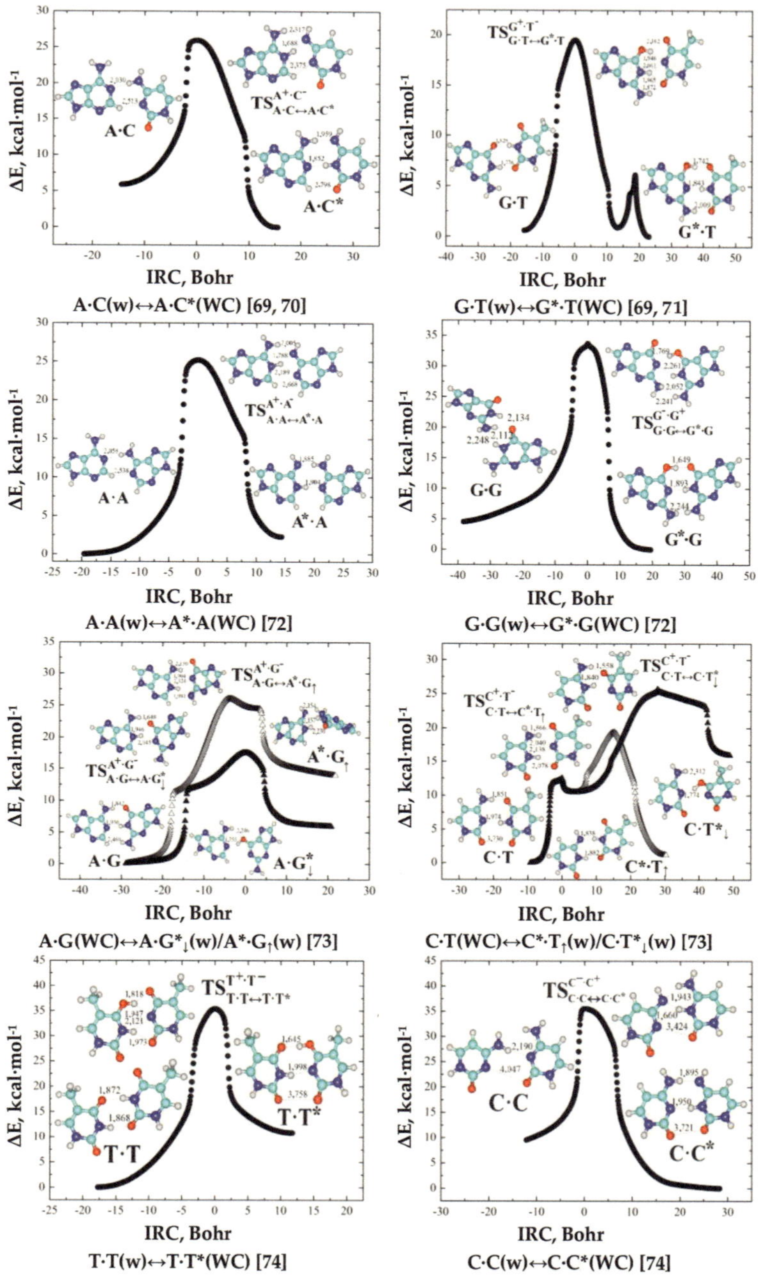

Figure 3. Energetic profiles and stationary structures on the potential energy hypersurface of the biologically important transformations *via* the PT, accompanied by the shifting of the bases relative to each other within a base pair into the sides of the DNA minor or major grooves, leading to the occurrence of the spontaneous transitions and transversions—incorporation and replication errors (B3LYP/6–311++G(d,p) level theory, $\varepsilon = 1$).

Notably, each of the discussed tautomerizations is realized precisely through four different topological and energetic pathways. The number of mobile protons (two in each pair) and number of wobbling directions of WC base pairs (two by the number of the grooves in DNA—minor and major) determines the number of tautomerization pathways. Characteristically, in

Tautomeric conversion	ΔG	ΔE	$\Delta\Delta G_{TS}$	$\Delta\Delta E_{TS}$	ΔΔG	ΔΔE	$\tau_{99.9\%}$ [a]	N[b]
MP2/aug-cc-pVDZ//B3LYP/6–311++G(d,p)								
A·T(WC)↔A*·T↑(w) [68]	9.90	9.59	16.72	16.02	6.82	6.43	1.1×10^{-7}	5.4×10^{-8}
A·T(WC)↔A·T*$_{O2}$↑(w) [68]	10.91	11.25	16.72	16.02	5.81	4.77	2.0×10^{-8}	9.9×10^{-9}
A·T(WC)↔A·T*↓(w) [68]	13.08	14.84	20.28	20.41	7.20	5.57	2.1×10^{-7}	2.5×10^{-10}
G·C(WC)↔G·C*↑(w) [68]	13.35	14.10	30.47	30.74	17.12	16.64	3.95	1.6×10^{-10}
G·C(WC)↔G*·C↓(w) [68]	15.10	16.49	31.08	31.53	15.98	15.04	0.58	1.3×10^{-11}
G·C(WC)↔G·C*↓(w) [68]	15.08	15.96	30.88	31.41	15.80	15.45	0.42	8.8×10^{-12}
G·C(WC)↔G*·C↑(w) [68]	14.85	17.22	24.87	25.64	10.02	8.42	2.5×10^{-5}	8.4×10^{-12}
MP2/cc-pVQZ//B3LYP/6–311++G(d,p)								
A·C(w)↔A·C*(WC) [69, 70]	4.87	6.77	19.98	18.85	24.84	25.62	4.9×10^{2}	–
G·T(w)↔G*·T(WC) [69, 71]	−1.69	−2.46	17.04	16.37	18.73	18.83	8.8	–
A·A(w)↔A*·A(WC) [72]	4.18	1.64	26.89	23.59	22.71	21.94	4.4×10^{4}	–
G·G(w)↔G*·G(WC) [72]	−4.96	−6.75	26.81	26.08	31.77	32.83	5.0×10^{7}	–
A·G(WC)↔A·G*↓(w) [73]	3.76	6.19	17.01	17.07	13.25	10.88	5.3×10^{-3}	–
A·G(WC)↔A*·G↑(w) [73]	14.29	14.09	25.29	24.39	11.00	10.30	1.2×10^{-4}	–
C·T(WC)↔C*·T↑(w) [73]	0.56	0.55	17.05	17.36	16.48	16.81	6.8×10^{-7}	–
C·T(WC)↔C·T*↓(w) [73]	12.07	14.57	26.64	25.32	14.57	10.75	5.4×10^{-2}	–
T·T(w)↔T·T*(WC) [74]	8.98	8.64	31.06	31.90	22.09	23.26	1.6×10^{4}	–
C·C(w)↔C·C*(WC) [74]	−8.90	−10.73	25.38	24.32	34.28	35.05	4.4×10^{6}	–

Note: for designations see **Table 1**.

[a]The time necessary to reach 99.9% of the equilibrium concentration between the reactant and the product of the tautomerization reaction, s.

[b]Populations of the wobble mispairs containing mutagenic tautomers.

Table 2. Energetic and kinetic characteristics of the tautomeric transformations of the classical Watson-Crick or wobble DNA base pairs, which are involved into the processes of the spontaneous point mutagenesis, *via* the DPT accompanied by the substantial changes of their geometry in the continuum with ε = 1.

each case mostly, one pathway is most probable at the origin of the spontaneous point mutations (**Figures 2** and **3**, **Table 2**).

Obtained results are crucial for understanding the microstructural mechanisms of spontaneous transitions and transversions, since they allow us to explain how incorrect purine·pyrimidine, purine·purine and pyrimidine·pyrimidine wobble pairs adapt to the enzymatically competent sizes in the recognition pocket of the high-fidelity DNA polymerase. In particular, established A·C(w) → A·C*(WC) [70] and G·T(w) → G*·T(WC) [71] transformations *via* the sequential PT allow us to interpret the X-ray [14, 15] and molecular dynamics simulations data [19] according the acquisition by the wobble A·C(w)/G·T(w) mispairs of the Watson-Crick geometry by their transformation to the A·C*(WC)/G*·T(WC) Watson-Crick-like base mispairs by the participation of the C* and G* mutagenic tautomers in the recognition pocket of the high-fidelity DNA polymerase. Moreover, we theoretically predicted the G·T(w) → G*·T(WC) transformation for the wobble G·T(w) base mispair, which was confirmed by an NMR experiment of a DNA duplex [16–18].

Mutagenic pressure of the analogues of DNA bases could be explained within the framework of the proposed model of the w↔WC mutagenic tautomerization. In particular, mutagenic action of the analogue of C-6H,8H-3,4-dihydropyrimido[4,5-c] [1, 2]oxazin-7-one [11, 12]—increases the population of the G·P*↑ (4.5×10^{-3}) and G·P*↓ (1.4×10^{-4}) base mispairs by its participation in comparison with the analogical values for the canonical C DNA base. Mutagenic activity of the halogen derivatives of the uracil base is associated with the decreasing of the transformation barriers of the wobble G·^{5}XU(w) (X = H, CH_3, Br, Cl, F) mispairs into the G·^{5}XU*(WC) mispairs with Watson-Crick geometry, thus inducing higher frequency of the transitions. The maximal effect is observed for the ^{5}BrU-calculated frequency of the induced mutations (35 [71]), which is in good accordance with experimental data (from 20 [75] to 29 [76]).

3.4. *Anti*↔*syn* conformational transitions of the long purine-purine DNA mismatches

All long purine·purine DNA base mispairs can acquire enzymatically competent conformations—A*·A_{syn}(TF), G·A_{syn}, A*·G^*_{syn} and G·G^*_{syn}—through the A*·A(WC)↔A*·A_{syn}(TF), G·A(WC)↔G·A_{syn}, A*·G*(WC)↔A*·G^*_{syn} and G·G*(WC)↔G·G^*_{syn} conformational transitions [77], eventually guaranteeing their chemical incorporation into the newly synthesized structure of the DNA double helix (TF-Topal-Fresco nucleobase pair [10]; *syn-syn*-orientation of the base according the sugar-phosphate moiety) (**Figure 4**). Characteristic time of these nondissociative conformational transitions (~10^{-7} s) is much less than the period of time the high-fidelity DNA polymerase spends on incorporating one nucleotide into the DNA double helix (~8.3×10^{-4} s [67]). So-called long A*·A(WC), G·A(WC), A*·G*(WC) and G·G*(WC) DNA base mispairs have been outlined as "node stations" on the way of the formation of the enzymatically competent conformations arising in the recognition pocket of the high-fidelity DNA polymerase at its transition from the open to closed state.

3.5. Physico-chemical scenarios of the origin of the replication and incorporation point errors in DNA

In the framework of such qualitatively new model conceptions, we were able to shed light on the microstructural mechanisms of the occurrence of point mutations—replication and incorporation point errors.

Thus, the spontaneous mutagenic tautomerization of the Watson-Crick pairs of nucleotide bases into the wobble base mispairs, which includes the A*, T*, G* and C* mutagenic tautomers, has been established to be the source of the generation of the mutagenic tautomers of the DNA bases arising at the separation of DNA strands. At this juncture, *replication errors* would arise in the following way (as an example, we would consider the case, when A* belongs to the template strand of DNA): A* + C → A*·C → A·C*, A* + A → A*·A → A*·A_{syn}, A* + G → A *·G → A·G → A*·G* → A*·G^*_{syn}. Similar schemes of structural transformations, which occur directly in the recognition pocket of the high-fidelity DNA polymerase, would take place also for three other cases, when G*, T* and C* belong to the template strand of DNA.

Incorporation errors would occur according to the following scenario: in the recognition pocket of the high-fidelity DNA polymerase, it would form the appropriate wobble base mispair

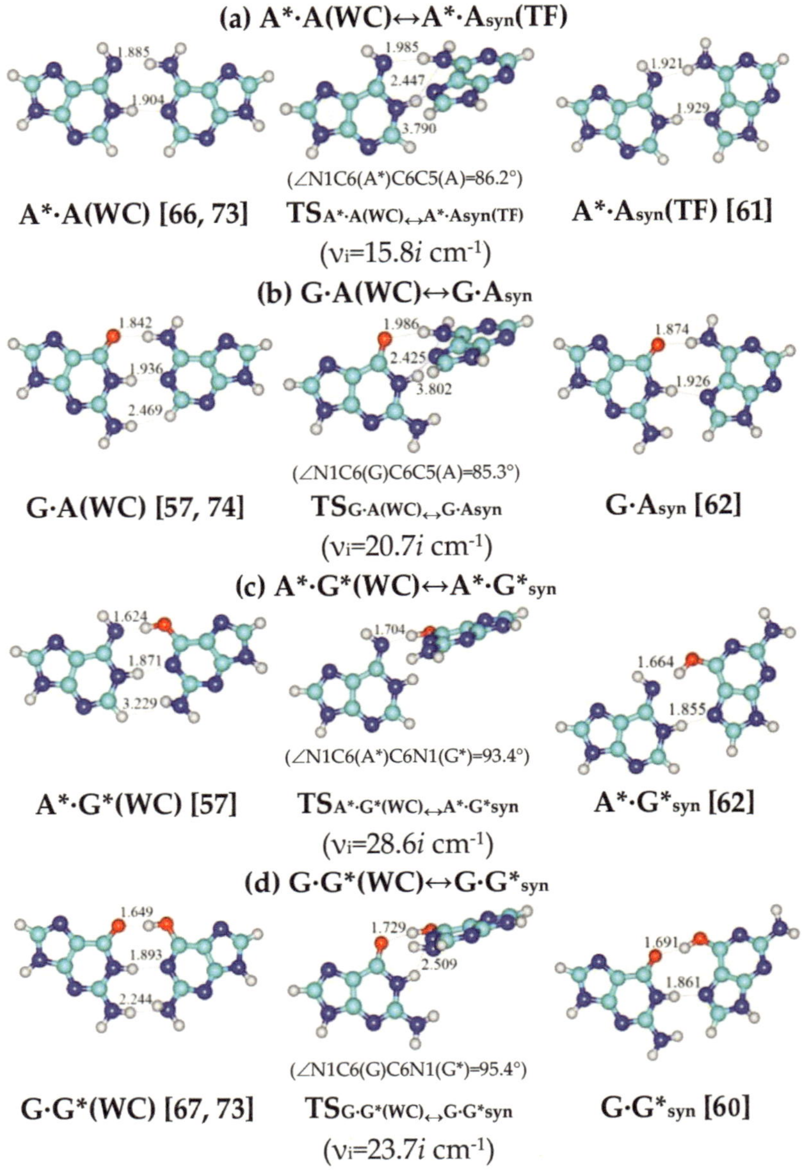

Figure 4. Structures corresponding to the stationary points on the reaction pathways of the (a) A*·A(WC)↔A*·A_{syn}(TF), (b) G·A(WC)↔G·A_{syn}, (c) A*·G*(WC)↔A*·G^*_{syn} and (d) G·G*(WC)↔G·G^*_{syn} *anti*↔*syn* conversions through the large-scale adjustments of the bases relative to each other, obtained at the B3LYP/6–311++G(d,p) level of theory, ε = 1 [77].

tautomerizing into the pair with Watson-Crick architecture of the binding. For the case, when A belongs to the template strand of DNA: A + C → A·C → A·C*, A + A → A·A → A*·A → A*·A_{syn}, A + G → A·G → A*·G* → A*·G^*_{syn}.

Both processes have two common features—they involve the same pairs, which play the role of intermediates on the path of formation of enzymatically competent conformations of some incorrect pairs, as well as the same set of terminal incorrect pairs, able to acquire the enzymatically competent conformations during the process of thermal fluctuations.

Finally, it becomes clear why spontaneous point errors occur quite rarely. This, in particular, is due to the fact that the mechanisms of their occurrence are kinetically controllable, with the time $\tau_{99.9\%}$, which is necessary to reach 99.9% of the equilibrium concentration of the reactant and product, significantly greater than the time that the DNA polymerase spends incorporating one nucleotide into the DNA double helix that is synthesized (~8.3×10^{-4} s [67]).

Based on our own theoretical data, which have been successfully confirmed by experimental data [16–18], one can make an assumption, why the DNA-repair enzymes, "sharpened" precisely for the wobble base mispairs, do not provide 100% accuracy. The reason consists in the ability of this pair to transform into a pair with Watson-Crick geometry, which, figuratively speaking, is a "hiding place" from the enzyme, because it is not recognized by it, thus restricting the ultimate accuracy of the repair process.

So, obtained data, in principle, enable to understand the mechanism of elimination from the genome of mutagenic tautomers, whose lifetime exceeds by orders of magnitude the time of cellular DNA replication.

Again, established ability of the wobble pair to be formed from the Watson-Crick-like pair involving mutagenic tautomer of the DNA bases enables DNA-repair complex to reveal and eliminate them from the genome during several cycles of DNA replication.

3.6. Profiles of the physico-chemical parameters along the IRC of tautomerizations *via* DPT and PT

We developed original methodology tracking the evolution of all physico-chemical parameters along the entire reaction pathways: in particular, the electronic energy, the first derivative of the electronic energy by the IRC-dE/dIRC, the dipole moment of the base pair, the distances and the angle of the intermolecular specific contacts (H-bonds or van der Waals contacts), electron density, the Laplacian of the electron density, ellipticity and the energy at the (3,-1) bond critical points of the intrapair specific contacts, the NBO charges of the hydrogen atoms involved in the tautomerization, the glycosidic angles and the distance between the glycosidic hydrogens. This works not only in the stationary structures such as reagent, product and transition state of the tautomerizations *via* the DPT and w↔WC tautomeric reactions *via* the PT [51–74, 78].

Additionally, for the first time, we have introduced the conception of the key points (KPs) based on the electron-topological characteristics of the intermolecular bonds, namely the value of the electron density and its Laplacian at the corresponding (3,-1) bond critical points. This approach allows us to comprehensively describe the mechanism of the tautomerization process. Thus, depending on the symmetry and nature of the system, maximum number of KPs could reach 9 and minimal—5, when KPs are degenerated (see **Figures 5** and **6** for illustration on the example of the 2AP·T(WC)↔2AP·T*(w)).

Arrangement of the extrema of the derivative of the energy by IRC—dE/dIRC—coincides with the second and penultimate KPs, where mutual transformations of the H-bond into a covalent bond and *vice versa* occur. These data allow us to separate the pathway of the tautomerization reaction into the zones of reagent, transition state and product of the reaction. In general, these key points could be considered as "fingerprints" of the tautomerization process *via* DPT or PT.

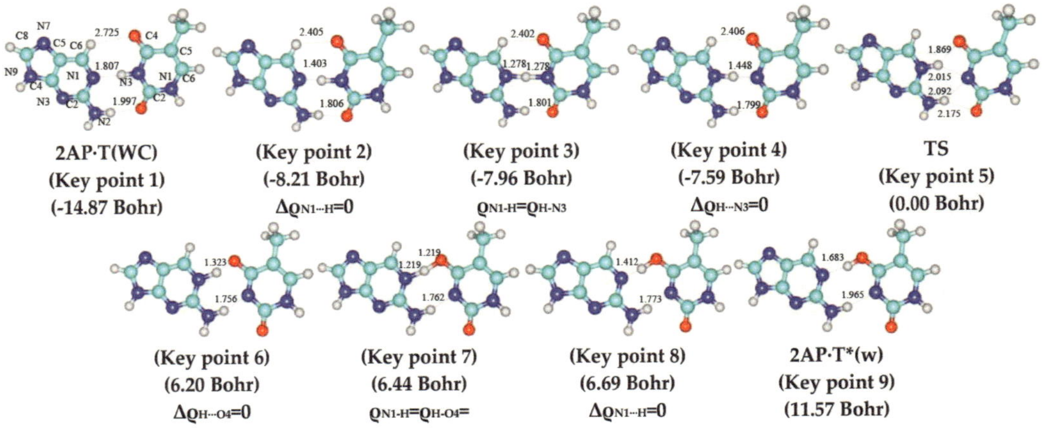

Figure 5. Geometric structures of the nine key points with their IRC coordinated describing the evolution of the 2AP·T(WC)↔2AP·T*(w) tautomerization *via* the single PT and sequential shifting of the bases relative to each other within the base pair into the minor groove side of the DNA helix along the IRC obtained at the B3LYP/6–311++G(d,p) level of theory, $\varepsilon = 1$ [79] tautomerization). At this point, three KPs correspond to the two abovementioned local minima (the first and the last KPs–reagent and product, respectively) and transition state of the tautomerization. Other KPs include two KPs, for which migrating proton is localized midway between the electronegative atoms involved in the specific contact and are characterized by the loosened A-H-B covalent bridge, and also four key points, in which the H-bonds begin to acquire the features of the covalent bond and *vice versa*, that is where the Laplacian of the electron density passes through zero: $\Delta\varrho = 0$.

This methodology enables to make an objective conclusion about the character of tautomerization (concerted, synchronous or asynchronous), quantitatively estimate the cooperativity of the specific intermolecular interactions (namely, H-bonds, in particular nonclassical CH···O/N or dihydrogen AH···HB H-bonds, loosened A-H-B covalent bridges and attractive A···B van der Waals contacts), sequentially changing each other along the IRC of the tautomerization, and trace how these interactions are grouped into the patterns (from 9 to 15) and how they successively substitute each other along the IRC of tautomerization.

3.7. Complete set of incorrect DNA base pairs responsible for the origin of spontaneous transitions and transversions in DNA

For the first time, we outline a complete set of the 12 incorrect DNA base pairs representing a primary cause of spontaneous point mutations and determining both incorporation and replication errors: A·C*/C*·A, G*·T/T·G*, G·A_{syn}, A*·G^*_{syn}, A*·A_{syn}, G·G^*_{syn}, C·T/T·C, C*·C/C·C* and T*·T/T·T* (three of these mispairs—G·A_{syn}, C·T and T·C—consist exclusively of the canonical tautomers of the DNA bases) (**Figure 7**). Precisely, these mismatches, which quite easily in the process of the thermal fluctuations acquire enzymatically competent conformations and do not cause steric constraints in the recognition pocket of the high-fidelity replication DNA polymerase (**Table 3**), should be experimentally observed in the closed conformation of the latter.

3.8. Key microstructural mechanisms of the 2-aminopurine (2AP) mutagenicity

Based on the mechanisms of the spontaneous point mutations [33, 34, 51–66, 68–74, 78], we established physico-chemical mechanisms of the mutagenic action of the classical mutagen

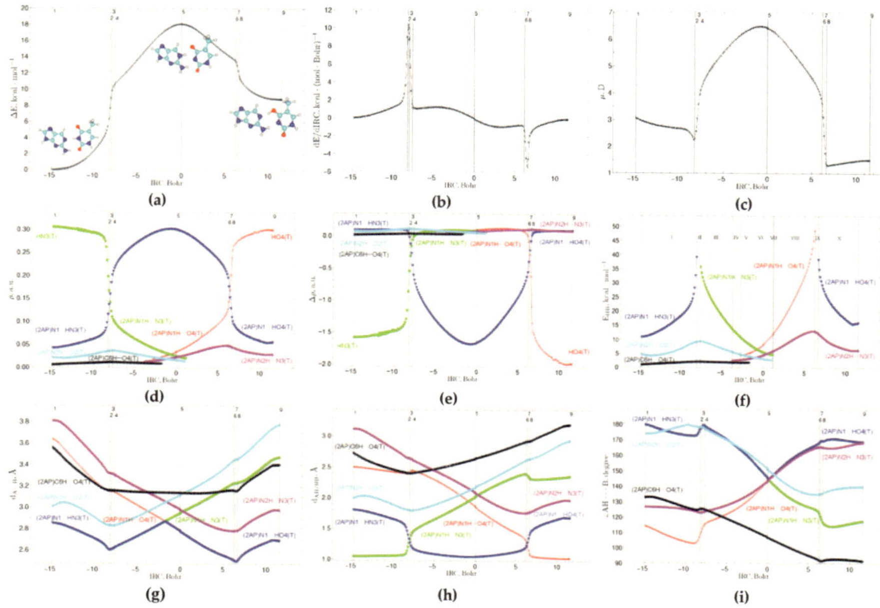

Figure 6. Profiles of: **(a)** the relative electronic energy ΔE, **(b)** the first derivative of the electronic energy with respect to the IRC (dE/dIRC), **(c)** the dipole moment μ, **(d)** the electron density ϱ, **(e)** the Laplacian of the electron density Δϱ, **(f)** the energy of the intermolecular H-bonds E_{HB} estimated by the EML formula [79] at the (3,-1) BCPs, **(g)** the distance $d_{A\cdots B}$ between the electronegative A and B atoms, **(h)** the distance $d_{AH/HB}$ between the hydrogen and electronegative A or B atoms and **(i)** the angle ∠AH···B of the covalent and hydrogen bonds along the IRC of the 2AP·T(WC)↔2AP·T*(w) tautomerization obtained at the B3LYP/6–311++G(d,p) level of theory, ε = 1.

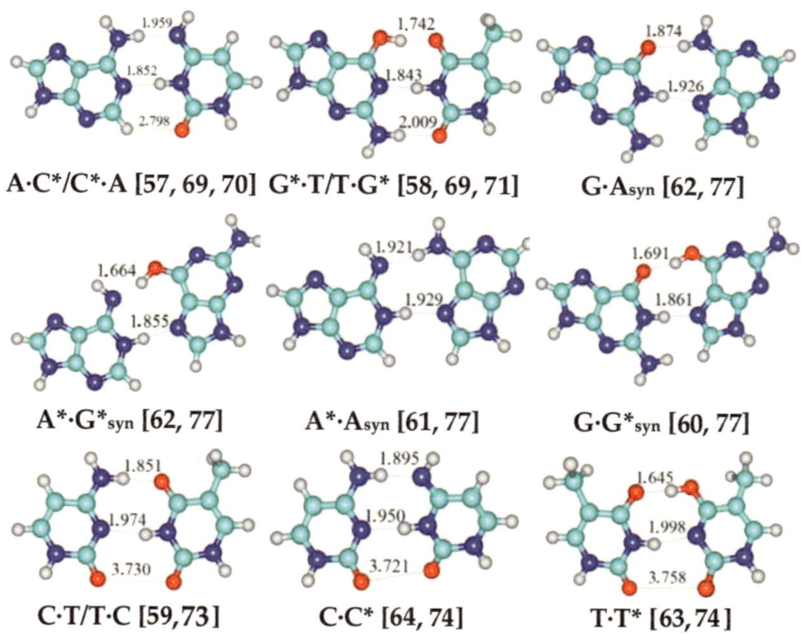

Figure 7. Geometrical structures of the 12 incorrect DNA base mispairs causing spontaneous point incorporation and replication errors (B3LYP/6–311++G(d,p) level of theory, ε = 1).

Mispairs	Geometrical parameters			Energetic parameters				
	$R(H_{N1/N9}\text{-}H_{N1/N9})^{a}$	α_1^{b}	α_2^{c}	ΔE_{def}^{d}		$-\Delta E_{int}^{e}$	$\Sigma E_{HB}/\lvert\Delta E_{int}\rvert^{f}$	$-\Delta G_{int}^{g}$
A·C*	9.996	55.3	58.2	0.10	0.29	15.73	91.8	2.27
A*·C	10.059	55.3	57.2	0.29	0.53	23.50	65.9	10.76
G*·T	10.291	51.5	51.1	0.14	0.40	19.79	87.7	7.09
G·T*	10.202	50.6	52.2	0.45	0.90	33.40	61.3	20.66
$G{\cdot}A_{syn}$	10.399	51.6	38.5	3.00	3.61	17.00	65.9	2.80
$A^{*}{\cdot}G^{*}_{syn}$	10.411	50.3	37.5	3.18	3.72	23.00	72.6	11.47
$A^{*}{\cdot}A_{syn}$	10.322	53.9	41.2	2.18	2.72	16.73	74.8	3.83
$G{\cdot}G^{*}_{syn}$	10.425	48.7	36.1	4.04	4.66	19.82	69.5	7.28
C·T	8.215	59.7	57.0	8.67	8.87	13.86	85.4	1.54
C·C*	8.086	60.3	59.5	8.57	8.76	14.75	91.2	2.34
T·T*	8.385	53.6	58.1	10.97	10.91	16.67	84.0	4.69
A·T	10.130	54.3	54.8	0.00	0.25	14.92	86.9	1.43
G·C	10.209	52.9	55.3	0.11	0.00	29.28	60.8	15.97

[a]The distance between the glycosidic protons at the N1/N9 atoms, Å.

[b]The glycosidic angles for the bases situated on the left and right within the base pair, respectively, degree.

[c]The glycosidic angles for the bases situated on the left and right within the base pair, respectively, degree.

[d]The electronic energy of deformation, necessary to apply to the mismatch to acquire the sizes of the A·T (in the left column) and G·C (in the right column) Watson-Crick DNA base pairs.

[e]The electronic energy of interaction.

[f]The contribution of the total energy of the intermolecular H-bonds to the electronic energy of interaction, %.

[g]The Gibbs free energy of interaction (T = 298.15 K).

Table 3. Selected structural and energetic (in kcal·mol^{-1}) characteristics of the canonical and noncanonical DNA base pairs, responsible for the origin of the spontaneous transitions and transversions (MP2/6-311++G(2df,pd)//B3LYP/6-311++G(d,p) level of theory, ε = 1).

2AP—high-energy structural isomer of A nucleotide base [75–77, 80–82]. In the literature, a great amount of experimental and theoretical phenomenological data on 2AP has been collected [83–87] without proper justification and substantiation.

We have found for the first time that the microstructural mechanism of the mutagenic action of 2AP, causing induced *replication errors*, generates with higher probability the mutagenic tautomer T* according to the 2AP·T(WC) → 2AP·T*(w) tautomeric reaction, than for the Watson-Crick A·T(WC) DNA base pair according to the A·T(WC) → A·T*(w) tautomerization reaction [68, 88]. At this point, the ratio of probabilities determining *replication errors* consists $P_{2AP{\cdot}T}/P_{A{\cdot}T} = 1.8{\cdot}10^{3}$. The mutagenic effect is achieved due to the greater stability of the 2AP·T*(w) complex by the participation of 2AP ($\Delta E_{int} = -20.95$ and $\Delta G_{int} = -9.18$ kcal·mol^{-1}) in comparison with the analogical A·T*(w) base mispair by the participation of A ($\Delta E_{int} = -13.44$ and $\Delta G_{int} = -1.61$ kcal·mol^{-1}) (**Figure 8a, Table 4**) [68, 88].

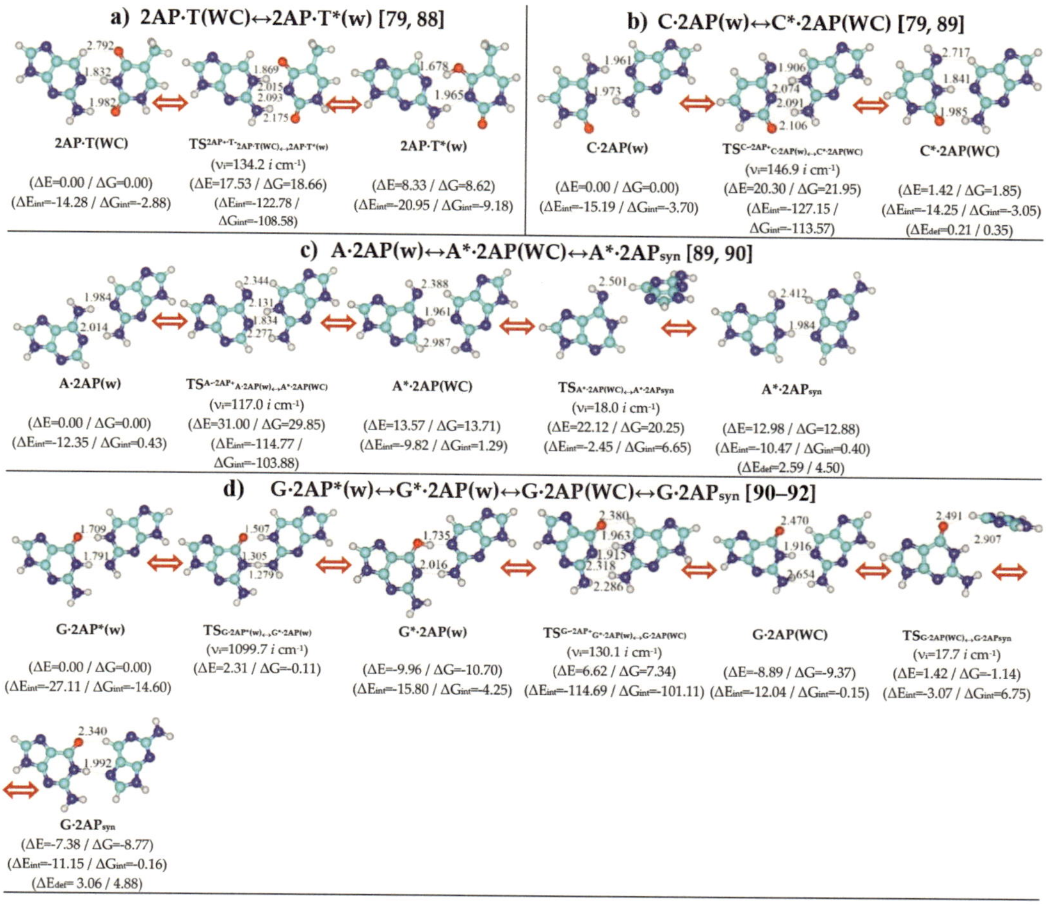

Figure 8. Reaction pathways of the biologically important tautomerizations and conformational transitions of the structures containing canonical DNA bases and 2AP in the main and rare tautomeric forms leading to the replication (**a**) and incorporation (**b, c, d**) errors—transitions and transversions. Relative electronic ΔE and Gibbs free ΔG energies, electronic ΔE_{int} and Gibbs free ΔG_{int} energies of interaction, the deformation energies ΔE_{def}(A·T)/ΔE_{def}(G·C) necessary to apply to the mismatch to acquire the sizes of the A·T(WC)/G·C(WC) Watson-Crick DNA base pairs (in kcal·mol^{-1}), imaginary frequencies ν_i (cm^{-1}) at the TSs of the interconversions are presented below them in brackets (MP2/aug-cc-pVDZ//B3LYP/6–311++G(d,p) level of theory in vacuum at T = 298.15 K). The base, belonging to the template strand of DNA, is situated on the left, while the base of the incoming nucleotide—on the right.

We have shown for the first time that 2AP very effectively produces induced *incorporation errors* by binding with C DNA base and forming the wobble C·2AP(w) mispair, which is tautomerized *via* the C·2AP(w) → C*·2AP(WC) tautomeric reaction into the Watson-Crick-like C*·2AP(WC) base mispair, which quite easily in the process of the thermal fluctuations acquires enzymatically competent conformation (estimated ratio of probabilities $P_{C\cdot 2AP}/P_{C\cdot A} = 1.92\cdot 10^4$) (**Figure 8b**, **Table 4**) [89].

By estimating the probability ratio $P_{A\cdot 2AP}/P_{A\cdot A} = 40.5$, we conclude that 2AP in the case of the A·2AP(w) → A*·2AP(WC) → A*·2AP$_{syn}$ structural transformations (**Figure 8c**, **Table 4**) causes transversion, when a pyrimidine base (in this case T) is substituted by a purine, in particular—A [89].

Tautomerization/ Conformational transition	ν_i	ΔG	ΔE	$\Delta\Delta G_{TS}$	$\Delta\Delta E_{TS}$	ΔΔG	ΔΔE	$\tau_{99.9\%}$	τ
a) 2AP·T(WC)↔2AP·T*(w) [79, 88]	134.2	8.62	8.33	18.66	17.53	10.04	9.21	$2.53 \cdot 10^{-5}$	3.7×10^{-6}
A·T(WC)↔A·T*(w) [51, 53, 68]	99.7	13.08	14.84	20.28	20.41	7.20	5.57	$2.09 \cdot 10^{-7}$	3.0×10^{-8}
b) C·2AP(w)↔C*·2AP(WC) [79, 89]	146.9	1.85	1.42	21.95	20.30	20.11	18.88	$5.87 \cdot 10^{2}$	8.9×10^{1}
C·A(w)↔C*·A(WC) [57, 70]	588.5	−6.07	−7.20	19.51	17.61	25.58	24.81	$1.74 \cdot 10^{2}$	7.1×10^{5}
c) A·2AP(w)↔A*·2AP(WC) [89, 90]	117.0	13.71	13.57	29.85	31.00	16.14	17.43	0.76	0.1
A*·2AP(WC)↔A*·$2AP_{syn}$ [89]	18.0	−0.83	−0.59	6.54	8.55	7.37	9.14	$5.59 \cdot 10^{-8}$	4.1×10^{-8}
A·A(w)↔A·A*(WC) [72]	152.4	3.63	1.09	25.86	22.56	22.24	21.47	$2.22 \cdot 10^{4}$	3.2×10^{3}
A·A*(WC)↔A*·A(WC) [65]	497.5	0.00	0.00	6.39	9.71	6.39	9.71	$2.28 \cdot 10^{-8}$	6.4×10^{-9}
A*·A(WC)↔A*·A_{syn}(TF) [61, 77]	15.8	0.56	1.23	8.09	8.09	7.53	6.85	$2.66 \cdot 10^{-7}$	5.3×10^{-8}
d) G·2AP*(w)↔G*·2AP(w) [91, 92]	1099.7	−10.70	−9.96	−0.11	2.31	10.59	12.26	$4.39 \cdot 10^{-13}$	4.5×10^{-6}
G*·2AP(w)↔G·2AP(WC) [90, 91]	130.1	1.33	1.07	18.04	16.58	16.70	15.51	1.77	0.3
G·2AP(WC)↔G·$2AP_{syn}$ [91]	17.7	0.60	1.51	8.23	10.31	7.63	8.80	$3.22 \cdot 10^{-7}$	6.4×10^{-8}
G·A*(w)↔G·A(WC) [73]	126.8	−6.93	−6.73	16.98	16.32	23.92	23.05	3.14	5.5×10^{4}
G·A(WC)↔G·A_{syn} [56, 62, 77]	20.7	0.76	0.58	8.39	8.89	7.64	8.31	$3.47 \cdot 10^{-7}$	6.4×10^{-8}

Note: see **Tables 1** and **2**.

Table 4. Energetic and kinetic characteristics of the biologically important tautomerizations and conformational transitions of the structures containing canonical DNA bases and 2AP in the main or rare tautomeric forms leading to replication and incorporation errors—transitions and transversions (MP2/aug-cc-pVDZ//B3LYP/6-311++G(d,p) level of theory, ε = 1).

We prove for the first time that 2AP* as a base of the incoming nucleotide may produce also another transversion, when 2AP* mutagenic tautomer pairs with G base and formed G·2AP*(w) mispair converts according to the route of the sequential tautomeric and conformational transformations—G·2AP*(w) → G*·2AP(w) → G·2AP(WC) → G·$2AP_{syn}$ (**Figure 8d**, **Table 4**) [91]. Estimated ratio of probabilities $P_{G\cdot 2AP*}/P_{G\cdot A*} = 1.90 \cdot 10^{7}$ points that this route of the tautomerically conformational transformations is mutagenic, generating appropriate transversions, when pyrimidine bases (in this case C) are replaced by the analogue of the purine base—2AP. This also causes low-probable transitions and transversions, since in the next rounds of the DNA replication, 2AP pairs not only with T, but also with the C and A DNA bases [91].

Our theoretical data are in good agreement with existing experimental results [80, 81, 83, 84] and also allow a unified physico-chemical interpretation of them.

By analyzing profiles of the physico-chemical characteristics for the tautomerization reactions *via* the DPT and PT involving 2AP, which are integral parts of the biologically important tautomerically conformational transformations, we have established that 2AP·T(WC)↔2AP·T*(w) [79], 2AP·C*(WC)↔2AP·C(w) [79], G*·2AP(w)↔G·2AP(WC) [90] and A·2AP(w)↔A*·2AP(WC) [90] tautomerization pathways proceed through the stepwise concerted mechanism *via* the sequential intrapair PT between the bases followed by the shifting of the 2AP relatively the T/C*/G*/A bases, accordingly, while the T·2AP*(w)↔T*·2AP(w) and G·2AP*(w)↔G*·2AP(w) [92] DPT tautomerization reactions proceed through the asynchronous concerted mechanism.

4. Conclusions

Reported results are crucial for understanding the microstructural mechanisms of the spontaneous transitions and transversions, since they allow us to explain, on one side, the origin of the mutagenic tautomers at the separation of the DNA strands before DNA replication and, on the other side, how incorrect purine·pyrimidine, purine·purine and pyrimidine·pyrimidine wobble mispairs adapt to enzymatically competent sizes in the recognition pocket of the high-fidelity DNA polymerase.

Obtained results allow us to explain biological experiments available in the literature, which still remain without proper theoretical justification:

- Numerical estimations of the frequencies of the mispair occurrence satisfactorily explain experimental data: ($10^{-3}\div10^{-4}$) G·T/T·G > > A·C/C·A > > C·T/T·C > A·A > G·A/A·G > > G·G ≈ C·C (10^{-6}) [93].
- Established A·C(w)↔A·C*(WC) and G·T(w)↔G*·T(WC) wobble(w)↔Watson-Crick(WC) transformations *via* the sequential PT allow us to explain the way of the acquisition by the A·C(w)/G·T(w) wobble mispairs of the Watson-Crick geometry in the active center of the high-fidelity DNA polymerase or DNA duplex and also to interpret X-ray [14, 15] and NMR [16–18] experiments.
- Presented approach allows us to clarify the microstructural mechanisms of the mutations induced by the classical mutagens, in particular 2-aminopurine, for which induced frequencies agree well with the experimental data.
- Ionization mechanism cannot entirely explain the nature of the spontaneous transitions [94].

These data clarify the nature of genome variability and reveals new facets of the Watson-Crick hypothesis of the spontaneous point mutagenesis arising during DNA replication and significantly expands the possibilities for rational design of chemical mutagens with targeted action, which could be interesting for synthetic biology and biotechnology.

Finally, authors believe that these principles could be extended without any constrains to the processes determining the protein synthesis.

In view of the prominent role, that play parallel and antiparallel Hoogsteen pairings in DNA:RNA helices, as it was reliably established by Prof. Seligmann [95, 96] for mitochondrial genomes, it is important to explore in future mutagenic tautomerization of these classical base pairs by the quantum-chemical methods.

Acknowledgements

The authors gratefully appreciate technical support and computational facilities of joint computer cluster of SSI "Institute for Single Crystals" of the National Academy of Sciences of Ukraine (NASU) and Institute for Scintillation Materials of the NASU incorporated into Ukrainian National Grid. This work was partially supported by the Grant of the NASU for young scientists, Grant of the President of Ukraine to support the research of young scientists [project number F70] from the State Fund for Fundamental Research of Ukraine of the Ministry of the Education and Science of Ukraine and by the Scholarship of Verkhovna Rada (Parliament) of Ukraine for the talented young scientists in 2017 year given to DrSci Ol'ha O. Brovarets'. O. O. B. expresses sincere gratitude to organizing committee for financial support of the participation in the "EMBO/FEBS Lecture Course Spetsai Summer School 2017 for Proteins and Organized Complexity" (September 24–October 1, 2017, Spetses, Greece), to Lawyers Association "AVER Lex "(Kyiv, Ukraine) for the sponsorship of presenting the plenary lecture as invited speaker at the "EMN Meeting on Computation and Theory" (November 6–10, 2017, Dubai, United Arab Emirates), to Max Planck Institute of Molecular Plant Physiology (MPI-MP) (hosted by Prof. Yariv Brotman) for the kind invitation and financial support of the invited talk (November 29, 2017, Potsdam, Germany), to organizing committee headed by Prof. Karl Kuchler (Medical University Vienna, Austria) for the kind invitation and financial support (ABC fellow) of the participation in the seventh FEBS Special Meeting "ATP-Binding Cassette (ABC) Proteins: from Multidrug Resistance to Genetic Disease" (March 6–12, 2018, Innsbruck, Austria) and to Chemistry Biological Interface Division of the Royal Society of Chemistry (RSC, UK) for the RSC Travel Grant for the participation at the "3rd Green and Sustainable Chemistry Conference" (May 13-16, 2018, Hotel Intercontinental, Berlin, Germany). The funders had no role in study design, data collection and analysis, decision to publish or preparation of the manuscript.

Conflict of interest

There are no conflicts to declare.

Dedication

This chapter is dedicated to 100th anniversary of the National Academy of Sciences of Ukraine.

Author details

Ol'ha O. Brovarets'[1,2]* and Dmytro M. Hovorun[1,2]

*Address all correspondence to: o.o.brovarets@imbg.org.ua

1 Department of Molecular and Quantum Biophysics, Institute of Molecular Biology and Genetics, National Academy of Sciences of Ukraine, Kyiv, Ukraine

2 Department of Molecular Biotechnology and Bioinformatics, Taras Shevchenko National University of Kyiv, Institute of High Technologies, Kyiv, Ukraine

References

[1] Cooper GM. The Cell: A Molecular Approach. 2nd ed. Boston University. Sunderland (MA): Sinauer Associates; 2000

[2] Freese EB. On the molecular explanation of spontaneous and induced mutations. Brookhaven Symposia in Biology. 1959;**12**:63-75

[3] von Borstel RC. Origins of spontaneous base substitutions. Mutation Research. 1994; **307**:131-140

[4] Friedberg EC, Walker GC, Siede W, Wood RD, Schultz RA, Ellenberger T. DNA Repair and Mutagenesis. Washington D.C: ASM Press; 2006

[5] Drake JW, Charlesworth B, Charlesworth D, Crow JF. Rates of spontaneous mutation. Genetics. 1998;**148**:1667-1686

[6] Lee H, Popodi E, Tang H, Foster PL. Rate and molecular spectrum of spontaneous mutations in the bacterium *Escherichia coli* as determined by whole-genome sequencing. Proceedings of the National Academy of Sciences of the United States of America. 2012;**109**:E2774-E2783

[7] Lynch M. Rate, molecular spectrum, and consequences of human mutation. Proceedings of the National Academy of Sciences of the United States of America. 2010;**107**:961-968

[8] Fijalkowska IJ, Schaaper RM, Jonczyk P. DNA replication fidelity in *Escherichia coli*: A multi-DNA polymerase affair. FEMS Microbiology Reviews. 2012;**36**:1105-1121

[9] Watson JD, Crick FHC. The structure of DNA. Cold Spring Harbor Symposia on Quantitative Biology. 1953;**18**:123-131

[10] Topal MD, Fresco JR. Complementary base pairing and the origin of substitution mutations. Nature. 1976;**263**:285-289

[11] Nedderman AN, Stone MJ, Lin PKT, Brown DM, Williams DH. Base pairing of cytosine analogues with adenine and guanine in oligonucleotide duplexes: Evidence for exchange between Watson-Crick and wobble base pairs using ^{1}H NMR spectroscopy. Journal of the Chemical Society, Chemical Communications. 1991;(19):1357-1359. http://pubs.rsc.org/en/content/articlelanding/1991/c3/c39910001357#!divAbstract

[12] Nedderman AN, Stone MJ, Williams DH, Lin PKY, Brown DM. Molecular basis for methoxyamine-initiated mutagenesis: ^{1}H nuclear magnetic resonance studies of oligonucleotide duplexes containing base-modified cytosine residues. Journal of Molecular Biology. 1993;**230**:1068-1076

[13] Harris VH, Smith CL, Jonathan Cummins W, Hamilton AL, Adams H, Dickman M, Hornby DP, Williams DM. The effect of tautomeric constant on the specificity of nucleotide incorporation during DNA replication: Support for the rare tautomer hypothesis of substitution mutagenesis. Journal of Molecular Biology. 2003;**326**:1389-1401

[14] Bebenek K, Pedersen LC, Kunkel TA. Replication infidelity *via* a mismatch with Watson–crick geometry. Proceedings of the National Academy of Sciences of the United States of America. 2011;**108**:1862–1867

[15] Wang W, Hellinga HW, Beese LS. Structural evidence for the rare tautomer hypothesis of spontaneous mutagenesis. Proceedings of the National Academy of Sciences of the United States of America. 2011;**108**:17644-17648

[16] Kimsey IJ, Petzold K, Sathyamoorthy B, Stein ZW, Al-Hashimi HM. Visualizing transient Watson-Crick-like mispairs in DNA and RNA duplexes. Nature. 2015;**519**:315-320

[17] Szymanski ES, Kimsey IJ, Al-Hashimi HM. Direct NMR evidence that transient tautomeric and anionic states in dG·dT form Watson–Crick-like base pairs. Journal of the American Chemical Society. 2017;**139**:4326-4329

[18] Kimsey IJ, Szymanski ES, Zahurancik WJ, Shakya A, Xue Y, Chu C-C, Sathyamoorthy B, Suo Z, Al-Hashimi HM. Dynamic basis for dG·dT misincorporation *via* tautomerization and ionization. Nature. 2018;**554**:195-201

[19] Maximoff SN, Kamerlin SCL, Florian J. DNA polymerase λ active site favors a mutagenic mispair between the enol form of deoxyguanosine triphosphate substrate and the keto form of thymidine template: A free energy perturbation study. The Journal of Physical Chemistry B. 2017;**121**:7813-7822

[20] Danilov VI, Anisimov VM, Kurita N, Hovorun D. MP2 and DFT studies of the DNA rare base pairs: The molecular mechanism of the spontaneous substitution mutations conditioned by tautomerism of bases. Chemical Physics Letters. 2005;**412**:285-293

[21] Fonseca Guerra C, Bickelhaupt FM, Saha S, Wang F. Adenine tautomers: Relative stabilities, ionization energies, and mismatch with cytosine. The Journal of Physical Chemistry A. 2006;**110**:4012-4020

[22] Löwdin P-O. Proton tunneling in DNA and its biological implications. Reviews of Modern Physics. 1963;**35**:724-732

[23] Löwdin P-O. Quantum genetics and the aperiodic solid: Some aspects on the biological problems of heredity, mutations, aging, and tumors in view of the quantum theory of the DNA molecule. In: Löwdin P-O, editor. Advances in Quantum Chemistry (2). New York, USA. London, UK: Academic Press; 1966. pp. 213-360

[24] Godbeer AD, Al-Khalili JS, Stevenson PD. Modelling proton tunneling in the adenine-thymine base pair. Physical Chemistry Chemical Physics. 2015;**17**:13034-13044

[25] Turaeva N, Brown-Kennerly V. Marcus model of spontaneous point mutation in DNA. Chemical Physics. 2015;**461**:106-110

[26] Padermshoke A, Katsumoto Y, Masaki R, Aida M. Thermally induced double proton transfer in GG and wobble GT base pairs: A possible origin of the mutagenic guanine. Chemical Physics Letters. 2008;**457**:232-236

[27] Strazewski P, Tamm C. Replication experiments with nucleotide base analogues. Angewandte Chemie International Edition. 1990;**29**:36-57

[28] Sowers LC, Shaw BR, Veigl ML, Sedwick WD. DNA base modification: Ionized base pairs and mutagenesis. Mutation Research. 1987;**177**:201-218

[29] Brown T, Kennard O, Kneale G, Rabinovich D. High-resolution structure of a DNA helix containing mismatched base pairs. Nature. 1985;**315**:604-606

[30] Rossetti G, Dans PD, Gomez-Pinto I, Ivani I, Gonzalez C, Orozco M. The structural impact of DNA mismatches. Nucleic Acids Research. 2015;**43**:4309-4321

[31] Kool ET. Active site tightness and substrate fit in DNA replication. Annual Review of Biochemistry. 2002;**71**:191-219

[32] Brovarets' OO, Kolomiets' IM, Hovorun DM. Elementary molecular mechanisms of the spontaneous point mutations in DNA: A novel quantum-chemical insight into the classical understanding. In: Tada T, editor. Quantum Chemistry—Molecules for Innovations. Rijeka, Croatia: InTech Open Access; 2012. pp. 59-102

[33] Brovarets' OO. Physico-chemical nature of the spontaneous and induced by the mutagens transitions and transversions [Ph.D. thesis]. Kyiv, Ukraine: Taras Shevchenko National University of Kyiv; 2010

[34] Brovarets' OO. Microstructural mechanisms of the origin of the spontaneous point mutations [DrSci thesis]. Kyiv, Ukraine: Taras Shevchenko National University of Kyiv; 2015

[35] Aguilera A, Gómez-González B. Genome instability: A mechanistic view of its causes and consequences. Nature Reviews. Genetics. 2008;**9**:204-217

[36] Rudd SG, Valerie NCK, Helleday T. Pathways controlling dNTP pools to maintain genome stability. DNA Repair. 2016;**44**:193-204

[37] Jordheim LP, Durantel D, Zoulim F, Dumontet C. Advances in the development of nucleoside and nucleotide analogues for cancer and viral diseases. Nature Reviews. Drug Discovery. 2013;**12**:447-464

[38] Galmarini CM, Mackey JR, Dumontet C. Nucleoside analogues and nucleobases in cancer treatment. The Lancet Oncology. 2002;**3**:415-424

[39] Del Grosso E, Dallaire A-M, Vallée-Bélisle A, Ricci F. Enzyme-operated DNA-based nanodevices. Nano Letters. 2015;**15**:8407-8411

[40] Liedl T, Sobey TL, Simmel FC. DNA-based nanodevices. NanoToday. 2007;**2**:36-41

[41] Piccolino M. Biological machines: From mills to molecules. Nature Reviews. Molecular Cell Biology. 2000;**1**:149-153

[42] Frisch MJ, Trucks GW, Schlegel HB, Scuseria GE, Robb MA, Cheeseman JR, Pople JA. GAUSSIAN 09 (Revision B.01). Wallingford CT: Gaussian Inc; 2010

[43] Tirado-Rives J, Jorgensen WL. Performance of B3LYP density functional methods for a large set of organic molecules. Journal of Chemical Theory and Computation. 2008; **4**:297-306

[44] Wiberg KB. Basis set effects on calculated geometries: 6-311++G** *vs.* aug-cc-pVDZ. Journal of Computational Chemistry. 2004;**25**:1342-1346

[45] Parr RG, Yang W. Density-Functional Theory of Atoms and Molecules. Oxford: Oxford University Press; 1989

[46] Hratchian HP, Schlegel HB. Finding minima, transition states, and following reaction pathways on *ab initio* potential energy surfaces. In: Dykstra CE, Frenking G, Kim KS, Scuseria G, editors. Theory and Applications of Computational Chemistry: The First 40 Years. Amsterdam: Elsevier; 2005. pp. 195-249

[47] Mertz EL, Krishtalik LI. Low dielectric response in enzyme active site. Proceedings of the National Academy of Sciences of the United States of America. 2000;**97**:2081-2086

[48] Petrushka J, Sowers LC, Goodman M. Comparison of nucleotide interactions in water, proteins, and vacuum: Model for DNA polymerase fidelity. Proceedings of the National Academy of Sciences of the United States of America. 1986;**83**:1559-1562

[49] Bader RFW. Atoms in Molecules: A Quantum Theory. Oxford: Oxford University Press; 1990

[50] Atkins PW. Physical Chemistry. Oxford: Oxford University Press; 1998

[51] Brovarets' OO, Hovorun DM. Can tautomerisation of the A·T Watson-Crick base pair *via* double proton transfer provoke point mutations during DNA replication? A comprehensive QM and QTAIM analysis. Journal of Biomolecular Structure and Dynamics. 2014;**32**:127-154

[52] Brovarets' OO, Hovorun DM. Why the tautomerization of the G·C Watson–Crick base pair *via* the DPT does not cause point mutations during DNA replication? QM and QTAIM comprehensive analysis. Journal of Biomolecular Structure and Dynamics. 2014;**32**:1474-1499

[53] Brovarets' OO, Hovorun DM. Proton tunneling in the A·T Watson-Crick DNA base pair: Myth or reality? Journal of Biomolecular Structure and Dynamics. 2015;**33**:2716-2720

[54] Brovarets' OO, Zhurakivsky RO, Hovorun DM. DPT tautomerisation of the wobble guanine·thymine DNA base mispair is not mutagenic: QM and QTAIM arguments. Journal of Biomolecular Structure and Dynamics. 2015;**33**:674-689

[55] Brovarets' OO, Yurenko YP, Dubey IY, Hovorun DM. Can DNA-binding proteins of replisome tautomerize nucleotide bases? *Ab initio* model study. Journal of Biomolecular Structure and Dynamics. 2012;**29**:1101-1109

[56] Brovarets' OO, Zhurakivsky RO, Hovorun DM. Is the DPT tautomerisation of the long A·G Watson-Crick DNA base mispair a source of the adenine and guanine mutagenic tautomers? A QM and QTAIM response to the biologically important question. Journal of Computational Chemistry. 2014;**35**:451-466

[57] Brovarets' OO, Hovorun DM. The physicochemical essence of the purine·pyrimidine transition mismatches with Watson-Crick geometry in DNA: A·C* *versa* A*·C. A QM and QTAIM atomistic understanding. Journal of Biomolecular Structure and Dynamics. 2015;**33**:28-55

[58] Brovarets' OO, Hovorun DM. The nature of the transition mismatches with Watson-Crick architecture: The G*·T or G·T* DNA base mispair or both? A QM/QTAIM perspective for the biological problem. Journal of Biomolecular Structure and Dynamics. 2015;**33**:925-945

[59] Brovarets' OO, Hovorun DM. Atomistic understanding of the C·T mismatched DNA base pair tautomerization *via* the DPT: QM and QTAIM computational approaches. Journal of Computational Chemistry. 2013;**34**:2577-2590

[60] Brovarets' OO, Hovorun DM. Does the G·G*$_{syn}$ DNA mismatch containing canonical and rare tautomers of the guanine tautomerise through the DPT? A QM/QTAIM microstructural study. Molecular Physics. 2014;**112**:3033-3046

[61] Brovarets' OO, Zhurakivsky RO, Hovorun DM. Does the tautomeric status of the adenine bases change upon the dissociation of the A*·A$_{syn}$ Topal-Fresco DNA mismatch? A combined QM and QTAIM atomistic insight. Physical Chemistry Chemical Physics. 2014;**16**:3715-3725

[62] Brovarets' OO, Hovorun DM. DPT tautomerisation of the G·A$_{syn}$ and A*·G*$_{syn}$ DNA mismatches: A QM/QTAIM combined atomistic investigation. Physical Chemistry Chemical Physics. 2014;**16**:9074-9085

[63] Brovarets' OO, Zhurakivsky RO, Hovorun DM. Structural, energetic and tautomeric properties of the T·T*/T*·T DNA mismatch involving mutagenic tautomer of thymine: A QM and QTAIM insight. Chemical Physics Letters. 2014;**592**:247-255

[64] Brovarets' OO, Hovorun DM. Atomistic nature of the DPT tautomerisation of the biologically important C·C* DNA base mispair containing amino and imino tautomers of cytosine: A QM and QTAIM approach. Physical Chemistry Chemical Physics. 2013;**15**:20091-20104

[65] Brovarets' OO, Hovorun DM. DPT tautomerization of the long A·A* Watson-Crick base pair formed by the amino and imino tautomers of adenine: Combined QM and QTAIM investigation. Journal of Molecular Modeling. 2013;**19**:4223-4237

[66] Brovarets' OO, Hovorun DM. How does the long G·G* Watson-Crick DNA base mispair comprising keto and enol tautomers of the guanine tautomerise? The results of a QM/QTAIM investigation. Physical Chemistry Chemical Physics. 2014;**16**:15886-15899

[67] Kirmizialtin S, Nguyen V, Johnson KA, Elber R. How conformational dynamics of DNA polymerase select correct substrates: Experiments and simulations. Structure. 2012;**20**:618-627

[68] Brovarets' OO, Hovorun DM. New structural hypostases of the A·T and G·C Watson-Crick DNA base pairs caused by their mutagenic tautomerisation in a wobble manner: A QM/QTAIM prediction. RSC Advances. 2015;**5**:99594-99605

[69] Brovarets' OO, Hovorun DM. Physicochemical mechanism of the wobble DNA base pairs Gua·Thy and Ade·Cyt transition into the mismatched base pairs Gua*·Thy and Ade·Cyt* formed by the mutagenic tautomers. Ukrainica Bioorganica Acta. 2009;**8**:12-18

[70] Brovarets' OO, Hovorun DM. Tautomeric transition between wobble A·C DNA base mispair and Watson-Crick-like A·C* mismatch: Microstructural mechanism and biological significance. Physical Chemistry Chemical Physics. 2015;**17**:15103-15110

[71] Brovarets' OO, Hovorun DM. How many tautomerisation pathways connect Watson-Crick-like G*·T DNA base mispair and wobble mismatches? Journal of Biomolecular Structure and Dynamics. 2015;**33**:2297-2315

[72] Brovarets' OO, Hovorun DM. Wobble↔Watson-Crick tautomeric transitions in the homo-purine DNA mismatches: A key to the intimate mechanisms of the spontaneous transversions. Journal of Biomolecular Structure and Dynamics. 2015;**33**:2710-2715

[73] Brovarets' OO, Hovorun DM. Novel physico-chemical mechanism of the mutagenic tautomerisation of the Watson–Crick-like A·G and C·T DNA base mispairs: A quantum-chemical picture. RSC Advances. 2015;**5**:66318-66333

[74] Brovarets' OO, Hovorun DM. A novel conception for spontaneous transversions caused by homo-pyrimidine DNA mismatches: A QM/QTAIM highlight. Physical Chemistry Chemical Physics. 2015;**17**:21381-21388

[75] Lasken RS, Goodman MF. A fidelity assay using "dideoxy" DNA sequencing: A measurement of sequence dependence and frequency of forming 5-bromouracil·guanine base mispairs. Proceedings of the National Academy of Sciences of the United States of America. 1985;**82**:1301-1305

[76] Kaufman ER, Davidson RL. Bromodeoxyuridine mutagenesis in mammalian cells: Mutagenesis is independent of the amount of bromouracil in DNA. Proceedings of the National Academy of Sciences of the United States of America. 1978;**75**:4982-4986

[77] Brovarets' OO, Hovorun DM. How do long improper purine-purine pairs of DNA bases adapt the enzymatically competent conformation? Structural mechanism and its quantum-mechanical grounds. Ukrainian Journal of Physics. 2015;**60**:748-756

[78] Brovarets' OO, Hovorun DM. By how many tautomerisation routes the Watson–Crick-like A·C* DNA base mispair is linked with the wobble mismatches? A QM/QTAIM vision from a biological point of view. Structural Chemistry. 2015;**27**:119-131

[79] Brovarets' OO, Voiteshenko I, Pérez-Sánchez HE, Hovorun DM. A QM/QTAIM detailed look at the Watson-Crick↔wobble tautomeric transformations of the 2-aminopurine·pyrimidine mispairs. Journal of Biomolecular Structure and Dynamics. 2018;**36**: 1649-1665

[80] Wacker A, Lodemann E, Gauri K, Chandra P. Synthesis and coding properties of 2-aminopurine polyribonucleotide. Journal of Molecular Biology. 1966;**18**:382

[81] Law SM, Eritja R, Goodman MF, Breslauer KJ. Spectroscopic and calorimetric characterization of DNA duplexes containing 2-aminopurine. Biochemistry. 1996;**35**:12329-12337

[82] Hovorun DM. A structural isomerism of nucleotide bases: AM1 calculation. Biopolymers and Cell. 1997;**13**:127-134

[83] Freese E. The specific mutagenic effect of base analogue on phage T4. Journal of Molecular Biology. 1959;**1**:87-105

[84] Pullman B, Pullman A. Electronic delocalization and biochemical evolution. Nature. 1962;**196**:1137-1142

[85] Danilov VI, Krugliak IA, Kuprievich VA, Shramko OV. O mekhanizme mutagennogo deistviia 2-aminopurina. Biofizika. 1967;**12**:726-729

[86] Brovarets' OO, Hovorun DM. Molecular mechanisms of the mutagenic action of 2-aminopurine on DNA. Ukrainica Bioorganica Acta. 2010;**9**:11-17

[87] Brovarets' OO, Hovorun DM. IR vibrational spectra of H-bonded complexes of adenine, 2-aminopurine and 2-aminopurine$^+$ with cytosine and thymine: Quantum-chemical study. Optics and Spectroscopy. 2010;**111**:750-757

[88] Brovarets' OO, Pérez-Sánchez HE, Hovorun DM. Structural grounds for the 2-aminopurine mutagenicity: A novel insight into the old problem of the replication errors. RSC Advances. 2016;**6**:99546-99557

[89] Brovarets' OO, Pérez-Sánchez HE. Whether 2-aminopurine induces incorporation errors at the DNA replication? A quantum-mechanical answer on the actual biological issue. Journal of Biomolecular Structure and Dynamics. 2017;**35**:3398-3411

[90] Brovarets' OO, Voiteshenko I, Hovorun DM. Physico-chemical profiles of the wobble↔Watson-Crick G*·2AP(w)↔G·2AP(WC) and A·2AP(w)↔A*·2AP(WC) tautomerisations: A QM/QTAIM comprehensive survey. Physical Chemistry Chemical Physics. 2018;**20**:623-636

[91] Brovarets' OO, Pérez-Sánchez HE. Whether the amino-imino tautomerism of 2-aminopurine is involved into its mutagenicity? Results of a thorough QM investigation. RSC Advances. 2016;**110**:108255-108264

[92] Brovarets' OO, Voiteshenko I, Pérez-Sánchez HE, Hovorun DM. A QM/QTAIM research under the magnifying glass of the DPT tautomerisation of the wobble mispairs involving 2-aminopurine. New Journal of Chemistry. 2017;**41**:7232-7243

[93] Huang MM, Arnheim N, Goodman MF. Extension of base mispairs by Taq DNA polymerase: Implications for single nucleotide discrimination in PCR. Nucleic Acids Research. 1992;**20**:4567-4573

[94] Brovarets OO, Zhurakivsky RO. Hovorun, D.M. Is there adequate ionization mechanism of the spontaneous transitions? Quantum-chemical investigation. Biopol Cell. 2010;**26**:398-405

[95] Seligmann H. Overlapping genes coded in the 3′-to-5′-direction in mitochondrial genes and 3′-to-5′ polymerization of non-complementary RNA by an 'invertase'. Journal of Theoretical Biology. 2012;**315**:38-52

[96] Seligmann H. Triplex DNA:RNA, 3′-to-5′ inverted RNA and protein coding in mitochondrial genomes. Journal of Computational Biology. 2013;**20**:660-671

Chapter 3

Directed Mutations Recode Mitochondrial Genes: From Regular to Stopless Genetic Codes

Hervé Seligmann

Additional information is available at the end of the chapter

http://dx.doi.org/10.5772/intechopen.80871

Abstract

Mitochondrial genetic codes evolve as side effects of stop codon ambiguity: suppressor tRNAs with anticodons translating stops transform genetic codes to stopless genetic codes. This produces peptides from frames other than regular ORFs, potentially increasing protein numbers coded by single sequences. Previous descriptions of marine turtle Olive Ridley mitogenomes imply directed stop-depletion of noncoding +1 gene frames, stop-creation recodes regular ORFs to stopless genetic codes. In this analysis, directed stop codon depletion in usually noncoding gene frames of the spiraling whitefly *Aleurodicus dispersus*' mitogenome produces new ORFs, introduces stops in regular ORFs, and apparently increases coding redundancy between different gene frames. Directed stop codon mutations switch between peptides coded by regular and stopless genetic codes. This process seems opposite to directed stop creation in HIV ORFs within genomes of immunized elite HIV controllers. Unknown DNA replication/edition mechanisms probably direct stop creation/depletion beyond natural selection on stops. Switches between genetic codes regulate translation of different gene frames.

Keywords: codon-amino acid reassignment, *Lepidochelys olivacea*, antitermination, ribosomal RNA, directional evolution, APOBEC

1. Introduction

Mitochondrial genetic code diversification frequently reassigns stop codons to amino acids [1]. This situation probably reflects ambiguity in roles of stop codons during translation in mitochondria. Indeed, phylogenetic reconstructions of the evolution of genetic codes based on differences between codons in amino acid and stop codon assignments resemble known phylogenies of organisms using these genetic codes, if ambiguity of stop codons in mitochondrial (but not nuclear) genetic codes is accounted [2].

These observations suggest translational activity of mitochondrial tRNAs with anticodons matching stop codons [3] templated by antisense strands of regular mitochondrial tRNAs [4, 5]. Predicted occurrences of mitochondrial stop suppressor (antiterminator) tRNAs coevolve with stop codon usages in predicted off-frame protein coding genes in all analyzed mitochondria (primates and Drosophila [6, 7], including their ribosomal RNAs [8], turtles [9] and Chaetognaths [10]), and in a peptide detected by specific monoclonal immunolocalization in human mitochondria [11]. Hence, there are probably more mitochondrion-encoded genes than usually accepted [12, 13]. Mitogenome size reduction probably causes gene multifunctionality, including mt tDNAs functioning as replication origins [14–21].

Translation of stop codons occurs in different organisms [22, 23], but seems particularly widespread in mitochondria [2, 3] as reflected by the evolution of mitochondrial genetic codes [1]. Nuclear genetic codes lacking dedicated stop codons have been described in protists [24–27] and fungi [28].

1.1. Alternative coding by expanded codons

Switching between regular and stopless genetic codes is not the only strategy increasing dramatically information encoded by genomes. Isolated tetracodons, codons expanded by a fourth silent nucleotide, are known since the dawn of molecular biology [29]. These are sometimes translated by tRNAs with expanded anticodons [30, 31]. It seems probable that systematic frameshifts produce stretches of tetracodons that code for (yet) undetected peptides ([32–34]). Some evidence suggests that tetracoding occurs especially at high environmental temperatures [35] and is predicted by genetic code optimization [36]: codon-anticodon interactions are more stable when four rather than only three base pairs hybridize. Other theoretical considerations suggest that the mitochondrial vertebrate genetic code evolved from a specific subset of 64 tetracodons, the tesserae, chosen on the basis of symmetry principles [37].

Indeed, analyses of mitochondrial mass spectra searching for peptides matching translations assuming tetra- and pentacodons, codons expanded by one or two silent nucleotides, detected numerous tetra- and pentacoded peptides [38–43].

1.2. Alternative coding by swinger polymerization

Further little known mechanisms increase numbers of proteins potentially coded by single sequences. Polymerization occasionally exchanges systematically between nucleotides during DNA replication [44–46] or RNA transcription [47–53] for long sequence stretches (23 exchange rules are possible, nine symmetric, e.g., A<>C, and fourteen asymmetric, e.g., A > C > G > A), producing swinger sequences. Swinger replication, in particular the double symmetric exchange A<>T + C<>G, seems most frequent for mitochondrial ribosomal RNAs [46]. This increases the coding potential of rRNAs, strengthening the hypothesis that rRNAs are modern remnants of protogenomes that templated for translational molecules (tRNA-like and rRNA-like) and protein coding genes [54–58] by dense overlap coding. This is compatible with the occurrence of protein coding regions within modern rRNAs [8, 59–61].

I stress here that the exchange A<>T + C<>G is not trivial: this creates the complement of the template sequence, which is not the regular inverse (or reverse) complement. "Complement" is frequently used as shortcut for inverse complement, but the A<>T + C<>G transformed sequence is a different sequence because it lacks the 3′-to-5′ inversion combined with nucleotide complementarity. The shortcut has been used because 3′-to-5′ inverted sequences had not been described previous to the description of A<>T + C<>G transformed sequences.

It seems regular transcription occasionally switches abruptly to swinger transcription (and vice versa), as indicated by chimeric RNAs. These RNAs correspond in part to regular DNA, and an adjacent part corresponds to DNA only if accounting for swinger transformation [62]. Corresponding chimeric peptides have also been detected [63]. Chimeric DNA also exists: the mitogenome of the stonefly *Kamimuria wangi* (NC_024033) is regular, beside its 16S rRNA, which is entirely swinger transformed along transformation A<>T + C<>G [46].

1.3. Regulation of alternative transcriptions by secondary structure

Secondary structures are important components of RNA function and evolution [64, 65]. Secondary structures formed by tRNA sequences punctuate posttranscriptional processing of mitochondrial transcripts [66–68]. Palindromes potentially forming secondary structures after sequence swinger-tranformation associate with detected mitochondrial swinger RNAs [69]. This is similar to what is known from regular RNA processing in mitochondria and, surprisingly, giant viruses [70] which bear also other striking resemblances with mitogenomes, including similar gene order [71]. Transcription sometimes deletes systematically mono- or dinucleotides after transcribing trinucleotides (del-transcription), translated into peptides that in part converge with peptides translated from regular RNAs by expanded anticodons [38]. Del-transcription, or at least detection of delRNAs, seems downregulated by secondary structures formed after transformation of the sequence by systematic deletions [72].

1.4. Mechanisms that switch between genetic codes?

Phenomena systematically exchanging nucleotides remind more specific mechanisms that alter the genetic code according to which a protein is coded, from a regular genetic code to a stopless genetic code, and/or vice versa. Indeed, previous analyses of mitogenomes revealed that in one GenBank mitogenome (from a marine turtle, the Olive Ridley, *Lepidochelys olivacea*), following GenBank's annotations, several regular protein coding genes do not code for the regular proteins essential for mitochondrial metabolism and usually encoded at these genomic locations. These essential proteins are indeed coded by the corresponding sequences, but only after a frameshift, and only if stops in that frame are translated, explaining the erroneous annotation of stopless ORFs (abbreviation for open reading frames) that do not code for recognized mitochondrial proteins [9].

This was originally interpreted as resulting from directed selection on stop codons. Observations of systematic mutations in contexts creating stop codons in ORFs of HIV genes specifically in elite controllers immune to HIV [73, 74] suggests that enzymatically directed mutagenesis during DNA replication and/or edition could transform ORFs coded according to a regular genetic code into one coded by a stopless genetic code, and vice versa, as observed in several mitochondrial genes of the Olive Ridley. For HIV, introducing stops presumably drastically reduces viral production and contributes to immunity.

This hypothesis of mutations directed at stop codons is in line with observations that polymerase errors are more frequent in stop codon contexts, interpreted as an adaptational bias to introduce mutations in stops [75]. In the next section, GenBank is explored to detect further mitogenomes in which genetic codes were switched by producing stop codons in ORFs and stop-depletion in other frames.

2. Methods

2.1. Exploring GenBank for genetic code switches

Previous Blastp searches found proteins already described in GenBank and aligning with hypothetical peptides translated from randomly chosen frameshifted vertebrate mitochondrial genes. These analyses detected the unusual proteins translated from ORFs of the mitogenome of *Lepidochelys olivacea* [9]. In these cases, the regular mitochondrial proteins are coded in frames that include stops, and hence were not recognized as the regular gene. The annotated frame is stopless, but codes for other, unknown peptides. These other peptides are homologous to peptides translated after frameshift from regular mitochondrial protein coding genes, from other mitogenomes that did not undergo stop codon depletion in non-ORF frames.

2.2. Choice of seed sequences for BLAST searches

The method described above only detects homologies for sequences sufficiently similar to "seed" sequences used for BLAST analyses of GenBank. Therefore, using as seed the human mitogenome, mainly vertebrate proteins were detected, as for the above-mentioned *Lepidochelys olivacea*. A similar situation occurs for detection of swinger DNA/RNA sequences: the original searches using as seed swinger transformed versions of the human mitogenome only detected vertebrate sequences [45], but BLAST analyses using a randomly chosen invertebrate mitogenome (from the North Pacific krill *Euphausia pacifica* (NC_016184)) detected numerous additional swinger sequences, from insect mitogenomes [38].

This search principle for insect nucleotide sequences can also be applied for proteins. I use as seed the five peptides translated from the five "noncoding" frames of the 13 regular protein coding genes of *Euphausia*'s previously randomly chosen invertebrate mitogenome. These 65 peptides were blasted to search GenBank for proteins already described and with high homologies with peptides translated from *Euphausia*'s noncoding frames.

3. Results

3.1. Preliminary results from *Aleurodicus dispersus*

Preliminary BLAST analyses of peptides translated from noncoding frames of *Euphausia*'s mitochondrial protein coding genes detected GenBank proteins from the mitogenome of *Aleurodicus dispersus*, a sap-sucking spiraling whitefly. These have high homology levels with peptides translated from the antisense sequence of several among *Euphausia*'s protein coding genes. These unusual CDs in this insect mitogenome remind previous descriptions of other unusual CDs in the mitogenome of the marine turtle *Lepidochelys olivacea*. This justifies detailed analyses of peptides translated from the six frames of the 13 protein coding genes of the mitogenomes of *Aleurodicus dispersus* (JX566506), and, for comparative purpose, of its closest relative with a complete mitogenome in GenBank, *Aleurodicus dugesii* (NC_005939), whose predicted proteome seems coded according to regular rules.

3.2. *Aleurodicus dispersus* protein coding genes

All six frames of the 13 mitochondrial protein coding genes of *Aleurodicus dispersus* were translated according to the regular invertebrate mitochondrial genetic code. First, BLAST analyzed peptides translated from GenBank-annotated, stopless ORFs to verify which of these peptides are "normal," i.e., have regular homologies with the corresponding protein predicted for the regular ORF of the mitogenome of *Aleurodicus dugesii*.

These analyses confirm that GenBank annotations of the six *Aleurodicus dispersus* mitogenes COI, COII, AT6, COIII, ND3, and ND2 code for typical invertebrate proteins homologous with corresponding proteins in regular insect mitogenomes, notably *Aleurodicus dugesii*. The remaining seven genes follow different coding structures described below, based on frameshifts and/or stop depletion/translation. Blastp does not detect any homologies for proteins predicted according to GenBank annotations for genes AT8, ND1, ND6, ND5, ND4, and ND4l, and only partial homology for CytB.

Mitochondrial metabolism without the regular proteins usually translated from these seven genes seems impossible. Regular analyses of the mitogenome of *Aleurodicus dugesii* detect these proteins as they are annotated in GenBank. The possibility that these genes were transferred in *Aleurodicus dispersus* to the nucleus and that proteins are imported to the mitochondrion seems unlikely as ORFs occur at positions corresponding to gene locations coding for the seven missing proteins in the predicted mitoproteome of *Aleurodicus dispersus*.

3.3. Recoding of mitogenes in *Aleurodicus dispersus*

3.3.1. Two ORFs on the same strand: AT8

The case of the missing ATP synthetase subunit 8 is solved by Blastp analysis of the peptide coded by the +2 frameshifted sequence of gene AT8. Residues at positions 8–48 (the gene has 49 codons including stop codon) in frame +2 have 75% similarity with congeneric mitochondrial ATP synthetase subunit 8 of *Aleurodicus dugesii* (YP_026055, e value 2×10^{-9}, see alignment in **Figure 1**). It seems likely that the regular AT8 gene codes for the corresponding protein. This frame does not contain stops, implying that this gene has two stopless ORFs. The GenBank-annotated ORF does not correspond to the regular AT8, which is the +2 frameshifted sequence of the annotated sequence.

3.3.2. Stop codon translation after frameshift: ND6

For gene ND6, the stopless ORF annotated in GenBank does not align with any ND6-like protein. This conundrum is solved by Blastp analysis of the peptide translated from the +1 frameshifted sequence of ND6 as it is annotated in GenBank. It aligns with 86% similarity with the mitochondrial NADH dehydrogenase subunit 6 of congeneric *Aleurodicus dugesii* (positions 33–137 in *Aleurodicus dispersus* and 32–129 in *Aleurodicus dugesii*, e value 1×10^{-37}, not shown). Hence, the annotated gene corresponds to a stopless frame that does not translate into a recognizable mitochondrial protein, while the +1 frame, which contains three stop codons codes for ND6. Only one of the stop codons is within the alignment, where it corresponds to a tyrosine in *Aleurodicus dugesii*. This implies translation of at least one stop codon, as previously described for other short mitochondrial protein coding genes where the protein coding region includes a programmed frameshift and translation of stops (ND3 in birds [76] and in turtles [77]). It seems plausible that ND6 translation starts in the 5′ region of the frame as annotated in GenBank, and then a programmed frameshift occurs in the vicinity of the 5′-starting point of the alignment. Translation of the stop codon by tyrosine is compatible with translation by tRNAs with near-cognate anticodons [78–80].

3.3.3. Frameshift with stop translation: CytB

The situation in CytB is similar and reminds again known cases of proteins coded by two frames. The ORF as annotated in GenBank has high homology (96% similarity) from residue 137 to 355 with the regular cytochrome B of *Aleurodicus dugesii* (YP_026063, e value 5×10^{-91}, **Figure 2**). The 5′ extremity of cytochrome B is coded by the +1 frameshifted sequence of the gene, as indicated by high similarity (88%) in the alignment from residues 6–136 with the regular cytochrome B of *Aleurodicus dugesii* (YP_026063, e value 5×10^{-54}, **Figure 2**). Position 131 is a stop that corresponds to a tyrosine in *Aleurodicus dugesii*. Hence, this gene's coding structure implies frameshift and probable stop translation, potentially by near cognate anticodon.

```
JX566506     8   MVIFVFFFFFFFFFLSFNFYYYKFYTFKNKKIYFDYYKIKW   48
YP_026055    8   MWLVLFFFFFFFFFLSLNFYYYKSYNFKMSKSNINYYKMKW   48
```

Figure 1. Alignment between peptide translated from the +1 frameshifted annotated GenBank sequence of gene AT8 in JX566506 with the protein translated from sequence AGA54141. Bold indicates similar residues, and underlined letters are for identical residues.

```
Frame +1
JX566506    6    KNLFLFTNLNGFIIDLGVPSYLYLWWNFGSLLGLVLVIQFLTGLFLTFHYASIVRVAFDRVIHIMRDVNWGWLLRYMHIDGASFFFIFIYIHIGR 100
YP_026063   6    KNLFLFKNLNDFIIDLGVPTNLYLWWNFGSLLGLIFMIQFMTGLFLTFHYASNINVAFDSVIHIMRDVNSGWLLRYMHINGASFFFIFIYIHIGR 100

JX566506    101  GLYYFSFTKKKVWIRGEIILLLLMKIAFMG*IFPWG  136
YP_026063   101  GLYYFSFKKKLVWISGVMILLLLMMIAFMGYILPWG  136

Frame 0 according to GenBank annotation of JX566506
JX566506    137  AKNHFEGPTVITNLLSAIPLSGNLIVNWIWGGFSVGNATLNRFYSFHFFFPFILIFLIFFHLLFLHIDGSSNSLGLNNTYDKIKFYPYYLLKDYM  231
YP_026063   136  GQMSFWGATVITNLLSAIPIWGDLIVSWIWGGFSVGNATLNRFYSFHFFFPFILIFLIFFHLLFLHIDGSSNSLGLNNTYDKIKFYPYYLLKDYM 230

JX566506    232  GFMFFFFFFIIIIFFNPLILSDSENFIMANSLITPIHIQPEWYYLFAYAILRSITSKLGGVMALFFSILILLIMLFLKSKFNGLMFYPILKIMFF  326
YP_026063   231  GFMFFFFFFIIIIFFNPLILSDSENFIMANSLITPIHIQPEWYYLFAYAILRSITSKLGGVMALFFSILILLIMLFLKSKFNGLMFYPILKIMFF 325

JX566506    327  FFFFIVLILTWLGSKQVEYPYLMLGSLMT  355
YP_026063   326  FFFFIVLILTWLGSKQVEYPYLMLGQLMT  354
```

Figure 2. Alignment between peptides translated from frame 0 and the +1 frameshifted annotated GenBank sequence of gene CytB in JX566506 with *Aleurodicus dugesii* cytochrome B, sequence YP_026063. Bold indicates similar residues, and underlined letters are for identical residues. Frame +1 of sequence annotated in GenBank JX566506.

http://dx.doi.org/10.5772/intechopen.80871

3.3.4. Stop codon depletion in antisense strand: ND1

The annotation in GenBank for ND1 does not correspond to a protein homologous to NADH dehydrogenase subunit 1. However, the peptide translated from the +1 frame of the opposite (antisense) strand has high homology with NADH dehydrogenase subunit 1 from *Aleurodicus dugesii* (YP_026064, 94% similarity for the complete length, e value 0). This implies regular encoding of that protein. The misannotation originates from depletion of all stops in one frame of the antisense strand of that gene. The corresponding antisense frame has 15 TAR stop codons in the regular ND1 of *Aleurodicus dugesii*. **Figure 3** aligns the peptide translated from this presumably noncoding antisense frame in *Aleurodicus dugesii* with the peptide translated from the GenBank-annotated frame. Stop codons correspond in this alignment mainly to serine (seven cases), then to tryptophan (two cases) and once each to leucine, lysine, methionine, and asparagine. This predicted translation is to much lower extents compatible with near cognate translation, and might be due to specific tRNA(s) with anticodon(s) matching stops.

The fact that this antisense frame is stop codon depleted in *Aleurodicus dispersus* so that it does not necessitate any special translational machinery for its expression suggests the possibility that this frame is translated in *Aleurodicus dugesii* (and in other species) and produces an unknown functional protein, and this is due to stop codon translation by antiterminator tRNAs. Indeed, the entirety of both mitochondrial strands is transcribed to RNA; hence, RNA corresponding to this supposedly noncoding strand necessarily exists and could be translated [81]. The alignment suggests that the amino acid most probably inserted by that stop-suppressor tRNA is serine. This is in line with previous observations from cytochrome c oxidase subunit I from the silkworm *Samia ricini* [7, 9], where stop codons in a usually noncoding frame systematically mutated to serine. This finding strengthens serine as the likely residue inserted at stop codons in insect mitochondria. This awaits confirmation by translation and tRNA aminoacylation experiments (as for example done for giant virus tRNAs [82]).

```
Dug  2    IFK*SLVLSFFLV*YNLNDKLKKKYSIVNGKNLIQVKYINLS*RNRGSVHRVQMNKKHKI  61
Dis  4    IFKSSLVLSFFLVWYNLNDKLKKKYSIVNGKNLIQVKYINLSSRNRGSVHRVQMNKKHKI  63
Dug  62   MNVKKKIIDLIFMLKNIVNVINLMIKMLEYSAKKMKAKENLLYSMLKPEINSDSPSEKSN  121
Dis  64   MNVKKKIIDLIFMLKNIVNVINLMIKMLEYSAKKMKAKENLLYSMMKPEINSDSPSEKSK  123
Dug  122  GVRLVSAKIVMIQM*NKNIKYK*NIMYFCMMNM*LKFNCSVKLTIVMMMIIKLISYEIIW  181
Dis  124  GVRLVSAKMVMIQMSNMKIKSMWNDKFFCIKNMLLKFICSVKLMMIMMMIIKLISYEIIW  183
Dug  182  AMDRISPIIA*LEFEDHLINMMMIMLIDIILINIKMLNLLKLKFQ*NG*IIHIIKEQMMF  241
Dis  184  AMERINPIMASLELEDHLIIMMMIMFMDIILMTIKMLNLLKLKFQMNGSIIHIINEQMMF  243
Dug  242  NNGNM**MM*FDLKFKFISLENNLMASLKGWSIPMINVLLGPLRFCM*LKILRSIKVKNA  301
Dis  244  NKGNKSSMMKLDLKFMFISLVNNLMASLNGCKIPKIMVLLGPLRFCMNLKILRSINVKNA  303
Dug  302  ILKKVLINNKIMIKK  316
Dis  304  ILKKMDNNKMIMFNK  318
```

Figure 3. Alignment between the peptide translated from the +1 frameshifted antisense sequence of ND1 in *Aleurodicus dugesii* (YP_026063) and the peptide translated from the ORF annotated in GenBank for ND1 in *Aleurodicus dispersus* (JX566506). Underlined asterisks indicate stops in the antisense sequence of *Aleurodicus dugesii*, which frequently correspond to serine in the stop-depleted ORF of *Aleurodicus dispersus*.

3.3.5. Stop codon depletion in antisense strand and stop codon translation: ND4l and ND5

Annotations in GenBank for *Aleurodicus dispersus'* ND4l and ND5 do not match proteins homologous to the corresponding NADH dehydrogenase subunits. For ND4l, the peptide translated from frame 0 of the antisense of that gene (this frame includes five stops) yields a short alignment with the regular protein in *Aleurodicus dugesii* (24 residues, 87% similarity, e value 8.5, not shown). Hence, the annotated ORF in *Aleurodicus dispersus* is probably a stop-codon-depleted antisense sequence (the corresponding frame in *Aleurodicus dugesii* has four stops), which does not code for the regular ND4l gene. This stop codon depletion in *Aleurodicus dispersus* introduced five stops in the sense strand frame that apparently codes for ND4l according to the above-described alignment.

For ND5, the peptide translated from the +1 frame of the antisense of the GenBank-annotated sequence is homologous over its complete length to NADH dehydrogenase subunit 5 of *Aleurodicus dugesii* (89% similarity, e value 0, not shown). This frame has a single stop codon that aligns with serine in *Aleurodicus dugesii* (see discussion of insertion of serine at stops in previous section).

3.3.6. Stop codon depletion in antisense strand, frameshift, and stop translation: ND4

A further mitochondrial gene for which the GenBank annotation does not produce the expected protein for *Aleurodicus dispersus* is ND4. Alignment analyses detect peptides homologous with regular NADH dehydrogenase subunit 4 when translating frames +1 and +2 of the antisense of the GenBank-annotated ND4 gene. Blastp alignment analyses detect homology with the regular ND4-encoded protein of *Aleurodicus dugesii*; the regular protein is encoded in antisense frame +1 until residue 297 (89% similarity, e value 3×10^{-126}, not shown). This alignment includes a single stop, matching tyrosine in *Aleurodicus dugesii*. Part of the remaining protein is coded by a stopless stretch of antisense strand frame +2, where residues 341–427 align with the regular protein from *Aleurodicus dugesii* (73% similarity, e value 2×10^{-21}). Hence, the annotated ORF in *Aleurodicus dispersus* is a stop-codon-depleted antisense frame that codes for an apparently different protein, the actual NADH dehydrogenase subunit 4 is encoded by two frames, one containing a stop, on the opposite strand.

4. General discussion

4.1. Genomic stop codon-depletion: overall analysis

Table 1 presents numbers of stops in all six frames of the mitochondrial genes of *Aleurodicus dugesii*, and of *Aleurodicus dispersus*, according to the strand presented in GenBank. The frame coding for the regular protein in *Aleurodicus dugesii* is always the only stopless frame, the frame(s) coding for the regular proteins are underlined in *Aleurodicus dispersus*, these are not necessarily stopless, and are not necessarily the only stopless frame.

In order to account for slight variations in gene sizes, I compare between percentages of stop codons averaged across all six frames in the two species, gene by gene. Mean stop

http://dx.doi.org/10.5772/intechopen.80871

	Aleurodicus dugesii							*Aleurodicus dispersus*						
	N	F0	F1	F2	R0	R1	R2	N	F0	F1	F2	R0	R1	R2
AT6	217	**0**	40	12	39	15	11	218	**0**	34	13	38	18	11
AT8	48	**0**	6	6	4	3	6	51	0	7	**0**	4	7	2
COI	515	**0**	65	31	64	61	11	518	**0**	59	35	68	60	13
COII	222	**0**	33	15	24	25	3	222	**0**	29	15	21	21	5
COIII	261	**0**	34	11	37	14	13	266	**0**	25	16	33	22	16
CytB	378	**0**	39	21	50	47	12	380	**0**	**27**	24	37	53	20
ND1	320	39	15	45	**0**	31	47	320	28	**0**	48	0	38	56
ND2	320	**0**	59	20	42	37	22	318	**0**	43	14	35	41	15
ND3	121	**0**	19	4	20	16	1	121	**0**	16	4	18	15	1
ND4l	101	8	3	22	**0**	7	16	100	**5**	9	11	0	14	16
ND4	426	44	8	83	**0**	42	60	434	39	**19**	**50**	0	43	64
ND5	559	49	16	86	**0**	53	102	558	64	**0**	99	0	41	100
ND6	140	**0**	17	10	25	16	17	142	11	0	**3**	14	20	16
12S	245	21	27	20	36	22	21	249	28	27	32	20	22	28
16S	396	34	35	51	42	56	50	396	41	56	51	50	36	31

Table 1. TAR stop codons in the six frames of mitogenome-encoded genes of *Aleurodicus dugesii* and *Aleurodicus dispersus*.

codon percentages decrease in 11 among 13 protein coding genes of *Aleurodicus dispersus*, as compared to *Aleurodicus dugesii*. This is a significant majority of cases according to a one tailed sign test using a binomial distribution and assuming equal probability of getting more or less stop codons in any of these mitogenes ($P = 0.00562$). This overall stop codon depletion occurs in all seven "recoded" genes. Stop codon depletion occurs qualitatively in four among the six genes with regular, unchanged coding structure. This tendency is not statistically significant for this subgroup of genes when using the robust, but blunt nonparametric sign test. A paired t test between mean percentages of stop codons averaged across frames indicates also for these six genes a statistically significant decrease in stops in *Aleurodicus dispersus*, as compared to *Aleurodicus dugesii*. This result suggests that stop codon depletion occurred across all or at least most of this genome, and for most frames, not only for genes whose coding structure was altered, and not only for frames who became ORFs.

Presumably, unknown mechanisms associated with replication depleted stop codons in this species' mitogenome, perhaps cumulatively over several replication or DNA edition cycles. Total stop codon depletion in some frames produced new ORFs. Natural selection against stop codons presumably enhanced unknown enzymatic phenomena, eliminating stop codons in these frames. It seems plausible that these frames in usual mitogenomes code for proteins translated by stop suppressor tRNAs. Specific unknown conditions in *Aleurodicus dispersus* may favor enhanced expression of peptides coded by frames that usually include stops in other mitogenomes, such as *Aleurodicus dugesii*. These constraints would have ultimately caused genomic stop codon depletion in *Aleurodicus dispersus*. In regular mitogenomes, stop codon translation downregulates expression of these unusual peptides in favor of proteins coded by regular ORFs, but in *Aleurodicus dispersus*, this hierarchy may be inexistent (when two stopless ORFs occur in a gene) or reversed (as in several mitogenes of *Lepidochelys olivacea* [9]), with translation of the unusual peptide not necessitating stop codon suppression, and translation of regular mitochondrial proteins requiring tRNAs with anticodons matching stop codons.

4.2. Coding redundancy between frames and tolerating ribosomal frameshifts

The original hypothesis of frame shiftability suggests that different frames of a gene code for somewhat similar peptides, presumably because the genetic code is optimized to tolerate frameshifts [83–85]. This hypothesis suggests that redundancy among frames in *Aleurodicus dispersus* should be greater than in the closely related *Aleurodicus dugesii* where coding seems regular, assuming that changes in coding structure increase redundancy among frames for coding protein variants with similar functions.

I used ClustalX to align the regular protein with peptides coded by the +1 and +2 frames of the same coding strand, for each *Aleurodicus dispersus* and *Aleurodicus dugesii*. Numbers of amino acids that were identical in the alignment were divided by total peptide lengths. This proportion for genes from *Aleurodicus dispersus* is plotted as a function of the corresponding proportion for *Aleurodicus dugesii* for alignments between frame 0 and frame +1 (**Figure 4**). Redundancy between frame 0 and + 1 is greater in mitogenes of *Aleurodicus dispersus* in nine among twelve genes (there was no difference between these species for gene COII), a statistically significant majority according to a one tailed sign test (P = 0.0365). This tendency however does not exist for alignments between frames 0 and +2 (redundancy in *Aleurodicus dispersus* greater in 6 among thirteen genes).

This analysis tentatively indicates that stop codon depletion and coding by frameshifting and translation of stop codons might associate with a phenomenon increasing tolerance to

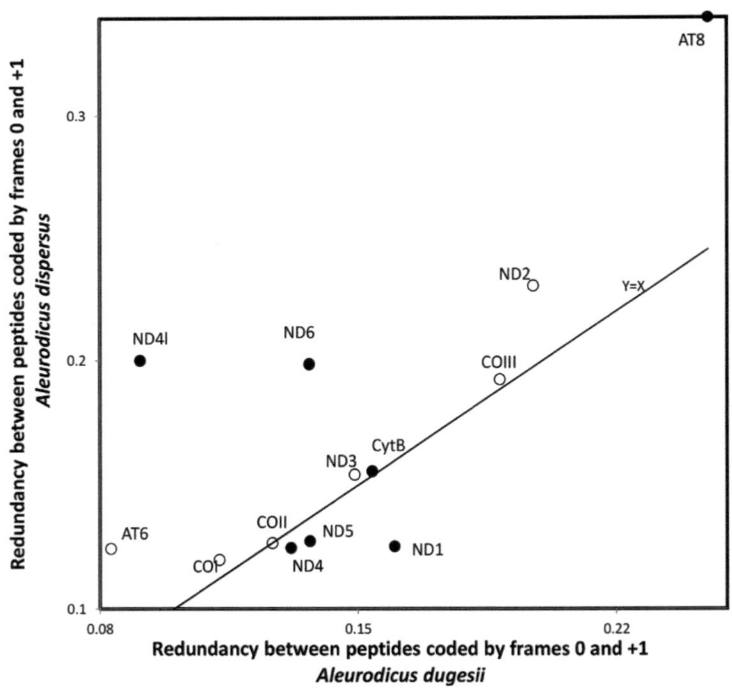

Figure 4. Redundancy between peptides coded by frames 0 and +1 for mitochondrial genes of *Aleurodicus dispersus* as a function of the corresponding redundancy for *Aleurodicus dugesii*. Filled symbols are for genes with unusual coding structure (frameshifts, stop depletion creating new ORFs, stop codon translation).

frameshifts during translation. Indeed, frequencies of off frame stop codons in mitochondrial genes are inversely correlated to predicted ribosomal RNA stability [86–88], suggesting that genes adapt to avoid negative effects of ribosomal frameshifts [44, 89, 90]. Stop codon-depletion may enable coding for more proteins, in addition to increasing redundancies between frames. Several effects could explain that results are not very strong statistically at the level of redundancy between frames. This hypothesis should be further tested, experimentally as done by Wang et al. [83–85] and by other bioinformatics analyses. For example, one can expect that frameshift tolerance biases exist for identity at amino acids that are not easily replaced by other amino acids (e.g., cysteine), but less for mutable ones (leucine, isoleucine, etc.). The preliminary tests presented here are not incompatible with the frameshift tolerance hypothesis [83–85].

It is important to understand in this context that the genetic code's discovery, among the greatest fundamental discoveries, is not over, but only in process. Indeed, coding sequences include much more information than generally believed, even beyond RNA editing (RDD [91]), systematic transformations during replication [44–46] and transcription [39, 47–51], and translation along expanded codons [32–43]. Cryptic codes [92, 93] such as the well-developed theory of the natural circular code [94–112] regulate the ribosomal translation frame [113–116], and protein cotranslational folding [117], remain to be described and decoded.

4.3. Sequencing artifacts and genome annotation

During the redescription of the recoded *Lepidochelys olivacea* mitogenome [9], an anonymous reviewer suggested that sequencing errors mimicked frameshifting mutations (insertion/deletion), producing the impression of frame recoding. This explanation is incompatible with the phenomena described in *Lepidochelys* and *Aleurodicus*, because these involve numerous specific changes/mutations in stop codon-specific nucleotide contexts, totally depleting stop codons in usually noncoding frames, and introducing stop codons in usually stopless, regular ORFs. Frameshifting mutations insert/delete a nucleotide within a regular ORF, which due to the frameshifting mutation is split between two frames. This does not deplete stop codons occurring in noncoding frames, nor introduce stops in the frameshifted ORF. ORF creation in usually noncoding frames by stop codon depletion in *Lepidochelys olivacea* [9] and *Aleurodicus dispersus* probably originates from natural, enzymatic, directed mutations [118] or other processes causing directed mutations, such as transposon-mediated directed mutations [119, 120].

Recoding probably occurs beyond mitogenomes. However, the short highly conserved mitogenomes [121] are most adequate to manual reannotation, a first necessary stage to detect events where genes are recoded from one to another genetic code. I suggest that annotations of genomes, and mitogenomes in particular, take systematically into account phenomena such as swinger sequences [51], and directed stop codon depletions that may result in ORFs that do not code for regular recognized proteins as presented here, especially in genomes/genes that seem unusual and remain in an unverified status in GenBank. **Figure 5** resumes the changes in coding structures that occurred in *Aleurodicus dispersus* due to recoding, as compared to the "ancestral" regular situation in *A. dugesii*. The proposed stopless genetic code in *Aleurodicus dispersus* presumably introduces serine at stops TAR and differs from previously described alternative arthropod mitochondrial genetic codes, which usually recode codons AGR [122, 123].

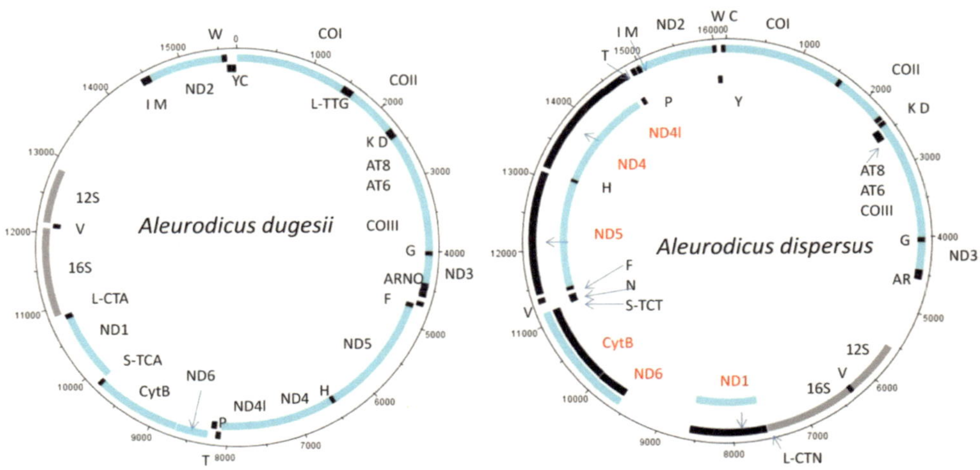

Figure 5. Classical and unusual mitogenome structures of whiteflies (*Aleurodicus dugesii; A. dispersus*). In *A. dispersus*, GenBank annotates genes ND1, ND4l, ND4, ND5, ND6 and CytB erroneously stopless frames coding for other proteins. A different frame with stops codes for the metabolically usual protein. CytB: both frames on same strand; other genes: opposite strands.

5. Conclusions

In vertebrate mitochondria, BLAST analyses of peptides translated from frames that are not recognized ORFs and contain stop codons align with high homology with proteins translated from regular mitochondrial ORFs in GenBank. Many such ORFs code for peptides matching usually noncoding sequences and occur in the mitogenome of *Lepidochelys olivacea* [9]. In this case, similar analyses are done for invertebrate mitochondria and a mitochondrial genome (JX566506, from *Aleurodicus dispersus*, Yu and Du, submitted in GenBank 2012, unpublished) considered as unverified are detected, probably because many protein-coding genes are undetectable with usual coding rules.

Several phenomena, and their combination, explain this situation. Alignment analyses detect the coding rules for these genes: frameshift, translation of stop codons, and depletion of stop codons in usually noncoding frames. Previous analyses detected in *Lepidochelys olivacea* CytB two stop-codon-deprived frames on the sense strand, among which one codes for the regular cytochrome B, and the other for an unknown protein. GenBank annotates erroneously the latter frame as coding for cytochrome B. A similar observation is reported here for the gene AT8 in *Aleurodicus dispersus*.

Some mitochondrial protein coding genes in *Aleurodicus dispersus* are unusual in the sense that the stop-codon-depleted frame erroneously annotated as the regular mitochondrial protein coding gene is on the strand opposite to the sense strand coding (with or without stop codons) for the actual usual protein: ND1, ND4l, ND4, ND5. The process depleting stop codons in these antisense frames is unknown and of particular interest. It is a probable combination of natural selection and enzymatically directed mutations to and from stop codons in the adequate nucleotide contexts, perhaps promoted by unknown conditions specific to *Aleurodicus dispersus*. In some genes, the protein usually coded by the regular genetic code necessitates translating stop codons (a stopless genetic code), while frames including stop codons and therefore not considered as ORFs become stop codon depleted, and hence corresponding peptides are coded by the regular invertebrate mitochondrial genetic code. This situation where peptides coded by regular and stopless genetic codes are swapped might reflect a reversal in hierarchies of needs for the expressions of the respective peptides, specific to *Aleurodicus dispersus*. The requirement for tRNAs translating stop codons would regulate these respective expressions, *de facto* swapping between regular and stopless genetic codes. I suggest that the enzymatically directed stop codon depletion is related to the process that caused directed introductions of stop codons in the coding frames of HIV proteins integrated in the nuclear genomes of "elite" HIV controller individuals [68, 69].

Acknowledgements

This study was supported by Méditerranée Infection and the National Research Agency under the program "Investissements d'avenir," reference ANR-10-IAHU-03, and the A*MIDEX project (no ANR-11-IDEX-0001-02).

Conflict of interest

The author declares no conflict of interest.

Author details

Hervé Seligmann[1,2]*

*Address all correspondence to: varanuseremius@gmail.com

1 Aix-Marseille University, URMITE, UM 63, CNRS UMR7278, IRD 198, INSERM U1095, Hospitalo-Universitary Institute, Méditerranée-Infection, Marseille, France

2 The National Natural History Collections, The Hebrew University of Jerusalem, Jerusalem, Israel

References

[1] Seligmann H. Phylogeny of genetic codes and punctuation codes within genetic codes. Bio Systems. 2015;**129**:36-43

[2] Seligmann H. Alignment-based and alignment-free methods converge with experimental data on amino acids coded by stop codons at split between nuclear and mitochondrial genetic codes. Bio Systems. 2018;**167**:33-46

[3] Seligmann H. Avoidance of antisense antiterminator tRNA anticodons in vertebrate mitochondria. Bio Systems. 2010;**101**:42-50

[4] Seligmann H. Undetected antisense tRNAs in mitochondrial genomes? Biology Direct. 2010;**5**:39

[5] Seligmann H. Pathogenic mutations in antisense mitochondrial tRNAs. Journal of Theoretical Biology. 2011;**269**:287-296

[6] Seligmann H. Two genetic codes, one genome: Frameshifted primate mitochondrial genes code for additional proteins in presence of antisense antitermination tRNAs. Bio Systems. 2011;**105**:271-285

[7] Seligmann H. An overlapping genetic code for frameshifted overlapping genes in Drosophila mitochondria: Antisense antitermination tRNAs UAR insert serine. Journal of Theoretical Biology. 2012;**298**:51-76

[8] Seligmann H. Putative protein-encoding genes within mitochondrial rDNA and the D-Loop region. In: Lin Z, Liu W, editors. Ribosomes: Molecular Structure, Role in Biological Functions and Implications for Genetic Diseases, Chapter 4. Nova Science Publisher. 2013. pp. 67-86

[9] Seligmann H. Overlapping genetic codes for overlapping frameshifted genes in Testudines, and *Lepidochelys olivacea* as a special case. Computational Biology and Chemistry. 2012;**41**: 18-34

[10] Barthélémy R-M, Seligmann H. Cryptic tRNAs in chaetognath mitochondrial genomes. Computational Biology and Chemistry. 2016;**62**:119-132

[11] Faure E, Delaye L, Tribolo S, Levasseur A, Seligmann H, Barthélémy R-M. Probable presence of an ubiquitous cryptic mitochondrial gene on the antisense strand of the cytochrome oxidase I gene. Biology Direct. 2011;**6**:56

[12] Breton S, Milani L, Ghiselli F, Guerra D, Stewart DT, Passamonto M. A resourceful genome: Updating the functional repertoire and evolutionary role of animal mitochondrial DNAs. Trends in Genetics. 2014;**30**:555-564

[13] Capt C, Passamonti M, Breton S. The human mitochondrial genome may code for more than 13 proteins. Mitochondrial DNA Part A, DNA mapping, sequencing, and analysis; **27**:3098-3101

[14] Seligmann H, Krishnan NM, Rao BJ. Possible multiple origins of replication in primate mitochondria: Alternative role of tRNA sequences. Journal of Theoretical Biology. 2006, 2015;**241**:321-332

[15] Seligmann H, Krishnan NM, Rao BJ. Mitochondrial tRNA sequences as unusual replication origins: Pathogenic implications for *Homo sapiens*. Journal of Theoretical Biology. 2006;**243**:375-385

[16] Seligmann H, Krishnan NM. Mitochondrial replication origin stability and propensity of adjacent tRNA genes to form putative replication origins increase developmental stability in lizards. Journal of Experimental Zoology Part B: Molecular and Developmental Evolution. 2006;**306**:433-4449

[17] Seligmann H. Hybridization between mitochondrial heavy strand tDNA and expressed light strand tRNA modulates the function of heavy strand tDNA as light strand replication origin. Journal of Molecular Biology. 2008;**379**:188-199

[18] Seligmann H. Mitochondrial tRNAs as light strand replication origins: Similarity between anticodon loops and the loop of the light strand replication origin predicts initiation of DNA replication. Biosystems. 2010;**99**:85-93

[19] Seligmann H. Mutation patterns due to converging mitochondrial replication and transcription increase lifespan, and cause growth rate-longevity tradeoffs. In: Seligmann H, editor. DNA Replication-Current Advances, Chapter 6. Rijeka, Croatia: InTech; 2011. pp. 151-180

[20] Seligmann H. Replicational mutation gradients, dipole moments, nearest neighbor effects and DNA polymerase gamma fidelity in human mitochondrial genomes. In: Stuart D, editor. The Mechanisms of DNA Replication, Chapter 10. Rijeka, Croatia: InTech; 2013. pp. 257-286

[21] Seligmann H, Labra A. The relation between hairpin formation by mitochondrial WANCY tRNAs and the occurrence of the light strand replication origin in Lepidosauria. Gene. 2014;**542**:248-257

[22] Atkins JF, Baranov PV. Translation: Duality in the genetic code. Nature. 2007;**448**:1004-1005

[23] Ivanova NN, Schwientek P, Tripp HJ, Rinke C, Pati A, Huntemann M, et al. Stop codon reassignments in the wild. Science. 2014;**344**:909-913

[24] Sánchez-Silva R, Villalobo E, Morin L, Torres A. A new noncanonical nuclear genetic code: Translation of UAA into glutamate. Current Biology. 2003;**13**:442-447

[25] Heaphy SM, Mariotti M, Gladyshev VN, Atkins JF, Baranov PV. Novel ciliate genetic code variants including the reassignment of all three stop codons to sense codons in *Condylostoma magnum*. Molecular Biology and Evolution. 2016;**33**:2885-2889

[26] Swart EC, Serra V, Petroni G, Nowacki M. Genetic codes with no dedicated stop codon: Context-dependent translation termination. Cell. 2016;**166**:691-702

[27] Záhonová K, Kostygov AY, Ševčíková T, Yurchenko V, Eliáš M. An unprecedented noncanonical nuclear genetic code with all three termination codons reassigned as sense codons. Current Biology. 2016;**26**:2364-2369

[28] Mühlhausen S, Findeisen P, Plessmann U, Urlaub H, Kollmar M. A novel nuclear genetic code alteration in yeasts and the evolution of codon reassignment in eukaryotes. Genome Research. 2016;**26**:945-955

[29] Riddle DL, Carbon J. Frameshift suppression: A nucleotide addition in the anticodon of a glycine transfer RNA. Nature: New Biology. 1973;**242**:230-234

[30] Sroga GE, Nemoto F, Kuchino Y, Bjork GR. Insertion (sufB) in the anticodon loop or base substitution (sufC) in the anticodon stem of tRNA(Pro)2 from *Salmonella typhimurium* induces suppression of frameshift mutations. Nucleic Acids Research. 1992;**20**:3463-3469

[31] Tuohy TM, Thompson S, Gesteland RF, Atkins JF. Seven, eight and nine-membered anticodon loop mutants of tRNA(2Arg) which cause +1 frameshifting. Tolerance of DHU arm and other secondary mutations. Journal of Molecular Biology. 1992;**228**:1042-1054

[32] Seligmann H. Putative mitochondrial polypeptides coded by expanded quadruplet codons, decoded by antisense tRNAs with unusual anticodons. Biosystems. 2012;**110**: 84-106

[33] Seligmann H. Pocketknife tRNA hypothesis: Anticodons in mammal mitochondrial tRNA side-arm loops translate proteins? Biosystems. 2013;**113**:165-175

[34] Seligmann H. Putative anticodons in mitochondrial tRNA sidearm loops: Pocketknife tRNAs? Journal of Theoretical Biology. 2014;**340**:155-163

[35] Seligmann H, Labra A. Tetracoding increases with body temperature in Lepidosauria. Biosystems. 2013;**114**:155-166

[36] Baranov PV, Venin M, Provan G. Codon size reduction as the origin of the triplet genetic code. PLoS One. 2009;**4**:e5708

[37] Gonzalez DL, Giannerini S, Rosa R. On the Origin of the Mitochondrial Genetic Code: Towards a Unified Mathematical Framework for the Management of Genetic Information. Nature Precedings; 2012. Available at: http://dx.doi.org/10.1038/npre.2012.7136.1

[38] Seligmann H. Codon expansion and systematic transcriptional deletions produce tetra-, pentacoded mitochondrial peptides. Journal of Theoretical Biology. 2015;**387**:154-165

[39] Seligmann H. Translation of mitochondrial swinger RNAs according to tri-, tetra- and pentacodons. Biosystems. 2016;**140**:38-48

[40] Seligmann H. Natural chymotrypsin-like-cleaved human mitochondrial peptides confirm tetra-, pentacodon, non-canonical RNA translations. Biosystems. 2016;**147**:78-93

[41] Seligmann H. Unbiased mitoproteome analyses confirm non-canonical RNA, expanded codon translations. Computational and Structural Biotechnology Journal. 2016;**14**:391-403

[42] Seligmann H. Natural mitochondrial proteolysis confirms transcription systematically exchanging/deleting nucleotides, peptides coded by expanded codons. Journal of Theoretical Biology. 2017;**414**:76-90

[43] Seligmann H. Reviewing evidence for systematic transcriptional deletions, nucleotide exchanges, and expanded codons, and peptide clusters in human mitochondria. Biosystems. 2017;**160**:10-24

[44] Seligmann H. Species radiation by DNA replication that systematically exchanges nucleotides? Journal of Theoretical Biology. 2014;**363**:216-222

[45] Seligmann H. Mitochondrial swinger replication: DNA replication systematically exchanging nucleotides and short 16S ribosomal DNA swinger inserts. Biosystems. 2014;**125**:22-31

[46] Seligmann H. Sharp switches between regular and swinger mitochondrial replication: 16S rDNA systematically exchanging nucleotides A<->T+C<->G in the mitogenome of *Kamimuria wangi*. Mitochondrial DNA Part A, DNA mapping, sequencing, and analysis. 2016;**27**:2440-2446

[47] Seligmann H. Overlapping genes in the 3′-to-5′-direction in mitochondrial genes and 3′-to-5′ polymerization of non-complementary RNA by an 'invertase'. Journal of Theoretical Biology. 2012;**315**:38-82

[48] Seligmann H. Triplex DNA:RNA, 3′-to-5′ inverted RNA and protein coding in mitochondrial genomes. Journal of Computational Biology. 2013;**20**:660-671

[49] Seligmann H. Polymerization of non-complementary RNA: Systematic symmetric nucleotide exchanges mainly involving uracil produce mitochondrial RNA transcripts coding for cryptic overlapping genes. Biosystems. 2013;**111**:156-174

[50] Seligmann H. Systematic asymmetric nucleotide exchanges produce human mitochondrial RNAs cryptically encoding for overlapping protein coding genes. Journal of Theoretical Biology. 2013;**324**:1-20

[51] Michel CJ, Seligmann H. Bijective transformation circular codes and nucleotide exchanging RNA transcription. Biosystems. 2014;**118**:39-50

[52] Seligmann H, Raoult D. Stem-loop RNA hairpins in giant viruses: Invading rRNA-like repeats and a template free RNA. Frontiers in Microbiology. 2018;**9**:101

[53] Warthi G, Seligmann H. Swinger RNAs in the human mitochondrial transcriptome. In: mitochondrial DNA-new insights, Seligmann H, Warthi G, editors. Chapter 4, InTech. ISBN: 978-953-51-6167-7

[54] Bloch DP, McArthur B, Widdowson R, Spector D, Guimaraes RC, Smith J. tRNA-rRNA sequence homologies: Evidence for a common evolutionary origin? Journal of Molecular Evolution. 1983;**19**:420-408

[55] Bloch DP, McArthur B, Widdowson R, Spector D, Guimaraes RC, Smith J. tRNA-rRNA sequence homologies: A model for the origin of a common ancestral molecule, and prospects for its reconstruction. Origins of Life. 1983;**14**:571-578

[56] Bloch DP, McArthur B, Guimaraes RC, Smith J, Staves MP. tRNA-rRNA sequence matches from inter- and intraspecies comparisons suggest common origins for the two RNAs. Brazilian Journal of Medical and Biological Research. 1983;**22**:931-944

[57] Root-Bernstein M, Root-Bernstein R. The ribosome as a missing link in the evolution of life. Journal of Theoretical Biology. 2015;**367**:130-158

[58] Root-Bernstein M, Root-Bernstein R. The ribosome as a missing link in the evolution II: Ribosomes encode ribosomal proteins that bind to common regions of their own mRNAs and rRNAs. Journal of Theoretical Biology. 2015;**397**:115-127

[59] Kermekchiev M, Ivanova L. Ribin, a protein encoded by a message complementary to rRNA, modulates ribosomal transcription and cell proliferation. Molecular and Cellular Biology. 2001;**21**:8255-8263

[60] Barthélémy R-M, Jaafari N, Galea P, Jule Y, Faure E. Immunodetection of ribin-like proteins in neuron-based cellular models. Journal of Medical Genetics and Genomics. 2010;**2**:44-56

[61] Caetano-Anollés D, Caetano-Anollés G. Piecemeal buildup of the genetic code, ribosomes, and genomes from primordial tRNA building blocks. Life (Basel, Switzerland). 2016;**6**:E43

[62] Seligmann H. Swinger RNAs with sharp switches between regular transcription and transcription systematically exchanging ribonucleotides: Case studies. Biosystems. 2015;**135**:1-8

[63] Seligmann H. Chimeric mitochondrial peptides from contiguous regular and swinger RNA. Computational and Structural Biotechnology Journal. 2016;**14**:283-297

[64] Seligmann H, Raoult D. Unifying view of stem-loop hairpin RNA as origin of current and ancient parasitic and non-parasitic RNAs, including in giant viruses. Current Opinion in Microbiology. 2016;**31**:1-8

[65] El Houmami N, Seligmann H. Evolution of nucleotide punctuation marks: From structural to linear signals. Frontiers in Genetics. 2017;**8**:36

[66] Ojala D, Montoya J, Attardi G. tRNA punctuation model of RNA processing in human mitochondria. Nature. 1981;**290**:470-474

[67] Stewart JB, Beckenbach AT. Characterization of mature mitochondrial transcripts in Drosophila, and the implications for the tRNA punctuation model in arthropods. Gene. 2009;**445**:49-57

[68] Shimpi GG, Vargas S, Poliseno A, Wörheide G. Mitochondrial RNA processing in absence of tRNA punctuations in octocorals. BMC Molecular Biology. 2017;**18**:16

[69] Seligmann H. Swinger RNA self-hybridization and mitochondrial non-canonical swinger transcription, transcription systematically exchanging nucleotides. Journal of Theoretical Biology. 2016;**399**:84-91

[70] Claverie JM, Abergel G. Mimivirus and its virophage. Annual Review of Genetics. 2009;**43**:49-66

[71] Seligmann H. Giant viruses as protein-coated mitochondria? Virus Research. 2018;**253**: 77-86

[72] Seligmann H. Systematically frameshifting by deletion of every 4th or 4th and 5th nucleotides during mitochondrial transcription: RNA self-hybridization regulates delRNA expression. Biosystems. 2016;**142-143**:43-51

[73] Colson P, Ravaux I, Tamalet C, Glazunova O, Baptiste E, Chabrière E, et al. HIV infection en route to endogenization: Two cases. Clinical Microbiology and Infection. 2014;**20**: 1280-1288

[74] Tamalet C, Colson P, Decroly E, Dhiver C, Ravaux I, Stein A, et al. Reevaluation of possible outcomes of infections with human immunodeficiency virus. Clinical Microbiology and Infection. 2016;**22**:299-311

[75] Jestin J-L, Kempf A. Chain termination codons and polymerase-induced frameshift mutations. FEBS Letters. 1997;**419**:153-156

[76] Mindell DP, Sorenson MD, Dimcheff DE. An extra nucleotide is not translated in mitochondrial ND3 of some birds and turtles. Molecular Biology and Evolution. 1998;**15**: 1568-1571

[77] Russell RD, Beckenback AT. Recoding of translation in turtle mitochondrial genomes: Programmed frameshift and evidence of a modified genetic code. Journal of Molecular Evolution. 2008;**67**:682-695

[78] Seligmann H. Do anticodons of misacylated tRNAs preferentially mismatch codons coding for the misloaded amino acid? BMC Molecular Biology. 2010;**11**:41

[79] Seligmann H. Error compensation of tRNA misacylation by codon-anticodon mismatch prevents translational amino acid misinsertion. Computational Biology and Chemistry. 2011;**35**:81-95

[80] Seligmann H. Coding constraints modulate chemically spontaneous mutational replication gradients in mitochondrial genomes. Current Genomics. 2012;**13**:37-54

[81] Chang DD, Clayton DA. Precise identification of individual promoters for transcription of each strand of human mitochondrial DNA. Cell. 1984;**36**:635-643

[82] Abergel C, Rudinger-Thirion J, Giegé R, Claverie JM. Virus-encoded aminoacyl-tRNA synthetases: Structural and functional characterization of mimivirus TyrRS and MetRS. Journal of Virology. 2007;**81**:12406-12417

[83] Wang X, Wang X, Chen G, Zhang J, Liu Y, Yang C. The shiftability of protein coding genes: The genetic code was optimized for frameshift tolerating. PeerJ PrePrints. 2015;**3**:e806v1

[84] Wang X, Dong Q, Chen G, Zhang J, Liu Y, Zhao J, et al. Why are frameshift homologs widespread within and across species? bioRxiv. 2016:067736. DOI: 10.1101/067736

[85] Geyer R, Mamlouk A. On the efficiency of the genetic code after frameshift mutations. PeerJ. 2018;**6**:e4825

[86] Seligmann H, Pollock DD. The ambush hypothesis: Hidden stop codons prevent off-frame gene reading. The MidSouth Computational Biology and Bioinformatics Society. 2003. Abstract 36

[87] Seligmann H, Pollock DD. The ambush hypothesis: Hidden stop codons prevent off-frame gene reading. DNA and Cell Biology. 2004;**23**:701-705

[88] Seligmann H. The ambush hypothesis at the whole-organism level: Off frame, 'hidden' stops in vertebrate mitochondrial genes increase developmental stability. Computational Biology and Chemistry. 2010;**34**:80-85

[89] Itzkovitz S, Alon U. The genetic code is nearly optimal for allowing additional information within protein-coding sequences. Genome Research. 2007;**17**:405-412

[90] Tse H, Cai JJ, Tsoi HW, Lam EP, Zuen KZ. Natural selection retains overrepresented out-of-frame stop codons against frameshift peptides in prokaryotes. BMC Genomics. 2010;**11**:491

[91] Bar-Yaacov D, Avital G, Levin L, Richards AL, Hachen N, Rebolledo Jaramillo B, et al. RNA–DNA differences in human mitochondria restore ancestral form of 16S ribosomal RNA. Genome Research. 2013;**23**:1789-1796. DOI: 10.1101/gr.161265.113

[92] Popov O, Segal D, Trifonov EN. Linguistic complexity of protein sequences as compared to texts of human languages. Biosystems. 1996;**38**:65-74

[93] Seligmann H. Bijective codon transformations show genetic code symmetries centered on cytosine's coding properties. Theory in Biosciences. 2018;**137**:17-31. DOI: 10.1007/s12064-017-0258-x

[94] Arquès DG, Michel CJ. A complementary circular code in the protein coding genes. Journal of Theoretical Biology. 1996;**182**:45-58

[95] Arquès DG, Lacan J, Michel CJ. Identification of protein coding genes in genomes with statistical functions based on the circular code. Bio Systems. 2002;**66**:73-92

[96] Frey G, Michel CJ. Circular codes in archaeal genomes. Journal of Theoretical Biology. 2003;**223**:413-431

[97] Ahmed A, Frey G, Michel CJ. Frameshift signals in genes associated with the circular code. In Silico Biology. 2007;**7**:155-168

[98] Ahmed A, Frey G, Michel CJ. Essential molecular functions associated with the circular code evolution. Journal of Theoretical Biology. 2010;**264**:613-622. DOI: 10.1016/j.jtbi.2010.02.006

[99] Gonzalez DL, Giannerini S, Rosa R. Circular codes revisited: A statistical approach. Journal of Theoretical Biology. 2011;**275**:21-28. DOI: 10.1016/j.jtbi.2011.01.028

[100] Michel CJ. Circular code motifs in transfer and 16S ribosomal RNAs: A possible translation code in genes. Computational Biology and Chemistry. 2012;**37**:24-37. DOI: 10.1016/j.compbiolchem.2011.10.002

[101] Michel CJ, Pirillo G. A permuted set of a trinucleotide circular code coding the 20 amino acids in variant nuclear codes. Journal of Theoretical Biology. 2013;**319**:116-121. DOI: 10.1016/j.jtbi.2012.11.023

[102] Michel CJ. A genetic scale of reading frame coding. Journal of Theoretical Biology. 2014;**355**:83-94. DOI: 10.1016/j.jtbi.2014.03.029

[103] Fimmel E, Strüngmann L. On the hierarchy of trinucleotide n-circular codes and their corresponding amino acids. Journal of Theoretical Biology. 2015;**364**:113-120. DOI: 10.1016/j.jtbi.2014.09.011

[104] Michel CJ. An extended genetic scale of reading frame coding. Journal of Theoretical Biology. 2015;**365**:164-174. DOI: 10.1016/j.jtbi.2014.09.040

[105] Michel CJ. The maximal C(3) self-complementary trinucleotide circular code X in genes of bacteria, eukaryotes, plasmids and viruses. Journal of Theoretical Biology. 2015;**380**:156-177. DOI: 10.1016/j.jtbi.2015.04.009

[106] Fimmel E, Strüngmann L. Codon distribution in error-detecting circular codes. Life (Basel, Switzerland). 2016;**6**(1). pii: E14. DOI: 10.3390/life6010014

[107] El Soufi K, Michel CJ. Circular code motifs in genomes of eukaryotes. Journal of Theoretical Biology. 2016;**408**:198-212. DOI: 10.1016/j.jtbi.2016.07.022

[108] El Soufi K, Michel CJ. Unitary circular code motifs in genomes of eukaryotes. Biosystems. 2017;**153-154**:45-62. DOI: 10.1016/j.biosystems.2017.02.001

[109] Michel CJ. The maximal C^3 self-complementary trinucleotide circular code X in genes of bacteria, archaea, eukaryotes, plasmids and viruses. Life (Basel, Switzerland). 2017;**7**. pii: E20. DOI: 10.3390/life7020020

[110] Michel CJ, Ngoune VN, Poch O, Ripp R, Thompson JD. Enrichment of circular code motifs in the genes of the yeast *Saccharomyces cerevisiae*. Life (Basel, Switzerland). 2017;**7**(4). pii: E52. DOI: 10.3390/life7040052

[111] Fimmel E, Michel CJ, Strüngmann L. Strong comma-free codes in genetic information. Bulletin of Mathematical Biology. 2017;**79**:1796-1819. DOI: 10.1007/s11538-017-0307-0

[112] Fimmel E, Strüngmann L. Mathematical fundamentals for the noise immunity of the genetic code. Biosystems. 2018;**164**:186-198. pii: S0303-2647(17)30237-X. DOI: 10.1016/j.biosystems.2017.09.007

[113] Michel CJ. Circular code motifs in transfer RNAs. Computational Biology and Chemistry. 2013;**45**:17-29. DOI: 10.1016/j.compbiolchem.2013.02.004

[114] El Soufi K, Michel CJ. Circular code motifs in the ribosome decoding center. Computational Biology and Chemistry. 2014;**52**:9-17. DOI: 10.1016/j.compbiolchem.2014.08.001

[115] El Soufi K, Michel CJ. Circular code motifs near the ribosome decoding center. Computational Biology and Chemistry. 2015;**59 Pt A**:158-176. DOI: 10.1016/j.compbiolchem.2015.07.015

[116] Fimmel E, Michel CJ, Starman M, Strüngmann L. Self-complementary circular codes in coding theory. Theory in Biosciences. 2018;**137**:51-65

[117] Seligmann H, Warthi G. Genetic code optimization for cotranslational protein folding: Codon directional asymmetry correlates with antiparallel betasheets, tRNA synthetase classes. Computational and Structural Biotechnology Journal. 2017;**15**:412-424. DOI: 10.1016/j.csbj.2017.08.001

[118] Hall BG. Spontaneous point mutations that occur more often when advantageous than when neutral. Genetics. 1990;**126**:5-16

[119] Li G-D. Natural site-directed mutagenesis might exist in eukaryotic cells. arXiv. 2016. arXiv:1603.06538

[120] Saier MH Jr, Zhang Z. Transposon-mediated directed mutation controlled by DNA binding proteins in *Escherichia coli*. Frontiers in Microbiology. 2014;**5**:390

[121] Satoh TP, Sato Y, Masuyama N, Miya M, Nishida M. Transfer RNA gene arrangement and codon usage in vertebrate mitochondrial genomes: A new insight into gene order conservation. BMC Genomics. 2010;**11**:479

[122] Abascal F, Posada D, Knight RD, Zardova R. Parallel evolution of the genetic code in arthropod mitochondrial genomes. PLoS Biology. 2006;**4**:e127

[123] Abascal D, Posada D, Zardova R. The evolution of the mitochondrial genetic code in arthropods revisited. Mitochondrial DNA. 2012;**23**:84-91. DOI: 10.3109/19401736.2011.653801

Chapter 4

Swinger RNAs in the Human Mitochondrial Transcriptome

Ganesh Warthi and Hervé Seligmann

Additional information is available at the end of the chapter

http://dx.doi.org/10.5772/intechopen.80805

Abstract

Transcriptomes include coding and non-coding RNAs and RNA fragments with no apparent homology to parent genomes. Non-canonical transcriptions systematically transforming template DNA sequences along precise rules explain some transcripts. Among these systematic transformations, 23 systematic exchanges between nucleotides, i.e. 9 symmetric (X ↔ Y, e.g. C ↔ T) and 14 asymmetric (X → Y → Z → X, e.g. A → T → G → A) exchanges. Here, comparisons between mitochondrial swinger RNAs previously detected in a complete human transcriptome dataset (including cytosolic RNAs) and swinger RNAs detected in purified mitochondrial transcriptomic data (not including cytosolic RNAs) show high reproducibility and exclude cytosolic contaminations. These results based on next-generation sequencing Illumina technology confirm detections of mitochondrial swinger RNAs in GenBank's EST database sequenced by the classical Sanger method, assessing the existence of swinger polymerizations.

Keywords: swinger RNA, non-canonical transcription, mitogenome, systematic nucleotide exchange, blast analyses

1. Introduction

Transcription is an intracellular mechanism that produces RNA by DNA-dependant RNA polymerisation. RNAs coding for polypeptide chains are mRNAs translated by other transcription products, tRNAs and ribosomal RNAs. Some RNAs do not correspond to any DNA sequence in the genome, suggesting in some cases spontaneous emergence [1]. These RNAs remain usually unreported and are ignored. Similarly, proteomic data include numerous peptides that do not match canonical translation of predicted ORFs, but imply translation of stop codons [2–8] by tRNAs with anticodons matching stops [9–11] or by tRNAs with expanded anticodons [12–14]. Assuming fusion of different transcripts explains the origins of some of these non-canonical RNAs [15]. Some human RNAs matching exons differ from their DNA by specific changes, called RDDs (RNA-DNA differences) [16]. RDDs can be single nucleotide substitutions or deletions [17–19], presumably resulting from post-transcriptional edition [20, 21]. Some short transcripts correspond to mitochondrial DNA at the condition that one assumes mono- or dinucleotide deletions after each transcribed nucleotide triplet [22, 23]. Formation of secondary structures by del-transformed sequences apparently downregulates del-transcription itself or its products, delRNAs [24].

Another type of systematic transformation consists of 23 systematic exchanges between nucleotides, 9 symmetric (X ↔ Y, e.g. A ↔ C,) [25, 26] and 14 asymmetric exchanges (X → Y → Z → X, e.g. A → C → G → A) [26, 27]. For example, in systematic transformation A ↔ C, nucleotide A is introduced in place of nucleotide C and vice versa. The two-headed arrow (↔) indicates that A and C replace each other during transcription. One-headed arrows (→) indicate asymmetric exchanges: in the example A → C → G → A, nucleotide A is systematically incorporated in place of every C; similarly, C replaces G and G replaces A during RNA polymerisation. Transcripts corresponding to systematic exchanges are called swinger RNAs. BLASTn analyses detect about 100 predicted swinger RNAs (longer than 100 nucleotides) in GenBank's EST database in addition to the (approximately) 10,000 canonical human mitochondrial RNAs in that database. Hence, about 1% of the human mitochondrial transcripts in GenBank's EST database correspond to 1 among 23 systematic nucleotide exchanges [25–28]. These systematic nucleotide exchanges (an expression that fits chemical contexts) are called bijective transformations in mathematical contexts [29–31]; swinger transcription fits biological contexts.

Mitogenomes are comparatively small, also because of the selection against multiple direct repeats [32–35] and invert repeats [15]: these form secondary structures that are frequently excised; such deletions are frequently deleterious. Vertebrate mitogenomes have densely packed coding and non-coding regions templating for RNAs. Non-canonical transformations greatly increase potential numbers of RNA products for single sequences: four and five RNA transcripts when assuming systematic deletions of mono- and dinucleotides for del-transcriptions, respectively, and 23 swinger RNAs when considering systematic nucleotide exchanges. Therefore, studies of swinger transformations focus on the human mitogenome, which is short (16,569 bp), hence reducing potential false-positive detections due to sheer genome size and because ample sequence data are available from several sources for this organism.

Note that swinger DNA has been detected (mainly corresponding to rRNA genes) for mitochondrial and nuclear sequences [36–38]. Hence, swinger RNAs result from canonical transcription of swinger-transformed DNA or swinger transcription of regular DNA [22]. Some mass spectra match predicted peptides translated from del- and swinger-transformed RNA [39–42]. Detection of chimeric RNAs, consisting of part regular, and part swinger-transformed contiguous sequences suggests that regular canonical and swinger-transformed RNA result from single polymerisation events, probably by the same polymerase [43]. Peptides corresponding to such chimeric RNAs also occur [44].

Secondary structure formation by swinger-transformed sequences associates with swinger RNA detection [45], suggesting regulation of swinger RNA processing by secondary structures, as observed for canonical mitochondrial RNAs, i.e. tRNA punctuation [46].

Abundances of human mitochondrial swinger RNAs detected in GenBank's EST database [25, 26], originating from various sources using Sanger sequencing, are proportional to those detected in transcriptomic data produced by next-generation sequencing, Illumina technology [47]. Similarly, abundances and lengths of swinger RNAs detected in *Mimivirus'* transcriptome sequenced by 454 technology are proportional to those detected when using SOLID sequencing [01]. These analyses confirmed that swinger RNAs are not sequencing artefacts due to specific sequencing technologies, but data sources do not exclude contamination by cytosolic RNA. Here, we compare the previously described human mitochondrial swinger transcriptome [39] from a complete human transcriptome (including cytosolic RNAs) with the swinger transcriptome as detected in purified human mitochondrial lines [48]. Reproducibility of swinger RNA coverages of the human mitogenome would exclude sequencing artefacts and cytosolic contaminations as alternative explanations for hypothetical swinger RNAs. We predict (1) the detection of swinger RNAs from transcriptomic data extracted from purified mitochondrial lines and (2) high similarities between mitogenomic swinger RNA coverages described here and previously [39].

2. Materials and methods

2.1. Detection of swinger RNAs

We used GenBank's BLASTn ('somewhat similar sequences' with default alignment parameters) [49] for in-silico alignment searches between each of the 23 swinger-transformed versions of the human mitogenome (NC_012920) and transcriptomic data in GenBank's Sequence Read Archive (SRA) (SRX084350-SRX084355 and SRX087285), sequenced by RNA-Seq, Illumina HiSeq 2500 technology [48]. Alignments with more than 80% identity were recorded and used as a swinger RNA candidate for further analysis.

2.2. Mitogenomic gene coverage by swinger RNAs

Locations of detected swinger RNAs were recorded by mapping these RNAs on the human mitogenome. We analyse separately 17 mitogenomic regions: the D-loop, 2 ribosomal RNAs (12S and 16S), 13 protein-coding genes involved in the electron transport chain and the WANCY region (intragenic region between ND2 and CO1 that templates for tRNAs with cognate amino acids W, A, N, C and Y). Percentage coverages by detected swinger RNAs were calculated for each swinger transformation in each selected mitogenomic region and used for further statistical analyses.

3. Results and discussion

3.1. Swinger RNAs in the human mitochondrial transcriptome

Table 1 summarises results from BLASTn analyses of the purified mitochondrial transcriptome [48] for the 23 swinger-transformed versions of the human mitogenome. In total 4120 reads aligned with the 23 swinger-transformed versions of the human mitogenome,

	Read	Contigs	Id	Coverage	Read	Contigs	Id	Coverage
Regular	700	142	99.76	8479	400	69	100	7658
A ↔ C	181	42	93.94	1239	163	10	89.12	389
A ↔ G	448	5	92.20	184	6	2	87.26	97
A ↔ T	98	48	94.34	1376	186	17	90.63	593
C ↔ G	319	7	89.99	227	28	8	85.01	343
C ↔ T	338	51	90.59	1599	253	26	92.47	937
G ↔ T	435	35	92.43	1614	400	5	88.36	249
A ↔ C + G ↔ T	123	25	89.79	730	11	2	86.23	76
A ↔ G + C ↔ T	63	34	92.63	982	69	8	89.3	257
A ↔ T + C ↔ G	126	36	92.87	1112	97	11	94.8	395
A → C → G → A	80	25	93.81	**778**	21	12	90.59	439
A → C → T → A	160	52	92.99	1474	31	12	90.79	453
A → G → C → A	98	58	91.70	1729	43	17	93.13	573
A → G → T → A	98	39	91.29	1245	28	12	88.49	469
A → T → C → A	218	50	93.12	1578	363	20	92.13	810
A → T → G → A	84	29	94.08	873	12	5	90.21	190
C → G → T → C	122	43	94.15	1167	21	4	88.44	247
C → T → G → C	165	57	91.90	2058	126	17	86.42	791
A → C → G → T → A	140	45	92.33	1306	38	15	89.53	575
A → C → T → G → A	157	35	95.32	971	54	10	92.65	327
A → G → C → T → A	211	26	92.63	713	99	15	87.35	530
A → G → T → C → A	78	27	93.60	777	30	11	91.29	369
A → T → C → G → A	195	17	88.94	463	60	9	92.1	321
A → T → G → C → A	183	55	94.14	1874	115	16	94.78	601

Current data are from purified mitochondrial lines, previous data are from complete human transcriptome, including cytosolic and mitochondrial transcriptomes. Columns 2–5: current analyses. Columns are (1) swinger transformation (includes lack of transformation), (2) aligning read numbers, (3) contig numbers, (4) mean identity between reads and transformed mitogenome and (5) total mitogenomic coverage by all swinger contigs. Columns 6–9 indicate corresponding data in the same order for the previous study.

Table 1. Total human mitogenome coverage by detected swinger RNAs from current (2018) and previous (2016) [39] analyses of two different datasets sequenced by Illumina.

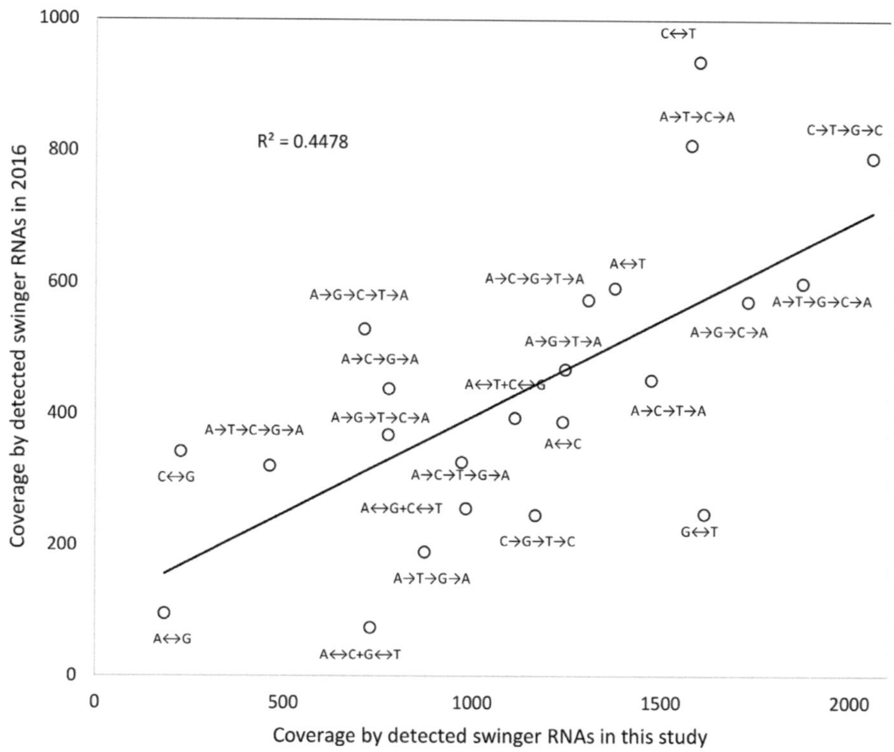

Figure 1. Total mitogenome coverages by swinger RNAs across the complete human mitogenome in previously analysed data [39] (y-axis) as a function of those obtained in current observations from purified mitochondrial lines.

producing 841 contigs. The highest detected identity between a theoretical mitogenome swinger transformation and a read was 95.32% for transformation A → C → T → G → A, and the lowest identity was 88.94% for transformation A → T → C → G → A. The overall identity averaged at 92.86%. A previous swinger analysis of other transcriptomic data [39] found swinger transformations A ↔ G and C ↔ T least and most frequent, respectively. Here, swinger transformation A ↔ G remains the least frequent; C ↔ T is the second most frequent, suggesting high reproducibility.

Total mitogenome coverages by swinger RNAs for each transformation were plotted as a function of corresponding coverages from a previous analysis published in 2016 [39]. Coverages are positively correlated (Pearson correlation coefficient $r = 0.669$, one-tailed $p = 0.0002$, **Figure 1**). Coverages for the purified mitochondrial line transcriptomes are systematically greater than for those for previous analyses (supplementary data and **Table 1**) [39].

3.2. Gene-level comparisons of swinger RNA coverages

Swinger RNA coverages of each of the 17 mitogenomic regions (D-loop, 2 rRNAs, 13 CDs and the WANCY region) are in **Tables 2** and **3**, for analyses of current and previous Illumina data [39], respectively. Pearson correlation coefficients between swinger coverages were calculated considering (1) genes, i.e. for each gene across the 23 different transformations, and (2) for each swinger transformation, across the 17 different mitogenomic regions.

Transformation	D-loop	12S	16S	ND1	ND2	W-Y	CO1	CO2	ATP8	ATP6	CO3	ND3	ND4L	ND4	ND5	ND6	Cytb
A ↔ C	6.4	5.6	9.1	0.0	15.1	25.0	5.8	0.0	9.2	3.7	7.3	11.8	0.0	8.3	7.9	26.7	3.7
A ↔ G	0.0	0.0	0.0	0.0	0.0	0.0	2.4	0.0	0.0	0.0	0.0	9.0	0.0	0.0	2.7	0.0	6.0
A ↔ T	9.4	2.8	8.3	3.2	15.9	11.5	1.7	3.1	22.2	0.0	7.7	7.5	8.4	20.4	10.6	20.2	2.5
C ↔ G	0.0	0.0	0.0	0.0	6.4	4.6	1.9	0.0	11.6	0.0	0.0	8.4	6.7	0.0	0.0	7.2	0.0
C ↔ T	13.9	2.5	9.9	11.3	8.8	0.0	0.1	1.5	28.5	13.5	6.8	9.5	0.0	5.4	17.9	41.5	11.4
G ↔ T	20.9	0.0	10.6	3.8	13.3	0.0	0.0	0.0	33.3	13.4	0.0	0.0	0.0	13.2	18.9	46.9	9.6
A ↔ C + G ↔ T	2.6	5.2	7.7	0.0	5.6	5.6	8.4	4.1	0.0	0.0	0.0	0.0	0.0	4.4	5.5	11.4	1.8
A ↔ G + C ↔ T	2.9	2.1	0.0	7.7	18.0	5.6	7.7	3.8	0.0	0.0	4.1	7.5	21.2	10.3	6.4	18.9	0.0
A ↔ T + C ↔ G	4.7	7.2	7.0	2.4	8.5	6.6	10.5	5.1	35.7	0.0	4.1	27.5	0.0	9.4	4.9	0.0	5.3
A → C → G → A	4.5	2.5	0.1	0.0	7.5	8.2	0.0	0.0	10.1	12.8	6.3	0.0	0.0	0.0	8.7	13.0	7.7
A → C → T → A	9.0	0.0	6.7	5.0	13.8	19.6	9.9	20.8	13.5	12.0	9.8	8.4	0.0	10.1	6.3	15.0	9.2
A → G → C → A	12.6	9.6	6.7	8.7	19.3	0.0	7.4	0.0	41.1	10.4	14.0	7.5	15.5	13.9	10.8	27.8	4.6
A → G → T → A	10.8	2.7	3.6	5.9	12.7	0.0	3.4	6.7	28.5	13.1	11.7	7.5	0.0	9.2	10.8	18.9	2.8
A → T → C → A	12.3	2.2	7.3	15.9	12.0	0.0	6.8	3.8	21.7	7.6	11.0	16.5	20.2	10.4	7.7	35.0	6.3
A → T → G → A	7.0	2.7	3.3	2.5	8.0	0.0	7.0	6.4	15.0	8.4	0.0	9.2	0.0	3.1	7.5	2.1	6.8
C → G → T → C	10.1	4.9	2.0	11.5	20.0	0.0	5.4	0.0	17.4	3.5	19.0	13.6	0.0	7.3	5.8	14.9	0.0
C → T → G → C	14.4	0.6	4.7	10.3	12.4	0.0	8.2	14.2	41.1	7.6	3.7	0.0	7.1	24.5	13.8	46.5	14.8
A → C → G → T → A	11.6	5.0	4.0	10.7	20.7	0.0	3.8	3.1	15.0	4.4	6.1	8.1	0.0	4.2	14.2	21.7	3.0
A → C → T → G → A	10.4	3.0	5.3	0.0	5.1	15.6	1.7	8.0	0.0	4.0	7.5	8.4	0.0	1.5	11.6	16.4	9.6
A → G → C → T → A	5.9	2.3	2.2	0.0	17.3	0.0	3.8	4.2	0.0	3.4	0.0	0.0	4.4	0.0	10.0	0.0	5.0
A → G → T → C → A	2.9	0.0	3.7	2.9	7.5	2.6	5.0	0.0	0.0	11.2	5.1	0.0	9.8	2.8	7.5	13.9	4.6
A → T → C → G → A	2.3	2.8	3.5	0.0	2.9	0.0	3.1	1.3	0.0	0.0	6.1	0.0	0.0	6.5	2.9	0.0	2.2
A → T → G → C → A	16.9	4.1	10.4	8.7	17.8	13.0	6.1	10.4	26.6	6.8	0.0	0.0	0.0	4.4	17.1	39.2	17.7

Table 2. Percentage coverage of mitogenomic regions by swinger RNAs in this study.

Transformation	1	2	3	4	5	6	7	8	9	10	11	12	13	14	15	16	17	r	P
A ↔ C	4.1	0.0	0.0	0.0	3.1	0.0	0.0	0.0	14.5	0.0	0.0	9.5	9.4	7.0	3.8	8.4	0.0	0.21	0.418
A ↔ G	0.0	0.0	0.0	0.0	0.0	0.0	3.2	0.0	0.0	0.0	0.0	0.0	0.0	0.0	2.6	0.0	0.0	0.198	0.446
A ↔ T	8.9	4.1	4.2	0.3	7.7	0.0	1.6	0.0	17.9	13.0	0.0	0.0	0.0	7.5	4.4	0.0	0.0	0.366	0.148
C ↔ G	5.1	0.0	0.0	0.0	9.8	0.0	3.2	0.0	13.5	0.0	0.0	0.0	0.0	0.0	0.0	6.7	0.0	0.66	0.004
C ↔ T	9.4	5.9	7.0	9.4	7.6	0.0	0.0	6.1	15.5	0.0	0.0	9.8	0.0	4.4	6.9	33.0	2.6	0.869	0.000
G ↔ T	3.7	0.0	0.0	5.0	4.7	0.0	0.0	0.0	24.2	0.0	0.0	0.0	0.0	0.0	0.0	10.1	4.3	0.696	0.002
A ↔ C + G ↔ T	0.0	0.0	0.0	0.0	0.0	0.0	2.7	0.0	0.0	0.0	0.0	9.8	0.0	0.0	0.0	0.0	0.0	−0.168	0.520
A ↔ G + C ↔ T	3.1	3.0	0.0	0.0	2.8	0.0	0.0	0.0	0.0	16.9	0.0	9.0	9.4	0.0	1.9	6.7	0.0	0.212	0.414
A ↔ T + C ↔ G	0.0	0.0	4.9	4.3	9.8	0.0	2.1	0.0	17.9	0.0	0.0	0.0	0.0	2.4	2.5	0.0	0.0	0.646	0.005
A → C → G → A	6.2	0.0	0.0	0.0	14.3	0.0	1.9	6.7	0.0	0.0	0.0	11.3	0.0	0.0	1.5	8.4	0.0	0.045	0.863
A → C → T → A	8.2	2.8	0.0	0.0	7.7	0.0	1.9	0.0	0.0	0.0	0.0	0.0	0.0	4.9	1.7	9.3	1.1	0.117	0.654
A → G → C → A	10.7	3.0	0.0	0.0	6.5	0.0	0.0	0.0	17.4	46.9	0.0	0.0	9.8	2.1	6.8	7.8	0.0	0.32	0.210
A → G → T → A	11.1	0.0	2.2	2.2	3.9	0.0	0.0	0.0	19.3	0.0	0.0	0.0	0.0	5.3	2.5	14.3	0.0	0.825	0.000
A → T → C → A	5.0	0.0	5.6	0.0	7.5	0.0	7.3	0.0	33.8	0.0	5.1	10.1	0.7	5.9	5.7	21.1	0.0	0.67	0.003
A → T → G → A	0.0	2.9	0.0	3.9	0.0	0.0	0.6	0.0	0.0	0.0	0.0	0.0	0.0	0.0	2.4	8.2	0.0	−0.263	0.308
C → G → T → C	4.5	4.5	1.8	3.1	0.0	0.0	0.0	0.0	0.0	0.0	3.6	0.0	0.0	0.0	0.0	6.9	0.0	0.335	0.189
C → T → G → C	7.9	0.0	2.2	4.8	3.8	12.0	2.3	0.0	30.0	0.0	0.0	0.0	0.0	0.0	7.0	40.2	6.6	0.833	0.000
A → C → G → T → A	8.8	0.0	2.2	1.4	6.6	7.4	0.0	0.0	24.2	0.0	0.0	0.0	0.0	4.4	6.0	10.1	0.0	0.571	0.017
A → C → T → G → A	5.4	2.5	4.1	0.0	0.0	8.7	0.0	0.0	0.0	0.0	0.0	0.0	0.0	0.0	4.2	12.8	0.0	0.765	0.000
A → G → C → T → A	4.5	0.0	4.7	0.0	3.1	0.0	2.1	4.4	19.3	0.0	9.3	9.2	0.0	0.0	7.5	0.0	0.0	−0.077	0.768
A → G → T → C → A	9.4	0.0	0.0	0.0	3.2	0.0	0.0	5.0	0.0	0.0	0.0	0.0	0.0	5.1	3.4	6.7	2.5	0.155	0.551

Transformation	1	2	3	4	5	6	7	8	9	10	11	12	13	14	15	16	17	r	P
A → T → C → G → A	2.9	0.0	0.0	3.6	7.8	0.0	0.0	1.2	0.0	0.0	0.0	10.4	8.8	1.7	0.0	0.0	0.0	−0.255	0.323
A → T → G → C → A	14.6	0.0	0.0	0.0	9.1	0.0	2.7	0.0	16.9	0.0	0.0	0.0	0.0	2.9	8.6	13.3	0.0	0.767	0.000
r	0.535	0.142	0.269	0.289	0.063	−0.017	0.21	−0.276	0.678	0.03	0.087	−0.156	0.393	0.294	0.586	0.752	0.522		
P	0.008	0.519	0.215	0.182	0.776	0.939	0.337	0.203	0.000	0.892	0.693	0.477	0.064	0.174	0.003	0.000	0.011		

Columns 1–17 areas in **Table 2**. r and P (last two columns and last two rows, respectively) indicate linear Pearson correlation coefficients between coverages across mitogenomic region/swinger transformations, comparing data in **Tables 2** and **3** by rows and columns, respectively.

Table 3. Percentage coverage of mitogenomic regions by swinger RNAs from analyses of complete human transcriptomic data [39].

Most correlations are positive along both genewise (columns) and transformation-wise (rows) analyses when comparing **Tables 2** and **3** (last rows and last columns in **Table 3**). Focusing on transformations and comparing coverages across genes for each transformation, correlations are positive between **Tables 2** and **3** for 19 among 23 transformations ($P = 0.00065$, one-tailed sign test) with 10 correlations statistically significant at $P < 0.05$. Analyses at the gene level across transformations detect 14 among 17 positive correlations ($P = 0.003$, one-tailed sign test), and six correlations at the gene level have $P < 0.05$ (one-tailed).

Across genes, at the transformation level, the strongest correlation was observed for transformation C ↔ T (**Figure 2**) with Pearson $r = 0.869$ and one-tailed $P = 0.0000029$. Across transformations, at the gene level, the strongest correlation was observed for the gene ND6 with Pearson $r = 0.752$ and one-tailed $P = 0.000017$ with highest coverage at C ↔ T transformation in both datasets (**Tables 2** and **3**). In order to test whether swinger coverage has more transformation than gene-specific effect, we calculated the combined P value using Fisher's method to combine P values, for the 23 swinger transformations and, separately, for the 17 mitogenome regions. The method sums $-2x\ln(P_i)$ where i ranges from 1 to k (k = 23 for transformations and k = 17 for genome regions/genes). This yield combined $P = 5.7 \times 10^{-21}$ for transformations and combined $P = 1.93 \times 10^{-7}$ for genes. This indicates a 3× stronger effect of transformation

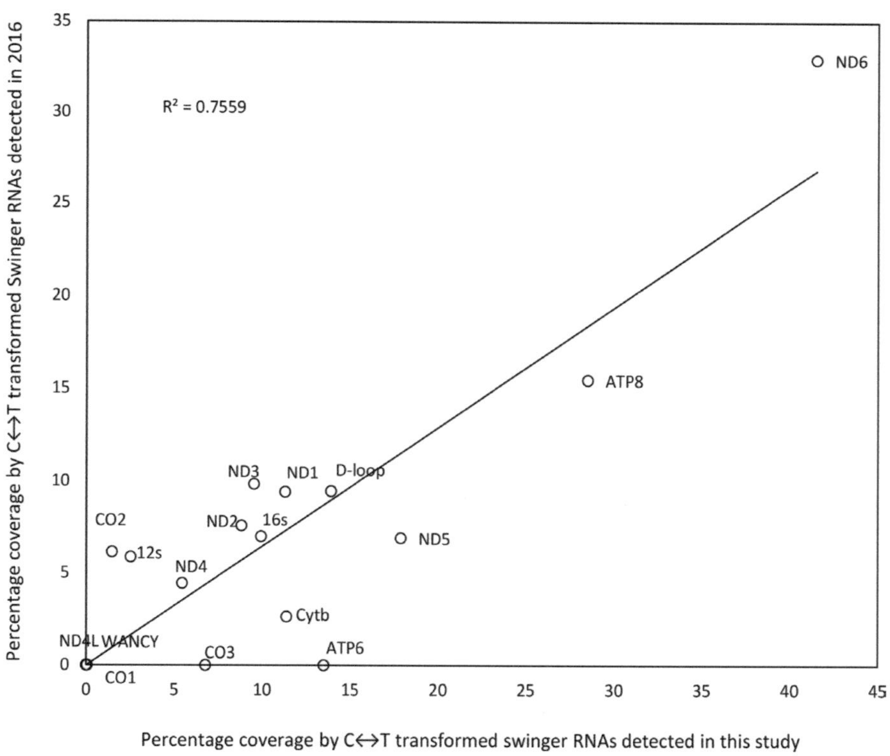

Figure 2. Percentage coverage of C ↔ T-transformed swinger RNAs across genes in this study as a function of their coverages in previously analysed data [39]. ND6 has the highest coverage among all transformations. Data from **Tables 2** and **3**.

across genes on coverage than a gene-specific effect across transformations. Hence, the most important unknown factor determines transformations. The genome region that is swinger-transcribed is important but secondary.

4. General conclusion

We find high reproducibility in swinger RNA coverage for the human mitogenome when comparing two independent transcriptomic datasets produced by Illumina sequencing. Positive correlations occur at each gene and transformation levels, reaffirming the reproducibility of the results, but are stronger at the transformation than gene level. The reproducibility of the swinger transcriptome in the giant virus *Mimivirus* and the ability to predict swinger RNA abundances from mathematical symmetry and error correcting principles [31, 50] together with present results from mitochondrial transcriptomes hint that swinger polymerizations are a universal phenomenon.

Acknowledgements

This work has been carried out thanks to the support of the A*MIDEX project (no ANR-11-IDEX-0001-02) funded by the 'Investissements d'Avenir' French government programme, managed by the French National Research Agency (ANR).

Author details

Ganesh Warthi[1]* and Hervé Seligmann[1,2,3]

*Address all correspondence to: g.warthi6791@gmail.com

1 Aix Marseille Univ, IRD, AP-HM, VITROME, IHU-Méditerranée Infection, Marseille, France

2 Aix-Marseille Univ, IRD, AP-HM, MEPHI, IHU-Méditerranée Infection, Marseille, France

3 The National Natural History Collections, The Hebrew University of Jerusalem, Jerusalem, Israel

References

[1] Seligmann H, Raoult D. Stem-loop RNA hairpins in giant viruses: Invading rRNA-like repeats and a template free RNA. Frontiers in Microbiology. 2018;**9**:101. Virology

[2] Seligmann H. Two genetic codes, one genome: Frameshifted primate mitochondrial genes code for additional proteins in presence of antisense antitermination tRNAs. Bio Systems. 2011;**105**(3):271-285. DOI: 10.1016/j.biosystems.2011.05.010

[3] Faure E, Delaye L, Tribolo S, Levasseur A, Seligmann H, Barthélémy RM. Probable presence of an ubiquitous cryptic mitochondrial gene on the antisense strand of the cytochrome oxidase I gene. Biology Direct. 2011;**6**:56. DOI: 10.1186/1745-6150-6-56

[4] Seligmann H. An overlapping genetic code for frame shifted overlapping genes in Drosophila mitochondria: Antisense antitermination tRNAs UAR insert serine. Journal of Theoretical Biology. 2012;**298**:51-76. DOI: 10.1016/j.jtbi.2011.12.026

[5] Seligmann H. Overlapping genetic codes for overlapping frameshifted genes in *Testudines*, and *Lepidochelys olivacea* as special case. Computational Biology and Chemistry. 2012;**41**:18-34. DOI: 10.1016/j.compbiolchem.2012.08.002

[6] Barthélémy RM, Seligmann H. Cryptic tRNAs in chaetognath mitochondrial genomes. Computational Biology and Chemistry. 2016;**62**:119-132. DOI: 10.1016/j.compbiolchem.2016.04.007

[7] Seligmann H. Putative protein-encoding genes within mitochondrial rDNA and the D-Loop region. In: Lin Z, Liu W, editors. Ribosomes: Molecular Structure, Role in Biological Functions and Implications for Genetic Diseases. Nova Publishers; 2013. pp. 67-86. chapter 4

[8] Seligmann H. Phylogeny of genetic codes and punctuation codes within genetic codes. Bio Systems. 2015;**129**:36-43. DOI: 10.1016/j.biosystems.2015.01.003

[9] Seligmann H. Avoidance of antisense, antiterminator tRNA anticodons in vertebrate mitochondria. Bio Systems. 2010;**101**(1):42-50. DOI: 10.1016/j.biosystems.2010.04.004

[10] Seligmann H. Undetected antisense tRNAs in mitochondrial genomes? Biology Direct. 2010;**5**:39 DOI: 10.1186/1745-6150-5-39

[11] Seligmann H. Pathogenic mutations in antisense mitochondrial tRNAs. Journal of Theoretical Biology. 2011;**269**(1):287-296. DOI: 10.1016/j.jtbi.2010.11.007

[12] Seligmann H. Putative mitochondrial polypeptides coded by expanded quadruplet codons, decoded by antisense tRNAs with unusual anticodons. Bio Systems. 2012;**110**(2):84-106. DOI: 10.1016/j.biosystems.2012.09.002

[13] Seligmann H, Labra A. Tetracoding increases with body temperature in *Lepidosauria*. Bio Systems. 2013;**114**(3):155-163. DOI: 10.1016/j.biosystems.2013.09.002

[14] Seligmann H. Putative anticodons in mitochondrial tRNA sidearm loops: Pocketknife tRNAs? Journal of Theoretical Biology. 2014;**340**:155-163. DOI: 10.1016/j.jtbi.2013.08.030

[15] Yang W, J min W, ding BA, Ou-yang CY, Shen HH, Chirn WG, et al. Possible formation of mitochondrial-RNA containing chimeric or trimeric RNA implies a post-transcriptional and post-splicing mechanism for RNA fusion. PLoS One. 2013;**8**(10):e77016. DOI: 10.1371/journal.pone.0077016

[16] Li M, Wang IX, Li Y, et al. Widespread RNA and DNA sequence differences in the human transcriptome. Science. 2011;**333**(6038):53-58. DOI: 10.1126/science.1207018

[17] Bar-Yaacov D, Avital G, Levin L Richards L, Hachen B, Rebolledo J, Nekrutenk A, et al. RNA-DNA differences in human mitochondria restore ancestral form of 16S ribosomal RNA. Genome Research. 2013;**23**(11):1789-1796. DOI: 10.1101/gr.161265.113

[18] Hodgkinson A, Idaghdour Y, Gbeha JC, Grenier E, Hip-Ki V, Bruat JP, et al. High-resolution genomic analysis of human mitochondrial RNA sequence variation. Science. 2014;**344**(6182):413-415. DOI: 10.1126/science.1251110

[19] Chen C, Bundschuh R. Systematic investigation of insertional and deletional RNA-DNA differences in the human transcriptome. BMC Genomics. 2012;**13**(1):616. DOI: 10.1186/1471-2164-13-616

[20] Moreira S, Valach M, Aoulad-Aissa M, Otto C, Burger G. Novel modes of RNA editing in mitochondria. Nucleic Acids Research. 2016;**44**(10):4907-4919. DOI: 10.1093/nar/gkw188

[21] Wang IX, Core LJ, Kwak H, Brady L, Bruzel A, McDaniel L, et al. RNA-DNA differences are generated in human cells within seconds after RNA exits polymerase II. Cell Reports. 2014;**6**(5):906-915. DOI: 10.1016/j.celrep.2014.01.037

[22] Seligmann H. Codon expansion and systematic transcriptional deletions produce tetra-, pentacoded mitochondrial peptides. Journal of Theoretical Biology. 2015;**387**:154-165. DOI: 10.1016/j.jtbi.2015.09.030

[23] El Houmami N, Seligmann H. Evolution of nucleotide punctuation marks: From structural to linear signals. Frontiers in Genetics. 2017;**8**:36. DOI: 10.3389/fgene.2017.00036

[24] Seligmann H. Systematically frameshifting by deletion of every 4th or 4th and 5th nucleotides during mitochondrial transcription: RNA self-hybridization regulates delRNA expression. Bio Systems. 2016;**142-143**:43-51. DOI: 10.1016/j.biosystems.2016.03.009

[25] Seligmann H. Replicational mutation gradients, dipole moments, nearest neighbor effects and DNA polymerase gamma fidelity in human mitochondrial genomes. In: Stuart D, editor. The Mechanisms of DNA Replication. Rijeka, Croatia: InTech; 2013a. pp. 257-286. chapter 10

[26] Seligmann H. Polymerization of non-complementary RNA: Systematic symmetric nucleotide exchanges mainly involving uracil produce mitochondrial RNA transcripts coding for cryptic overlapping genes. Biosystems. 2013b;**111**:156-174

[27] Seligmann H. Systematic asymmetric nucleotide exchanges produce human mitochondrial RNAs cryptically encoding for overlapping protein coding genes. Journal of Theoretical Biology. 2013c;**324**:1-20

[28] Seligmann H. Coding constraints modulate chemically spontaneous mutational replication gradients in mitochondrial genomes. Current Genomics. 2012;**13**:37-54

[29] Almeida JS, Vinga S. Biological sequences as pictures – A generic two dimensional solution for iterated maps. BMC Bioinformatics. 2009;**10**:100. DOI: 10.1186/1471-2105-10-100

[30] Fimmel E, Giannerini S, Gonzalez DL, Strüngmann L. Circular codes, symmetries and transformations. Journal of Mathematical Biology. 2015;**70**(7):1623-1644. DOI: 10.1007/s00285-014-0806-7

[31] Michel CJ, Seligmann H. Bijective transformation circular codes and nucleotide exchanging RNA transcription. Bio Systems. 2014;**118**(1):39-50. DOI: 10.1016/j.biosystems.2014.02.002

[32] Samuels DC. Mitochondrial DNA repeats constrain the life span of mammals. Trends in Genetics. 2004;**20**(5):226-229. DOI: 10.1016/j.tig.2004.03.003

[33] Samuels DC. Life span is related to the free energy of mitochondrial DNA. Mechanisms of Ageing and Development. 2005;**126**(10):1123-1129. DOI: 10.1016/j.mad.2005.05.003

[34] Samuels DC, Schon EA, Chinnery PF. Two direct repeats cause most human mtDNA deletions. Trends in Genetics. 2004;**20**(9):393-398. DOI: 10.1016/j.tig.2004.07.003

[35] Khaidakov M, Siegel ER, Shmookler Reis RJ. Direct repeats in mitochondrial DNA and mammalian lifespan. Mechanisms of Ageing and Development. 2006;**127**(10):808-812. DOI: 10.1016/j.mad.2006.07.008

[36] Seligmann H. Mitochondrial swinger replication: DNA replication systematically exchanging nucleotides and short 16S ribosomal DNA swinger inserts. Bio Systems. 2014;**125**:22-31. DOI: 10.1016/j.biosystems.2014.09.012

[37] Seligmann H. Species radiation by DNA replication that systematically exchanges nucleotides? Journal of Theoretical Biology. 2014;**363**:216-222. DOI: 10.1016/j.jtbi.2014.08.036

[38] Seligmann H. Sharp switches between regular and swinger mitochondrial replication: 16S rDNA systematically exchanging nucleotides A ↔ T+C ↔ G in the mitogenome of Kamimuria wangi. Mitochondrial DNA. 2016;**27**(4):2440-2446. DOI: 10.3109/19401736.2015.1033691

[39] Seligmann H. Translation of mitochondrial swinger RNAs according to tri-, tetra- and pentacodons. Bio Systems. 2016;**140**:38-48. DOI: 10.1016/j.biosystems.2015.11.009

[40] Seligmann H. Unbiased mitoproteome analyses confirm non-canonical RNA, expanded codon translations. Computational and Structural Biotechnology Journal. 2016;**14**:391-403. DOI: 10.1016/j.csbj.2016.09.004

[41] Seligmann H. Natural chymotrypsin-like-cleaved human mitochondrial peptides confirm tetra-, pentacodon, non-canonical RNA translations. Bio Systems. 2016;**147**:78-93. DOI: 10.1016/j.biosystems.2016.07.010

[42] Seligmann H. Natural mitochondrial proteolysis confirms transcription systematically exchanging/deleting nucleotides, peptides coded by expanded codons. Journal of Theoretical Biology. 2017;**414**:76-90. DOI: 10.1016/j.jtbi.2016.11.021

[43] Seligmann H. Swinger RNAs with sharp switches between regular transcription and transcription systematically exchanging ribonucleotides: Case studies. Bio Systems. 2015;**135**:1-8. DOI: 10.1016/j.biosystems.2015.07.003

[44] Seligmann H. Chimeric mitochondrial peptides from contiguous regular and swinger RNA. Computational and Structural Biotechnology Journal. 2016;**14**:283-297. DOI: 10.1016/j.csbj.2016.06.005

[45] Seligmann H. Swinger RNA self-hybridization and mitochondrial non-canonical swinger transcription, transcription systematically exchanging nucleotides. Journal of Theoretical Biology. 2016;**399**:84-91. DOI: 10.1016/j.jtbi.2016.04.007

[46] Ojala D, Montoya J, Attardi G. tRNA punctuation model of RNA processing in human mitochondria. Nature. 1981;**290**(5806):470-474. DOI: 10.1038/290470a0

[47] Garzon R, Volinia S, Papaioannou D, et al. Expression and prognostic impact of lncRNAs in acute myeloid leukemia. Proceedings of the National Academy of Sciences of the United States of America. 2014;**111**(52):18679-18684. DOI: 10.1073/pnas.1422050112

[48] Mercer TR, Neph S, Dinger ME, et al. The human mitochondrial transcriptome. Cell. 2011;**146**(4):645-658. DOI: 10.1016/j.cell.2011.06.051

[49] Altschul SF, Madden SF, Schaeffer AA, Zhang J, Zhang Z, Miller W, et al. Gapped BLAST and PSI-BLAST: A new generation of protein database search programs. Nucleic Acids Research. 1991;**25**:3389-3402

[50] Seligmann H. Bijective codon transformations show genetic code symmetries centered on cytosine's coding properties. Theory in Biosciences. 2017:1-15

Section 2

Phylogeny Using Mitogenomes

Expanding the Coding Potential of Vertebrate Mitochondrial Genomes: Lesson Learned from the Atlantic Cod

Tor Erik Jørgensen and Steinar Daae Johansen

Additional information is available at the end of the chapter

http://dx.doi.org/10.5772/intechopen.75883

Abstract

Vertebrate mitochondrial genomes are highly conserved in structure, gene content, and function. Most sequenced mitochondrial genomes represent bony fishes, and that of the Atlantic cod (*Gadus morhua*) is the best characterized among the fishes. In addition to the well-characterized 37 canonical gene products encoded by vertebrate mitochondrial genomes, new classes of gene products representing peptides and noncoding RNAs have been discovered. The Atlantic cod encodes at least two peptides (MOTS-c and humanin (HN)), two long noncoding RNAs (lncCR-L and lncCR-H), and a number of small RNAs. Here, we review recent research in the Atlantic cod focusing on putative mitochondrial-derived peptides, the mitochondrial transcriptome, and noncoding RNAs.

Keywords: *Gadus morhua*, long noncoding RNA, mitogenome, mitochondrial-derived peptide, mitochondrial transcriptome, mitochondrial small RNA, mtDNA

1. Introduction

The mitochondrial genome (mitogenome) is highly conserved among vertebrates [1]. All species investigated to date contain mitogenomes encoding the same 37 canonical gene products, organized in a highly similar gene order in most species. Complete mitogenome sequences have been determined from almost 5000 vertebrate species, where about 50% is represented by the bony fishes [2].

The Atlantic cod (*Gadus morhua*) is a benthopelagic fish in the Gadidae family, belonging to the order of Gadiformes [3, 4]. The 16.7 kb circular mitogenome was one of the first to be

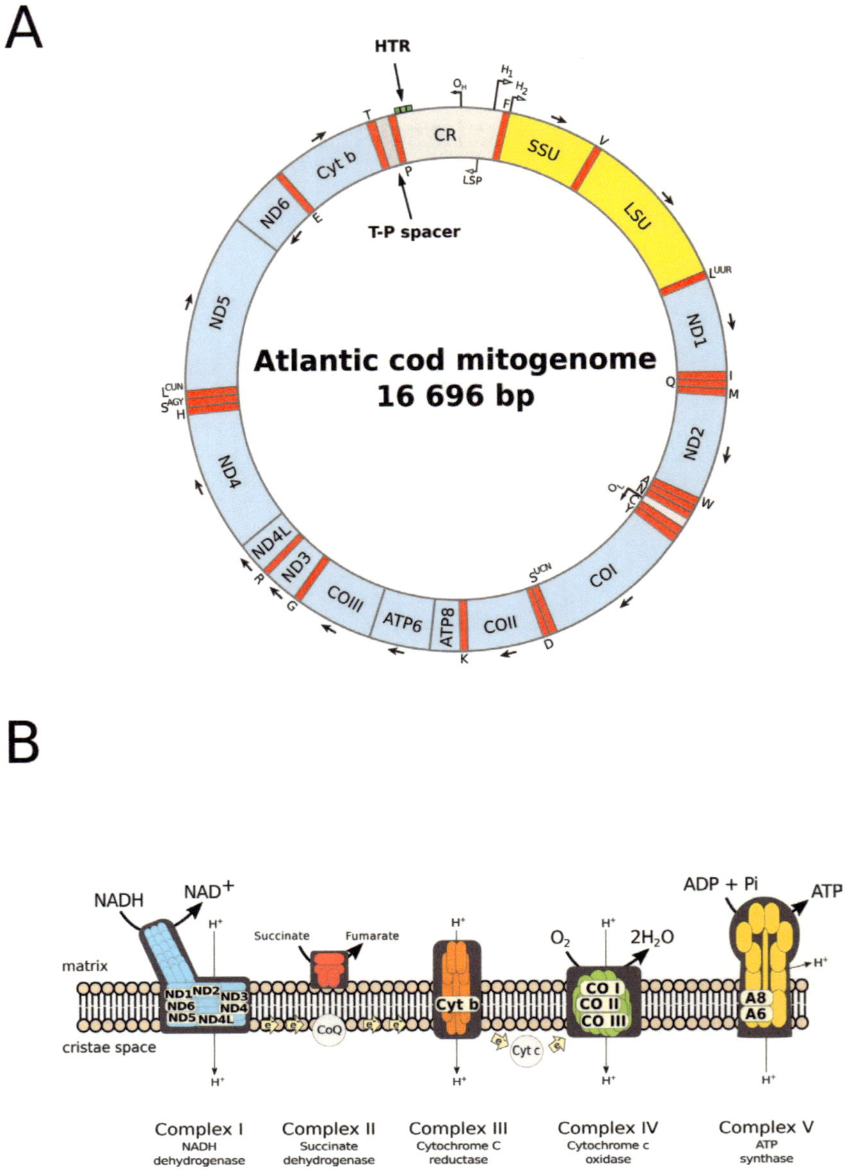

Figure 1. The Atlantic cod mitochondrial genome. (A) Circular map presenting gene content and organization. The mitochondrial genome harbors 13 protein-coding genes (light blue), 2 rRNA genes (yellow), 22 tRNA genes (red), and noncoding regions (gray). CR, control region; H_1 and H_2, H-strand promoters; LSP, L-strand promoter; O_H and O_L, origins of heavy- and light-strand replication, respectively; HTR, heteroplasmic tandem repeat; T–P spacer, intergenic noncoding spacer. tRNA genes are indicated by the standard one-letter symbols for amino acids. All genes are H-strand encoded, except Q, A, N, C, Y, S_1, E, P, and ND6 (L-strand encoded). mtSSU and mtLSU, mitochondrial small- and large-subunit rRNA genes; ND1–ND6, NADH dehydrogenase subunit 1–6; COI–COIII, cytochrome c oxidase subunit I–III; Cyt b, cytochrome b; ATP6 and ATP8, ATPase subunit 6 and 8. (B) Schematic view of the OxPhos complexes embedded in the inner mitochondrial membrane. ATP is generated by oxidative phosphorylation. The mitochondrial genome encodes 13 of the approximately 85 subunits, belonging to complex I (blue), complex III (orange), complex IV (green), and complex V (yellow).

completely sequenced from a fish species [5–7]. Atlantic cod possesses the same mitogenome organization as most vertebrate species, including that of humans and vertebrate model systems like mouse, rat, *Xenopus*, and zebrafish (**Figure 1A**).

Among the canonical gene products encoded by the Atlantic cod mitogenome, 13 represent hydrophobic proteins essential for oxidative phosphorylation (OxPhos), two are ribosomal RNAs (rRNAs) of the mitochondrial ribosome, and 22 are transfer RNAs (tRNAs) necessary for mitochondrial translation. The OxPhos system consists of five large protein complexes embedded in the inner mitochondrial membrane. However, only 13 of the approximately 85 OxPhos proteins are encoded by the mitogenome (**Figure 1B**) [8].

Both strands (H- and L-strands) have coding potential (**Figure 1A**). Most mitochondrial genes are encoded by the H-strand and include the small and large subunit rRNAs (mtSSU rRNA and mtLSU rRNA), 14 tRNAs, and 12 protein-coding genes. The L-strand, however, encodes only eight tRNAs and one protein. The control region (CR), located between the genes of $tRNA^{Pro}$ and $tRNA^{Phe}$, is the major noncoding region in the mitogenome and constitutes approximately 1000 bp in Atlantic cod [7, 9]. The CR harbors the genetic control elements for H-strand replication origin (OriH), the transcription initiation sites for H- and L-strands, as well as the displacement loop (D-loop) located between OriH and the termination associated sequence (TAS) [7, 9, 10]. Furthermore, a 30-bp spacer located between the genes of $tRNA^{Asp}$ and $tRNA^{Cys}$ contains the origin of L-strand synthesis. OriL appears functionally conserved in most vertebrates [11, 12], including the Atlantic cod [5].

Hallmarks of Atlantic cod mitogenomes are the noncoding intergenic T–P spacer, and the heteroplasmic tandem repeat (HTR) array at the 5′ domain of CR (**Figure 1A**). The 74-bp Atlantic cod T–P spacer [5, 13], located between the $tRNA^{Thr}$ and $tRNA^{Pro}$ genes, represents an evolutionary preserved feature present in all gadiform species [10, 13]. The T–P spacer is variable in sequence and size among gadiforms but still harbors two conserved 17-bp sequence motifs forming potential hairpin structures at the RNA level [10]. The HTR array consists of a 40-bp sequence motif usually present in two to five copies within an individual [5, 14, 15] and thus results in size heterogeneity and heteroplasmy of Atlantic cod mitogenomes. Here, we review recent developments in the characterization of Atlantic cod mitogenomes with focus on interindividual sequence variation, mitochondrial transcriptome, noncoding RNAs, and putative mitochondrial-derived peptides.

2. Sequence variation among Atlantic cod mitochondrial genomes

Complete mitogenome sequences have been obtained from approximately 200 specimens representing major ecotypes and geographic locations of Atlantic cod. In one study, based on SOLiD deep sequencing, we performed pooled sequencing of 44 specimens from each of the migratory northeast arctic cod (NA) and the stationary Norwegian coastal cod (NC) [16]. The sequencing represented more than 1100 times mitogenome coverage of each ecotype and 25 times coverage of each individual. We found a total of 365 SNP loci in the dataset, where 121 SNPs were shared between the ecotypes. One hundred fifty-one SNPs and ninety-three SNPs were specific to NA and NC cod, respectively. From the dataset we determined the mitochondrial substitution rate to be 14 times higher compared to that of the nuclear genome [16, 17].

More recently we analyzed 156 Atlantic cod mitogenomes at the individual level [18], including 32 specimens previously reported by Carr and Marshall [19]. We found 1034 SNPs in total among the sequences, which were not evenly distributed throughout the mitogenome. The ND2 gene (Complex I) and the COII gene (Complex IV) were the least and most conserved, respectively, among the protein-coding genes. Furthermore, rRNA and tRNA genes showed a significantly lower density of overall SNPs per site compared to protein-coding genes. Thus, the Atlantic cod mitogenome follows a similar pattern of conservation as seen for other vertebrates like zebrafish and human [20–23] and corroborates the observation that mutation rate constrains in vertebrate mitogenomes appear linked to the position of genes in relation to OriH and OriH [24, 25].

The noncoding regions of the Atlantic cod mitogenome showed a mosaic pattern of sequence conservation. Whereas the OriL and the central domain of CR were almost invariant among specimens, the T–P spacer and 5′ domain of CR contain significant sequence variation [7, 10, 13, 18]. The 74-bp T–P spacer was found to contain 16 variable sites and 26 haplotypes among 225 specimens assessed, including a 29-bp sequence duplication in three individuals [10]. Similarly, the 5′ domain of CR was the most variable region within the mitochondrial genome (more than three times that of average substitution rate). The elevated sequence variation was due to hot-spot substitution sites, homopolymeric heterogeneity, and the HTR array [18].

3. Mitochondrial-derived peptides

Vertebrate mitogenomes have the potential of encoding several short peptides (mitochondrial-derived peptides (MPDs)) [26–28]. The best characterized peptides among the MDPs are MOTS-c and humanin (HN). Genes coding for MOTS-c and HN are found as small open reading frames within the mitochondrial small subunit (mtSSU) and large subunit (mtLSU) ribosomal DNA, respectively [29, 30]. Studies in mammals indicate that MDPs are circulating signaling molecules with a number of proposed roles. While HN is involved in cellular stress resistance, apoptosis, and metabolism [29, 31–34], MOTS-c apparently represents an MDP hormone that regulates metabolic homeostasis and insulin sensitivity [30, 35].

The Atlantic cod open reading frames encoding MOTS-c and HN were identified at the exact same locations as in human, within the domain 3’M and domain IV of the mtLSU rRNA and mtSSU rRNA, respectively (**Figure 2A** and **B**). Comparative analysis revealed MOTS-c and HN to be invariant among Atlantic cod specimens [18] and well conserved between Atlantic cod and human (**Figure 2C**). Here, 8 of 16 amino acid residues in MOTS-c and 13 of 21 amino acid residues of HN were shared. Furthermore, when comparing gadiform species representing seven diverse families, we noted 10 of 16 and 15 of 21 amino acid residues to be shared in MOTS-c and HN, respectively (**Figure 2C**). The conserved features seen between gadiform species and human suggest related MDP functions.

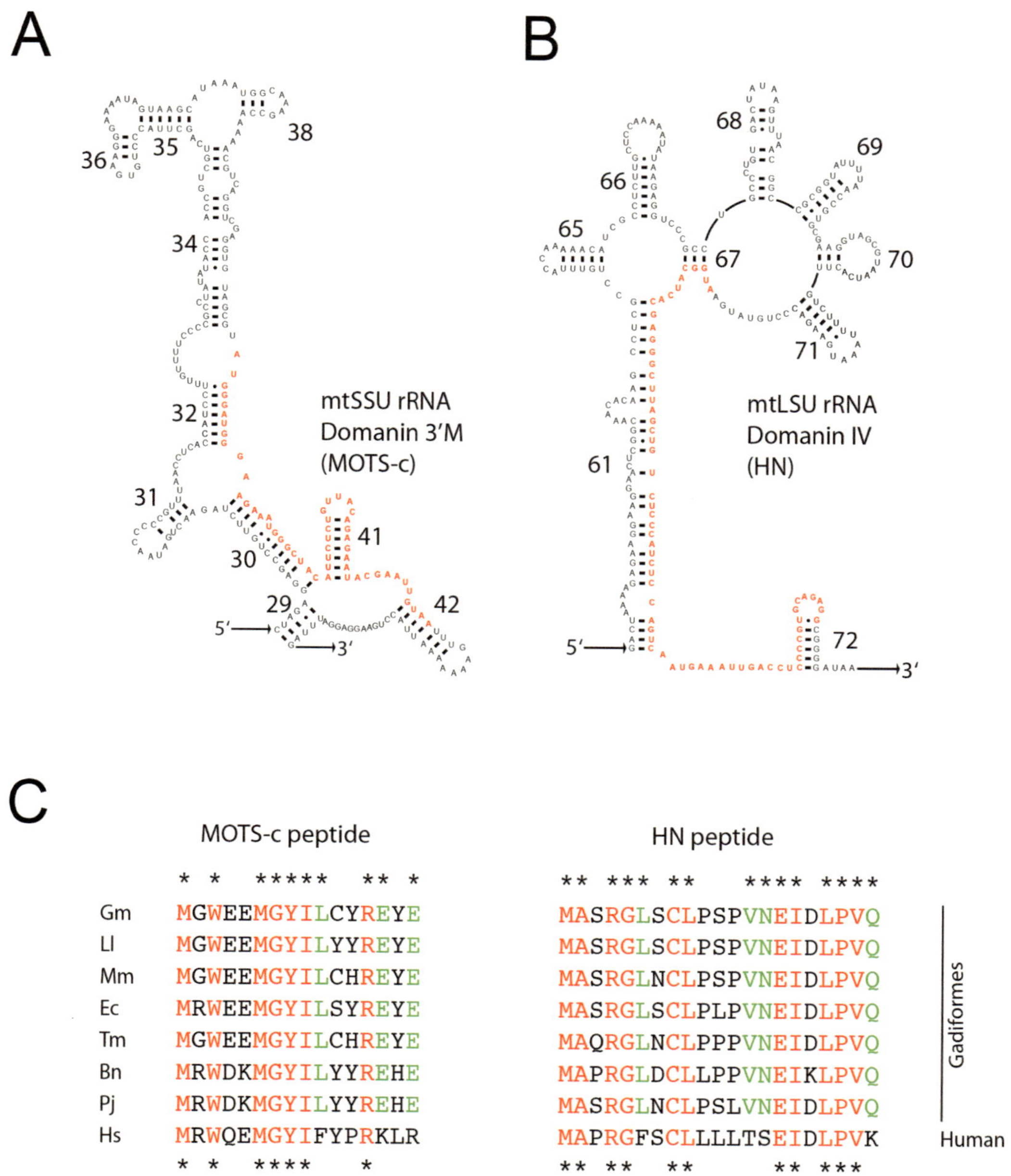

Figure 2. Putative mitochondrial-derived peptides in Atlantic cod. (A) Secondary structure diagram of the Atlantic cod mtSSU rRNA domain 3'M coding for the putative MOTS-c peptide (red letters). (B) Secondary structure diagram of the Atlantic cod mtLSU rRNA domain IV coding for the putative HN peptide (red letters). (C) Alignment of MDP (MOTS-c and HN) sequences from seven gadiform species representing different families (gm, *Gadus morhua*, Gadidae, HG514359; Ll, *Lota lota*, Lotidae, AP004412; mm, *Merluccius merluccius*, Merlucciidae, FR751402; Ec, *Enchelyopus cimbrius*, Phycidae, AJ315624 and FJ215015; tm, *Trachyrincus murragi*, Macrouridae, AP008990; Bn, *Bregmaceros nectabanus*, Bregmacerotidae, AP004409; Pj, *Physiculus japonicus*, Moridae, AP004409) and human (Hs, *Homo sapiens*, NC_012920). Stars above and below the alignment represent conserved residues among gadiforms and between gadiforms and human, respectively.

4. Mitochondrial transcriptome

Vertebrate mitochondrial transcriptomes have mainly been studied in human cells and tissues [36, 37]. Mature mitochondrial RNAs are generated from three polycistronic transcripts initiated within CR from two H-strand promoters (HSP_1 and HSP_2) and a single L-strand promoter (LSP) (**Figure 3A**) [36, 38–40]. The HSP_1-specific transcript is highly abundant and generates mtSSU rRNA, mtLSU rRNA, as well as $tRNA^{Val}$ and $tRNA^{Phe}$ [41, 42]. HSP_1-specific tRNAs have recently been proposed to perform a second role as a mitochondrial rRNA, substituting the lacking 5S rRNA in vertebrate mitochondrial ribosomes [43, 44]. While $tRNA^{Val}$ appears associated with the mitochondrial ribosomes in human and rat, $tRNA^{Phe}$ has been identified in porcine and bovine [45].

Ten H-strand-specific mRNAs are posttranscriptionally processed from the HSP_2 transcript, together with 13 tRNAs and the two rRNAs (**Figure 3A**) [46]. Most HSP_2 mRNAs are monocistronic, but two of the mRNAs are bicistronic (ND4/4 L mRNA and ATPase8/6 mRNA). Finally, the L-strand-specific transcript gives rise to the ND6 mRNA and eight tRNAs (**Figure 3A**).

4.1. Atlantic cod mitochondrial mRNAs

Similar to that of human cells, 11 mature mRNAs were readily expressed from the Atlantic cod mitogenome [47]. There are, however, some minor differences in mitochondrial mRNA maturation and modification between human and Atlantic cod. Mapping of the 5′ ends in mitochondrial mRNAs by pyrosequencing revealed that 10 of the 11 mRNAs contain no, or very short (1–2 nt), 5′ untranslated regions (UTRs) [47]. The only exception is the 5′ UTR of the COII mRNA, which contained a short hairpin structure. In Atlantic cod and all other Gadidae species, this hairpin structure is capped by a GAAA tetra-loop (**Figure 3B**) [47]. GAAA tetra-loops are known to frequently participate in long-range RNA:RNA tertiary interactions [48].

Most Atlantic cod mRNAs lack 3′ UTRs, but the COI mRNA has a 3′ UTR of 76 nt corresponding to the complete mirror sequence of $tRNA^{Ser(UCN)}$ (**Figure 3B**) [47]. A very similar 3′ UTR (72 nt) has been reported in the human COI mRNA [49], indicating a conserved role in vertebrates. The 3′ UTR of the ND5 mRNA is highly variable in length in vertebrates but is lacking completely in Atlantic cod [40, 47]. However, the closely related Gadidae species *Pollachius virens* (Saithe) contains an ND5 mRNA 3′ UTR of 16 nucleotides [47]. In humans, mitochondrial mRNAs contain short polyA tails of 40–50 adenosines at their 3′ ends [40, 45]. PolyA tails were identified in all mRNAs, except for ND6 mRNA [40], and seven UAA termination codons were created in the human mitochondria by polyA posttranscriptional editing [50]. Similarly, all mitochondrial mRNAs (except the ND6 mRNA) were found to be polyadenylated in Atlantic cod, and six UAA termination codons were generated by polyA addition [47].

4.2. Atlantic cod mitochondrial structural RNAs

The 22 mitochondrial tRNAs were found to be highly conserved in Atlantic cod, both in structure and sequence [5, 18], and some tRNAs ($tRNA^{Ile}$, $tRNA^{Ser(UCN)}$, $tRNA^{Ser(AGY)}$, and $tRNA^{Cys}$)

http://dx.doi.org/10.5772/intechopen.75883

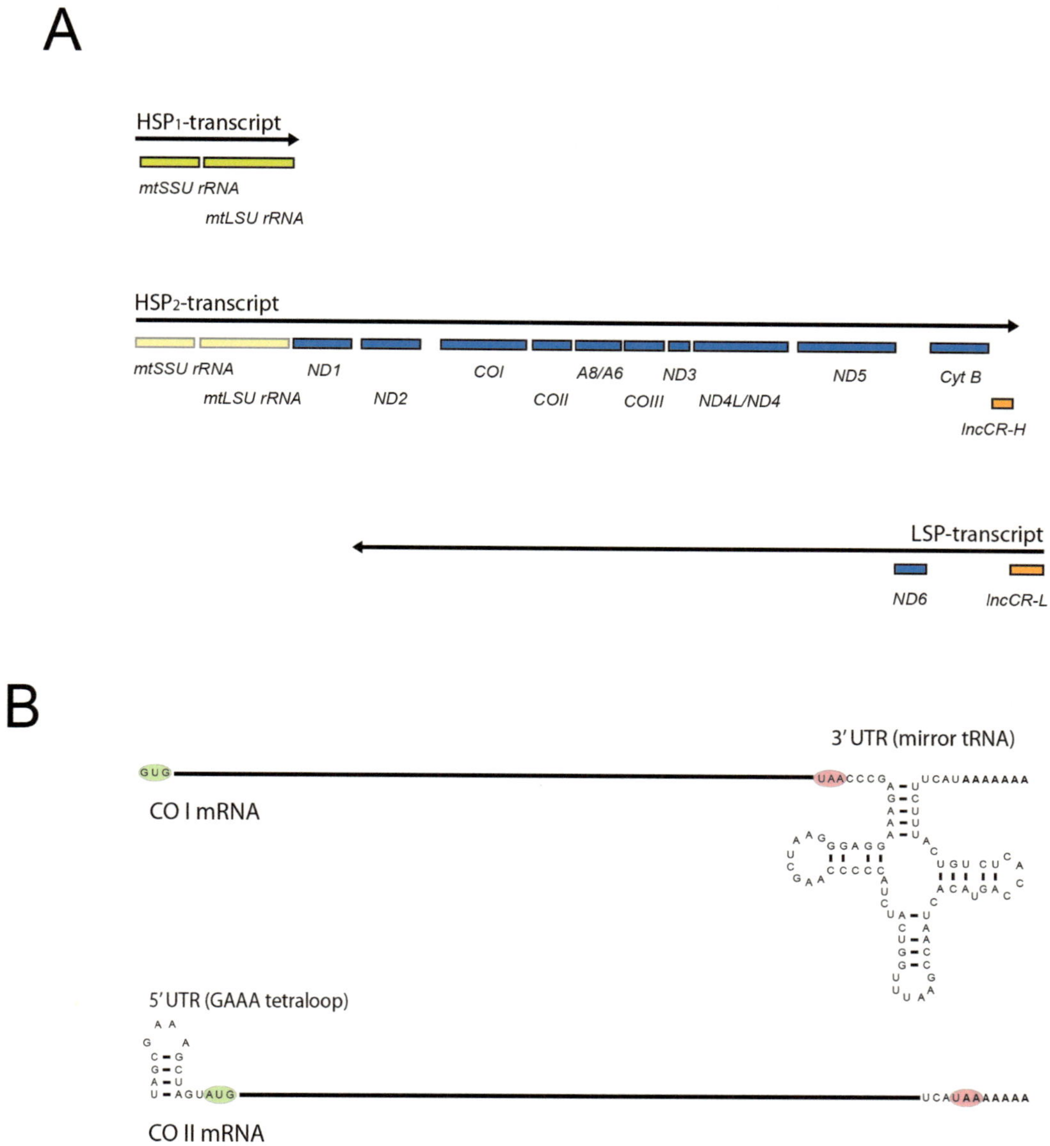

Figure 3. The mitochondrial transcriptome in Atlantic cod. (A) Schematic map of mitochondrial ribosomal RNA, messenger RNA, and long noncoding RNA generated from HSP_1, HSP_2, and LSP transcripts. mtSSU rRNA and mtLSU rRNA, mitochondrial small- and large-subunit ribosomal RNA (yellow boxes); ND1, ND2, ND3, ND4L/ND4, ND5, and ND6, NADH dehydrogenase subunit mRNAs; COI, COII, and COIII, cytochrome c oxidase subunit mRNAs; A8/A6, ATPase subunit bicistronic mRNA; Cyt B, cytochrome b mRNA (all mRNAs indicated by blue boxes); lncCR-H and lncCR-L, long noncoding RNAs (orange boxes). (B) 3′ untranslated region (UTR) and 5′ UTR in COI and COII mRNAs, respectively. Translation initiation codons (GUG and AUG) and termination codons (UAA) are indicated by green and red circles, respectively. The 3′ UTR of COI mRNA contains a mirror $tRNA^{Ser}$ motif, and the 5′ UTR of COII mRNA contains a GAAA tetra-loop hairpin motif.

were invariant in the 200 specimens investigated. SOLiD deep sequencing confirmed a non-template CCA addition at the 3′ ends of tRNAs (our unpublished results). Thus, mitochondrial tRNA processing and probably modification are highly similar in human and Atlantic cod [47].

The annotated mtSSU rRNA and mtLSU rRNA genes in Atlantic cod are 952 and 1664 bp, respectively [7]. The corresponding rRNAs are highly conserved within the species [18] and well conserved between different fish species [7, 51]. The 5′ and 3′ ends of Atlantic cod mitochondrial rRNAs have been precisely mapped using different approaches. Primer extension and pyrosequencing confirmed the 5′ ends to correspond to the annotated features based on comparative sequence alignments [47, 51]. The 3′ ends were mapped by pyrosequencing and by RNA ligation sequencing [51]. Interestingly, non-template adenosines were added at both rRNAs. Whereas the 3′ end of mtSSU rRNA was found to be homogenous and mono-adenylated, the corresponding end of mtLSU rRNA was heterogeneous and oligo-adenylated [51]. The observed mtLSU rRNA heterogeneity is consistent with the notion that mitochondrial rRNAs are transcribed and processed from two different precursor RNAs, the HSP_1 and HSP_2 primary transcripts (**Figure 3A**).

5. Mitochondrial noncoding RNAs

In addition to the canonical mitochondrial genes and the newly proposed MDPs, vertebrate mitogenomes encode several noncoding RNAs [36]. The first discovered mitochondrial long noncoding RNA (lncRNA) was the human L-strand-specific 7S RNA (lncCR-L) [52, 53].

At least eight vertebrate mitochondrial lncRNAs have now been proposed and characterized [54]. Two lncRNAs correspond to the H-strand and L-strand of CR (lncCR-H and lncCR-L) [10, 18, 47, 52, 55, 56], one is an antisense chimer to partial regions of the CytB and COI mRNAs (LIPCAR) [57–59], three are mRNA antisense RNAs (lncND5, lncND6, and lncCytB) [60], and two are chimeric RNAs that involve sense and antisense mtLSUrRNAs (SncmtRNA and ASncmtRNA) [61–63]. So far, LIPCAR, rRNA chimers, and lncCR-H have been associated with human diseases [56, 57, 61, 63–66]. There are apparently a large number of small noncoding RNAs (mitosRNAs) generated from vertebrate mitochondrial transcripts [36, 67–69]. None of these mitosRNAs have been assigned to a specific function funded on experimental evidence. However, in a recent study by Riggs and Podrabsky [70], mitosRNAs were associated to a hypoxia stress response in killifish embryos.

5.1. Atlantic cod mitochondrial long noncoding RNAs

Two lncRNAs (lncCR-H and lncCR-L) have been identified and investigated in Atlantic cod mitochondria (**Figure 4**) [10, 18, 47]. Both lncRNAs were found to be polyadenylated but transcribed from opposite strands within the CR [10]. We showed that the Atlantic cod lncCR-L has a mutation rate and an expression level corresponding to that of Complex I mRNAs [10, 18, 47]. The lncCR-L apparently corresponds to the 7S RNA in human mitochondria [52], and recently we showed that lncCR-L is differentially expressed in a human cancer-matched cell line pair [56].

The lncCR-H was found to be highly variable in sequence and structure, both between and within Atlantic cod specimens [10, 18]. A schematic overview of the lncCR-H RNA is presented in **Figure 4**. Here, the noncoding T–P spacer is present at the 5′ end and includes two potential RNA hairpin structures. The T–P spacer domain is followed by a mirror $tRNA^{Pro}$, before entering the HTR array motifs. The HTR copy numbers vary between 2 (80 bp)

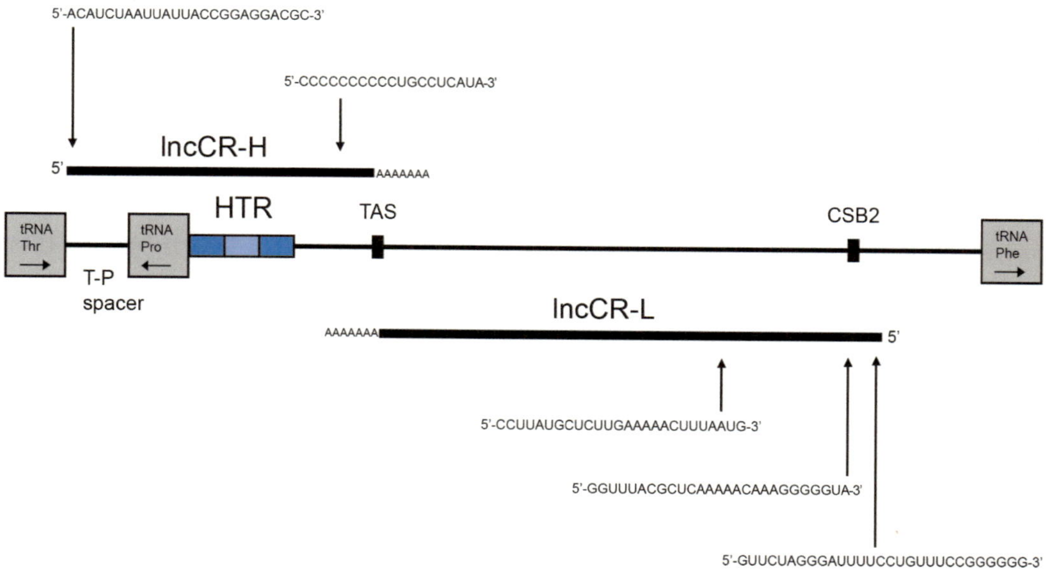

Figure 4. Schematic view of CR and corresponding noncoding RNAs in Atlantic cod. tRNA genes (tRNA^{Thr}, tRNA^{Pro}, tRNA^{Phe}), T–P spacer, HTR (heteroplasmic tandem repeat array), TAS (termination associated sequence), and CSB2 (conserved sequence box 2) are indicated. The H-strand-specific lncCR-H is located at the 5′ domain of CR and is the precursor of two enriched small RNAs (above CR map). The L-strand-specific lncCR-L is located at the central domain of CR and is the precursor of three enriched small RNAs (below CR map).

and more than 8 (>320 bp) [5, 14, 15, 18], rendering lncCR-H highly variable in size. Finally, lncCR-H terminates in a short polyA tail at TAS. Thus, lncCR-H has apparently no fixed length in Atlantic cod mitochondria and varies in size between approximately 300 and 500 nt. Interestingly, the TAS motif consists of a perfect palindromic sequence motif (**TTTATACAT**ATGTATAAA). We found lncCR-L to terminate with a polyA tail at the same site as lncCR-H but on the opposite strand [10].

5.2. Atlantic cod mitochondrial small RNAs

The Atlantic cod mitogenomes express a number of small RNAs, revealed by SOLiD small RNA sequencing experiments (our unpublished results). Here, the majority of mitosRNA was identified as mitochondrial tRNA-derived fragments (tRFs; see [69, 70]). Interestingly, most Atlantic cod mitochondrial tRFs correspond to H-strand tRNAs, and some tRFs were differentially expressed during early developmental stages (our unpublished results). Many of the same tRF species detected in Atlantic cod have recently been noted in rainbow trout egg cells [69] and in killifish embryos [70], suggesting a conserved feature at least among some bony fishes.

The SOLiD experiments also detected several abundant small RNAs mapping to the mitochondrial CR [17]. We found three small RNA candidates generated from lncCR-L, suggesting this lncRNA to be a precursor for mitosRNA (**Figure 4**). Similarly, two mitosRNA were generated from lncCR-H, one corresponded to a pyrimidine-rich motif and the other to tRF-1 derived from tRNA^{Thr} (**Figure 4**). What functions these small RNAs may serve in the mitochondria are not currently known, but we speculate that regulatory roles related to transcription elongation, mtDNA replication, or ribosome functions are likely.

6. Concluding remarks

The mitochondrial gene content and organization are highly conserved between Atlantic cod and human and strongly support a common functional platform. Similarly, the mitochondrial transcripts generating canonical mRNAs and structural RNAs are surprisingly similar. What about the newly proposed MDPs and noncoding RNAs? Are there any lineage-specific differences? Research is still in its infancy, but recent findings suggest conservations between fish and mammals. More experimental studies in Atlantic cod and model systems like zebrafish are highly encouraged, including investigations of the fascinating mitochondrial swinger RNAs [24, 71, 72]. Mitochondrial-derived noncoding RNAs need to be profiled and further investigated in adult tissue types during normal and stress conditions, as well as at various developmental stages. A first step could be to study the intracellular location by in situ RNA hybridization and then ask if the noncoding RNAs are confined to the mitochondrial compartment or exported to the cytoplasm or other cellular compartments. Our studies in Atlantic cod indicate that at least two of the mitochondrial lncRNAs may serve as precursors for small RNAs. We conclude that vertebrate mitogenomes encode a significant number of gene products in addition to the 37 canonical OxPhos proteins, rRNAs, and tRNAs.

Acknowledgements

We thank the current and former members of the mitochondrial DNA research team at the Genomics Group, Nord University, for the discussion and support. This work was supported by Nord University, Bodø, Norway.

Conflict of interest

The authors declare that they have no conflict of interest.

Author details

Tor Erik Jørgensen and Steinar Daae Johansen*

*Address all correspondence to: steinar.d.johansen@nord.no

Faculty of Biosciences and Aquaculture, Genomics Group, Nord University, Bodø, Norway

References

[1] Boore JL. Animal mitochondrial genomes. Nucleic Acids Research. 1999;**27**:1767-1780. DOI: 10.1093/nar/27.8.1767

[2] NCBI Public Database. 2018. Available from: https://www.ncbi.nml.nih.gov/genome/organelle/ [Accessed: Februrary 10, 2018]

[3] Bakke I, Johansen SD. Molecular phylogenetics of Gadidae and related Gadiformes based on mitochondrial DNA sequences. Marine Biotechnology. 2005;**7**:61-69. DOI: 10.1007/s10126-004-3131-0

[4] Johansen SD, Coucheron DH, Andreassen M, Karlsen BO, Furmanek T, Jørgensen TE, Emblem Å, Breines R, Nordeide JT, Moum T, Nederbragt AJ, Stenseth NC, Jakobsen KS. Large-scale sequence analyses of Atlantic cod. New Biotechnology. 2009;**25**:263-271. DOI: 10.1016/j.nbt.2009.03.014

[5] Johansen S, Guddal PH, Johansen T. Organization of the mitochondrial genome of Atlantic cod. Nucleic Acids Research. 1990;**18**:411-419. DOI: 10.1093/nar/18.3.411

[6] Johansen S, Johansen T. Sequence analysis of 12 structural genes and a novel non-coding region from mitochondrial DNA of Atlantic cod. Biochimica et Biophysica Acta. 1994;**1218**:213-217. DOI: 10.1016/0167-4781(94)90015-9

[7] Johansen S, Bakke I. The complete mitochondrial DNA sequence of Atlantic cod (*Gadus morhua*): Relevance to taxonomic studies among codfishes. Molecular Marine Biology and Biotechnology. 1996;**5**:203-214

[8] Kühlbrandt W. Structure and function of mitochondrial membrane protein complexes. BMC Biology. 2015;**13**:89. DOI: 10.1186/s12915-015-0201-x

[9] Johansen S, Johansen T. The putative origin of heavy strand replication (oriH) in mitochondrial DNA is highly conserved among teleost fishes. DNA Sequence – Journal of DNA Sequencing and Mapping. 1993;**3**:397-399. DOI: 10.3109/10425179309020843

[10] Jørgensen TE, Bakke I, Ursvik A, Andreassen M, Moum T, Johansen SD. An evolutionary preserved intergenic spacer in gadiform mitogenomes generates a long noncoding RNA. BMC Evolutionary Biology. 2014;**14**:182. DOI: 10.1186/s12862-014-0182-3

[11] Wanrooij S, Miralles Fusté J, Stewart JB, Wanrooij PH, Samuelsson T, Larsson N-G, Gustafsson CM, Falkenberg M. In vivo mutagenesis reveals that OriL is essential for mitochondrial DNA replication. EMBO Report. 2012;**13**:1130-1137. DOI: 10.1038/embor.2012.161

[12] Bailey LJ, Doherty AJ. Mitochondrial DNA replication: A PrimPol perspective. Biochemical Society Transactions. 2017;**45**:513-529. DOI: 10.1042/BST20160162

[13] Bakke I, Shields GF, Johansen S. Sequence characterization of a unique intergenic spacer in gadiformes mitochondrial DNA. Marine Biotechnology. 1999;**1**:411-415. DOI: 10.1007/PL00011797

[14] Arnason E, Rand DM. Heteroplasmy of short tandem repeats in mitochondrial DNA of Atlantic cod. Genetics. 1992;**132**:211-220. DOI: 10.3109/19401736.2010.551659

[15] Kijewska A, Burzynski A, Wenne R. Variation in the copy number of tandem repeats of mitochondrial DNA in the North-East Atlantic cod populations. Marine Biology Research. 2009;**5**:186-192. DOI: 10.1080/17451000802277408

[16] Karlsen BO, Emblem Å, Jørgensen TE, Klingan KA, Nordeide JT, Moum T, Johansen SD. Mitogenome sequence variation in migratory and stationary ecotypes of North-East Atlantic cod. Marine Genomics. 2014;**15**:103-108. DOI: 10.1016/j.margen.2014.01.001

[17] Karlsen BO, Klingan K, Emblem Å, Jørgensen TE, Jueterbock A, Furmanek T, Hoarau G, Johansen SD, Nordeide JT, Moum T. Genomic divergence between the migratory and stationary ecotypes of Atlantic cod. Molecular Ecology. 2013;**22**:5098-5111. DOI: 10.1111/mec.12454

[18] Jørgensen TE. Molecular and evolutionary characterization of the Atlantic cod mitochondrial genome [PhD thesis]. Norway: Nord University; 2018

[19] Carr SM, Marshall HD. Intraspecific phylogeographic genomics from multiple complete mtDNA genomes in Atlantic cod (*Gadus morhua*): Origins of the 'codmother,' transatlantic vicariance and midglacial population expansion. Genetics. 2008;**180**:381-389. DOI: 10.1534/genetics.108.089730

[20] Ingman M, Gyllensten U. Analysis of the complete human mtDNA genome: Methodology and inferences for human evolution. The Journal of Heredity. 2001;**92**:454-461. DOI: 10.1093/jhered/92.6.454

[21] Ingman M, Gyllensten U. mtDB: Human mitochondrial genome database, a resource for population genetics and medical sciences. Nucleic Acids Research. 2006;**34**:D749-D751. DOI: 10.1093/nar/gkj010

[22] Diroma MA, Calabrese C, Simone D, Santorsola M, Calabrese FM, Gasparre G, Attimonelli M. Extraction and annotation of human mitochondrial genomes from 1000 genomes whole exome sequencing data. BMC Genomics. 2014;**15**(Supp 13):S2. DOI: 10.1186/1471-2164-15-S3-S2

[23] Flynn T, Signal B, Johnson SL, Gemmell NJ. Mitochondrial genome diversity among six laboratory zebrafish (*Danio rerio*) strains. Mitochondrial DNA Part A. 2016;**27**:4364-4371. DOI: 10.3109/19401736.2015.1089536

[24] Seligmann H. Coding constraints modulate chemically spontaneous mutational replication gradients in mitochondrial genomes. Current Genomics. 2012;**13**:37-43. DOI: 10.2174/138920212799034802

[25] Seligmann H. Chap. 6: Mutation patterns due to converging mitochondrial replication and transcription increase lifespan, and cause growth rate-longevity tradeoffs. In: Seligmann H, editor. DNA Replication – Current Advances. Rijeka: InTech; 2011. pp. 137-166. DOI: 10.5772/791

[26] Kim S-J, Xiao J, Wan J, Cohen P, Yen K. Mitochondrially derived peptides as novel regulators of metabolism. The Journal of Physiology. 2017;**595**:6613-6621. DOI: 10.1113/JP274472

[27] Cobb LJ, Lee C, Xiao J, Yen K, Wong RG, Nakamura HK, Mehta HH, Gao Q, Ashur C, Huffman DM, Wan J, Muzumdar R, Barzilai N, Cohen P. Naturally occurring mitochondrial-derived peptides are age-dependent regulators of apoptosis, insulin sensitivity, and inflammatory markers. Aging. 2016;**8**:796-809. DOI: 10.18632/aging.100943

[28] Seligmann H. Chimeric mitochondrial peptides from contiguous regular and swinger RNA. Computational and Structural Biotechnology Journal. 2016;**14**:283-297. DOI: 10.1016/j.csbj.2016.06.005

[29] Lee C, Yen K, Cohen P. Humanin: A harbinger of mitochondrial-derived peptides? Trends in Endocrinology and Metabolism. 2013;**24**:222-228. DOI: 10.1016/j.tem.2013.01.005

[30] Lee C, Zeng J, Drew BG, Sallam T, Martin-Montalvo A, Wan J, Kim S-J, Mehta H, Hevener AL, de Cabo R, Cohen P. The mitochondrial-derived peptide MOTS-c promotes metabolic homeostasis and reduces obesity and insulin resistance. Cell Metabolism. 2015;**21**:443-454. DOI: 10.1016/j.cmet.2015.02.009

[31] Hashimoto Y, Niikura T, Tajima H, Yasukawa T, Sudo H, Ito Y, Kita Y, Kawasumi M, Kouyama K, Doyu M, Sobue G, Koide T, Tsuji S, Lang J, Kurokawa K, Nishimoto I. A rescue factor abolishing neuronal cell death by a wide spectrum of familial Alzheimer's disease genes and Aβ. Proceedings of the National Academy of Sciences of the United States of America. 2001;**98**:6336-6341. DOI: 10.1073/pnas.101133498

[32] Guo B, Zhai D, Cabezas E, Welsh K, Nouraini S, Satterthwait AC, Reed JC. Humanin peptide suppresses apoptosis by interfering with Bax activation. Nature. 2003;**423**:456-461. DOI: 10.1038/nature01627

[33] Paharkova V, Alvarez G, Nakamura H, Cohen P, Lee K-W. Rat Humanin is encoded and translated in mitochondria and is localized to the mitochondrial compartment where it regulates ROS production. Molecular and Cellular Endocrinology. 2015;**413**:96-100. DOI: 10.1016/j.mce.2015.06.015

[34] Capt C, Passamonti M, Breton S. The human mitochondrial genome may code for more than 13 proteins. Mitochondrial DNA Part A. 2016;**27**:3098-3101. DOI: 10.3109/19401736.2014.1003924

[35] Ming W, Lu G, Xin S, Huanyu L, Yinghao J, Xiaoying L, Chengming X, Banjun R, Li W, Zifan L. Mitochondria related peptide MOTS-c suppresses ovariectomy-induced bone loss via AMPK activation. Biochemical and Biophysical Research Communications. 2016;**476**:412-419. DOI: 10.1016/j.bbrc.2016.05.135

[36] Mercer TR, Neph S, Dinger ME, Crawford J, Smith MA, Shearwood A-MJ, Haugen E, Bracken CP, Rackham O, Stamatoyannopoulos JA, Filipovska A, Mattick JS. The human mitochondrial transcriptome. Cell. 2011;**146**:645-658. DOI: 10.1016/j.cell.2011.06.051

[37] Gustafsson CM, Falkenberg M, Larsson N-G. Maintenance and expression of mammalian mitochondrial DNA. Annual Review of Biochemistry. 2016;**85**:133-160. DOI: 10.1146/annurev-biochem-060815-014402

[38] Fernandez-Silva P, Acin-Perez R, Fernandez-Vizarra E, Perez-Martos A, Enriques JA. In vivo and in organelle analyses of mitochondrial translation. Methods in Cell Biology. 2007;**80**:571-588. DOI: 10.1016/S0091-679X(06)80028-2

[39] Falkenberg M, Larsson N-G, Gustafsson CM. DNA replication and transcription in mammalian mitochondria. Annual Review of Biochemistry. 2007;**76**:679-699. DOI: 10.1146/annurev.biochem.76.060305.152028

[40] Temperley RJ, Wydro M, Lightowlers RN, Chrzanowska-Lightowlers ZM. Human mitochondrial mRNAs-like members of all families, similar but different. Biochimica et Biophysica Acta. 1797;**2010**:1081-1085. DOI: 10.1016/j.bbabio.2010.02.036

[41] Shutt TE, Lodeiro MF, Cotney J, Cameron CE, Shadel GS. Core human mitochondrial transcription apparatus is a regulated two-component system in vitro. Proceedings of the National Academy of Sciences of the United States of America. 2010;**107**:12133-12138. DOI: 10.1073/pnas.0910581107

[42] Suzuki T, Nagao A, Suzuki T. Human mitochondrial tRNAs: Biogenesis, function, structural aspects, and diseases. Annual Review of Genetics. 2011;**45**:299-329. DOI: 10.1146/annurev-genet-110410-132531

[43] Brown A, Amunts A, Bai XC, Sugimoto Y, Edwards PC, Murshudov G, Scheres SHW, Ramakrishnan V. Structure of the large ribosomal subunit from human mitochondria. Science. 2014;**346**:718-722. DOI: 10.1126/science.1258026

[44] Ott M, Amunts A, Brown A. Organization and regulation of mitochondrial protein synthesis. Annual Review of Biochemistry. 2016;**85**:77-101. DOI: 10.1146/annurev-biochem-060815-014334

[45] Rorbach J, Minczuk M. The post-transcriptional life of mammalian mitochondrial RNA. Biochemical Journal. 2012;**444**:357-373. DOI: 10.1042/BJ20112208

[46] Asin-Cayuela J, Gustafsson CM. Mitochondrial transcription and its regulation in mammalian cells. Trends in Biochemical Sciences. 2007;**32**:111-117. DOI: 10.1016/j.tibs.2007.01.003

[47] Coucheron DH, Nymark M, Breines R, Karlsen BO, Andreassen M, Jørgensen TE, Moum T, Johansen SD. Characterization of mitochondrial mRNAs in codfish reveals unique features compared to mammals. Current Genetics. 2011;**57**:213-222. DOI: 10.1007/s00294-011-0338-2

[48] Abramovitz DL, Pyle AM. Remarkable morphological variability of a common RNA folding motif: The GNRA tetraloop-receptor interaction. Journal of Molecular Biology. 1997;**266**:493-506

[49] Slomovic S, Laufer D, Geiger D, Schuster G. Polyadenylation and degradation of human mitochondrial RNA: The prokaryotic past leaves its mark. Molecular and Cellular Biology. 2005;**25**:6427-6435. DOI: 10.1128/MCB.25.15.6427-6435.2005

[50] Hällberg BM, Larsson N-G. Making proteins in the powerhouse. Cell Metabolism. 2014;**20**:226-240. DOI: 10.1016/j.cmet.2014.07.001

[51] Bakke I, Johansen S. Characterization of mitochondrial ribosomal RNA genes in gadiformes: Sequence variation, secondary structure features, and phylogenetic implications. Molecular Phylogenetics and Evolution. 2002;**25**:87-100. DOI: 10.1016/S1055-7903(02)00220-8

[52] Ojala D, Crews S, Montoya J, Gelfand R, Attardi G. A small polyadenylated RNA (7S RNA), containing a putative ribosome attachment site, maps near the origin of human mitochondrial DNA replication. Journal of Molecular Biology. 1981;**150**:303-314. DOI: 10.1016/0022-2836(81)90454-X

[53] Chang DD, Clayton DA. Precise identification of individual promoters for transcription of each strand of human mitochondrial DNA. Cell. 1984;**36**:635-643. DOI: 10.1016/0092-8674(84)90343-X

[54] Dietrich A, Wallet C, Iqbal RK, Gualberto JM, Lotfi F. Organellar non-coding RNAs: Emerging regulation mechanisms. Biochimie. 2015;**117**:48-62. DOI: 10.1016/j.biochi.2015.06.027

[55] Gao S, Tian X, Chang H, Sun Y, Wu Z, Cheng Z, Dong P, Zhao Q, Ruan J, Bu W. Two novel lncRNAs discovered in human mitochondrial DNA using PacBio full-length transcriptome data. Mitochondrion. 2018;**38**:41-47. DOI: 10.1016/j.mito.2017.08.002

[56] Hedberg A, Knutsen E, Løvhaugen AS, Jørgensen TE, Perander M, Johansen SD. Cancer-specific SNPs originate from low-level heteroplasmic variants in human mitochondrial genomes of a matched cell line pair. Mitochondrial DNA Part A. 2018;29. DOI: 10.1080/24701394.2018.1461852

[57] Kumarswamy R, Bauters C, Volkmann I, Maury F, Fetisch J, Holzmann A, Lemesle G, de Groote P, Pinet F, Thum T. Circulating long noncoding RNA, LIPCAR, predicts survival in patients with heart failure. Circulation Research. 2014;**114**:1569-1575. DOI: 10.1161/CIRCRESAHA.114.303915

[58] de Gonzalo-Calvo D, Kenneweg F, Bang C, Toro R, van der Meer RW, Rijzewijk LJ, Smit JW, Lamb HJ, Llorente-Cortes V, Thum T. Circulating long-noncoding RNAs as biomarkers of left ventricular diastolic function and remodelling in patients with well-controlled type 2 diabetes. Scientific Reports. 2016;**6**:37354. DOI: 10.1038/srep37354

[59] Zhang Z, Gao W, Long QQ, Zhang J, Li YF, Liu DC, Yan JJ, Yang ZJ, Wang LS. Increased plasma levels of lncRNA H19 and LIPCAR are associated with increased risk of coronary artery disease in a Chinese population. Scientific Reports. 2017;**7**:7491. DOI: 10.1038/s41598-017-07611-z

[60] Rackham O, Shearwood A-MJ, Mercer TR, Davies SMK, Mattick JS, Filipovska A. Long noncoding RNAs are generated from the mitochondrial genome and regulated by nuclear-encoded proteins. Ribonucleic Acid. 2011;**17**:2085-2093. DOI: 10.1261/rna.029405.111

[61] Burzio VA, Villota C, Villegas J, Landerer E, Boccardo E, Villa LL, Martinez R, Lopez C, Gaete F, Toro V, Rodriguez X, Burzio LO. Expression of a family of noncoding mitochondrial RNAs distinguishes normal from cancer cells. Proceedings of the National Academy of Sciences of the United States of America. 2009;**106**:9430-9434. DOI: 10.1073/pnas.0903086106

[62] Landerer E, Villegas J, Burzio VA, Oliveira L, Villota C, Lopez C, Restovic F, Martinez R, Castillo O, Burzio LO. Nuclear localization of the mitochondrial ncRNAs in normal and cancer cells. Cellular Oncology. 2011;**34**:297-305. DOI: 10.1007/s13402-011-0018-8

[63] Vidaurre S, Fitzpatrick C, Burzio VA, Briones M, Villita C, Villegas J, Echenique J, Oliveira-Cruz L, Araya M, Borgna V, Socias T, Lopez C, Avila R, Burzio LO. Down-regulation of the antisense mitochondrial non-coding RNAs (ncRNAs) is a unique vulnerability of cancer cells and a potential target for cancer therapy. The Journal of Biological Chemistry. 2014;**289**:27182-27198. DOI: 10.1074/jbc.M114.558841

[64] Rivas A, Burzio V, Landerer E, Borgna V, Gatica S, Avila R, Lopes C, Villota C, de la Fuente R, Echenique J, Burzio LO, Villegas J. Determination of the differential expression of mitochondrial long non-coding RNAs as a noninvasive diagnosis of bladder cancer. BMC Urology. 2012;**12**:37. DOI: 10.1186/1471-2490-12-37

[65] Villota C, Campos A, Vidaurre S, Oliveira-Cruz L, Boccardo E, Burzio VA, Varas M, Villegas J, Villa LL, Valenzuela PDT, Socias M, Roberts S, Burzio LO. Expression of mitochondrial non-coding RNAs (ncRNAs) is modulated by high risk human papillomavirus (HPV) oncogenes. The Journal of Biological Chemistry. 2012;**287**:21303-21315. DOI: 10.1074/jbc.M111.326694

[66] Varas-Godoy M, Lladser A, Farfan N, Villota C, Villegas J, Tapia JC, Burzio LO, Burzio VA, Valenzuela PDT. In vivo knockdown of antisense non-coding mitochondrial RNAs by a lentiviral-encoded shRNA inhibits melanoma tumor growth and lung colonization. Pigment Cell and Melanoma Research. 2018;**31**:64-72. DOI: 10.1111/pcmr.12615

[67] Sripada L, Tomar D, Prajapati P, Singh R, Singh AK, Singh R. Systematic analysis of small RNAs associated with human mitochondria by deep sequencing: Detailed analysis of mitochondrial associated miRNA. PLoS One. 2012;**7**:e44873. DOI: 10.1371/journal.pone.0044873

[68] Ro S, Ma HY, Park C, Ortogero N, Song R, Hennig GW, Zheng H, Lin YM, Moro L, Hsieh JT, Yan W. The mitochondrial genome encodes abundant small noncoding RNAs. Cell Research. 2013;**23**:759-774. DOI: 10.1038/cr.2013.37

[69] Ma H, Weber GM, Wei H, Yao J. Identification of mitochondrial genome-encoded small RNAs related to egg deterioration caused by postovulatory aging in rainbow trout. Marine Biotechnology. 2016;**18**:584-597. DOI: 10.1007/s10126-016-9719-3

[70] Riggs CL, Podrabsky JE. Small noncoding RNA expression during extreme anoxia tolerance of annual killifish (*Austrofundulus limnaeus*) embryos. Physiological Genomics. 2017;**49**:505-518. DOI: 10.1152/physiolgenomics.00016.2017

[71] Seligmann H. Sharp switches between regular and swinger mitochondrial replication: 16S rDNA systematically exchanging nucleotides A ↔ T + C ↔ G in the mitogenome of *Kamimuria wangi*. Mitochondrial DNA Part A. 2016;**27**:2440-2446. DOI: 10.3109/19401736.2015.1033691

[72] Seligmann H. Reviewing evidence for systematic deletions, nucleotide exchange, and expanded codons, and peptide clusters in human mitochondria. Bio Systems. 2017;**160**:10-24. DOI: 10.1016/j.biosystems.2017.08.002

Chapter 6

Paleogenetics of Northern Iberian from Neolithic to Chalcolithic Time

Montserrat Hervella and Concepcion de-la-Rua

Additional information is available at the end of the chapter

http://dx.doi.org/10.5772/intechopen.76438

Abstract

Dynamics of the Neolithic transition across Europe using ancient DNA datasets have established that Neolithic European populations received a limited amount of admixture from resident hunter-gatherers. However, the genetic diversity of Neolithic and Chalcolithic human populations was shaped predominantly by local processes. In the Iberian Peninsula, the Cantabrian fringe showed different proportions of local hunter-gatherers' ancestry through time. The objective of this chapter is to analyze the mitochondrial variation of populations from the northern Iberian Peninsula from Neolithic to Chalcolithic time using new data from El Aramo mine (Asturias), in the context of the debate about the origin and dispersion of the Beaker culture in Europe.

Keywords: paleogenetic, northern Iberia, El Aramo mine, Bell Beaker culture, Chalcolithic

1. Introduction

1.1. State of the art

Ancient mitochondrial DNA (mtDNA) provides important insights into the movement and spread of human populations. In particular, European populations exhibit some remarkable changes after the end of the last glacial maximum (after 20,000 YBP). The changes in the early postglacial period are thought to be the result of the arrival of new human population groups to Europe [1]. These new populations brought to Europe new mitochondrial DNAs that caused a change in the frequency of the indigenous mtDNA lineages. By reconstructing the variability of the mtDNA of past populations, it is possible to infer population movements that shaped the current genetic variability of our species.

One of the most studied population movements is Neolithization, the transition from a nomadic hunter-gatherer to an agro-pastoralist lifestyle. The debate on the mechanisms of the Neolithic transition has been framed within a dichotomy based on either a demic (DD) or a cultural diffusion (CD). According to the DD model, the migrating people bringing new knowledge experienced some gene flow with the local hunter-gatherer groups. On the other hand, the CD model postulates that the Neolithic transition was mediated mainly through the transmission of the agro-pastoralist system without substantial movement of people [2].

However, several DNA studies on different ancient European populations indicated a more complex pattern for the Neolithic transition. Unlike the initial proposal based on classical genetic markers that suggested a major migration wave [3], further studies have shown that the Neolithization process varied in different regions, occurring along several different routes into and across Europe, and having a different genetic impact on the various regions and at various times [4–17].

The mtDNA frequency distribution observed in hunter-gatherers and farmers from Europe provides support for a random dispersion model for Neolithic farmers, with different impacts on the various geographic regions (Central Europe, Mediterranean Europe, and the Cantabrian fringe) [9].

The transition from the Neolithic to the Chalcolithic period in Europe has been debated. Previous mitochondrial DNA analyses on ancient Europeans have suggested that the current distribution of haplogroup H was modeled by the expansion of the Bell Beaker culture (BBC) out of Iberia during the Chalcolithic period. In addition, it has been suggested that these groups with Bell Beaker (BB) culture in Central Europe represented a population movement from the Iberian Peninsula [16]. However, according to the mtDNA variability in Chalcolithic groups from the Cantabrian fringe of Iberia, no genetic relationships have been detected between these Iberian and Central European groups [17]. This suggestion has been confirmed by the recent study [18] about the Beaker phenomenon and genomic data of Europe.

1.2. Paleogenetics and paleogenomics

Paleogenetics consists of the recovery and analysis of DNA obtained from the remains of individuals from the past, through polymerase chain reaction (PCR) and Sanger sequencing (ancient DNA—aDNA). These techniques are mainly applied in the analysis of mtDNA and fragments of nuclear DNA [9, 10, 19–22]. Since 2005, with the development of next-generation sequencing (NGS) technologies, it has been possible to retrieve also genomic data (*Paleogenomics*) from prehistoric European humans [23, 24]. This technology has allowed overcoming the apparently insurmountable difficulties associated with the deficient preservation of genetic material and the contamination of ancient DNA samples by modern DNA. NGS allows sequencing all those molecules that are present in DNA extracts (intact, contaminant, and damaged molecules, DNA from other organisms, etc.). The subsequent bioinformatic analysis allows discriminating endogenous sequences from exogenous sequences.

Massive sequencing has allowed important achievements in the field of human evolution, such as the "Neanderthal Genome" project, the discovery of new species (e.g., denisovans), and the recovery of the genome of very ancient humans (remains of La Sima de los Huesos—Atapuerca, Spain—dated to more than 400,000 years BP) [25–31].

The first paleogenomic studies about modern humans was the 7x coverage genome of the exceptionally well-preserved Tyrolean Ice man, Ötzi, dated to about 5300 years BP [32]. Currently, there are complete genomes from over 90 humans that inhabited Eurasia between 50,000 and 5000 years BP (hunter-gatherers and Neolithic farmers), shedding light on the migratory movements that shaped the genetic variability of modern humans and validating hypotheses proposed from the inference of modern genomes or partial sequences of these individuals [11, 13–15, 23, 24, 33–39]. These paleogenomic studies will enlarge the possibilities of selective and demographic analyses of the European prehistoric populations. The genomic data from European hunter-gatherers and farmers show that there is no evidence that the first modern humans in Europe (~45,000–37,000 years ago) contributed to the genetic makeup of current Europeans; these data rather suggest that individuals between ~37,000 and ~14,000 years descended from a single-founder population that is part of the ancestry of today's Europeans. During the period of greatest warming after ~14,000 years ago, a genetic component related to the inhabitants of the Middle East region became widespread in Europe. These results document how population rotation and migration have been recurring themes of European prehistory [23].

Recently, 400 European individuals ranging from the Neolithic period to the Bronze Age were analyzed using paleogenomic techniques, including 226 individuals associated to Beaker complex artifacts [18]. Limited genetic affinity between BBC-associated individuals from the Iberian Peninsula and Central Europe was observed, and thus the authors excluded migration as an important mechanism of spread between these regions [18]. This result rejects the hypothesis of the migratory movement of humans from the Iberian Peninsula to Central Europe in the Chalcolithic period accompanied by the BB culture [16].

In the debate about the biological influence of the dispersion of the Beaker culture in Europe, we have analyzed the mtDNA of remains recovered in El Aramo Mine in Asturias (Cantabrian fringe) from the Late Chalcolithic period that were not accompanied by BB cultural artifacts [41]. This human group is contemporaneous to other Iberian Chalcolithic populations both without Beaker complex artifacts associated and with Beaker culture associated. Sites without BBC associated are those of Longar and San Jaun Ante Portam Latinam (SJAPL) in the Basque Country [9]. Contemporaneous sites with Beaker complex culture associated are the central and southern Iberian and central European groups published by [18, 40]. The aim of this study is to contribute new mtDNA data variability of the Chalcolithic site from El Aramo Mine (Asturias) and to determine whether there is either a common genetic signal or a heterogeneous genetic landscape among Chalcolithic European groups (with and without BBC culture).

2. Material and methods

In this chapter, we have analyzed the human remains from El Aramo Mine discovered in 1888, a mine located in the Asturias region in the Cantabrian fringe of the Iberian Peninsula [41].

The direct ^{14}C analysis of the human remains from this mine indicated a dating between the Late Chalcolithic period and the Early Bronze Age. The anthropological remains from El Aramo Mine consists of 9 skulls and 12 skeletal remains. We have isolated DNA mainly from dental pieces (since it is the material that offers the greatest guarantees when recovering DNA). However, in some cases, we had to pulverize bone remains in order to perform DNA extraction, since it was the only anthropological material available.

In the case of teeth, we have selected those without caries or deep fissures that might extend into the dental pulp. The surface of the teeth was thoroughly cleaned with acids and ultraviolet (UV) irradiation to eliminate any possible DNA contaminants [42]. In the case of bones, the surface was thoroughly cleaned by abrasion and pulverized using a Freezer miller. Then we extracted DNA from bone and dental tissue by means of the phenol/chloroform method with some modifications [20–22, 43].

The sequencing of a 399 bp (nps 16,000–16,399) segment of HVS-I and 394 bp (nps1–394) of HVS-II of the mtDNA as per [44] was conducted by amplifying 6 overlapping fragments of 93–133 bp in length. The protocol followed and the primers used are described in [9, 45]. Likewise, in order to verify the obtained mtDNA haplogroups, the nucleotide position of the coding region of mtDNA was determined by means of PCR-restriction fragment length polymorphisms (RFLPs) [43, 46].

The extraction of DNA and the preparation of samples for PCR were performed in a sterile chamber with positive pressure, free of modern DNA, in which no post-PCR process had ever been carried out. Ancient DNA results were validated through the application of the following criteria [47, 48]: (1) suitable clothing was used (disposable cap, gloves, mask and laboratory coat), (2) controls were applied to detect contamination during the extraction process and in each one of the amplifications, (3) Real-time PCR quantification of amplifiable DNA to quantify one mtDNA fragment of 113 bp was conducted [9, 49], (4) a duplicate analysis was performed on the greatest possible number of individuals, and (5) Cloning of PCR products was performed with subsequent sequencing of the clones. The cloning was carried out using TOPO TA Cloning® Kits (Invitrogen), following the supplier's instructions.

The mitochondrial variability resulted from El Aramo Mine was compared with other ancient and present-day populations. With respect to hunter-gatherers, three groups were considered: one from Scandinavia, one from Central Europe [13, 14, 50, 51], and one from the Cantabrian fringe of the Iberian Peninsula [9, 17, 33, 52]. Regarding the Neolithic DNA, 14 populations were selected: 3 from the Near East [15], 4 from Central and Eastern Europe [16, 45], 5 from the Mediterranean area of Europe (Hungary, Romania, Catalonia and France) [6, 7, 10, 12], and 2 from northern Iberia [9, 11]. With regard to the Chalcolithic groups, we considered one from Central Europe with BB artifacts associated [16, 18], one from the Cantabrian fringe of Iberia without BC culture (Longar and SJAPL sites) [9] and another two from Iberia, one with BB culture, and another one without BB culture [BBC: Arroyal (Burgos), Camino de las Yeseras (Madrid), Humanajes (Madrid), La Magdalena (Madrid), and Paris Street (Barcelona). Without BBC: Camino del Molino (Murcia), Bolares (Extremadura), el Sotillo, chabola de la Hechicera (Alava), el Mirador (Burgos), La Mina, Trocs (Huesca), and El Portalón (Burgos)] [18]. The Bronze Age period is represented by three groups from Siberia, Kazakhstan, and

Romania [10, 53, 54]. The present-day populations database corresponds to that described in [10], to which the present-day population of Asturias, where El Aramo Mine is located, has been added [55, 56].

The F_{ST} distance matrix between present and ancient populations was calculated from the mtDNA haplogroup frequencies using Arlequin 3.11 [57]. Relationships between populations were studied through Multidimensional Scaling analysis (MDS), based on the F_{ST} distance matrix, using SPSS 20 Software. Median Joining Network (MJN) for certain haplogroups was generated to infer phylogenetic relationships between the mitochondrial lineages from the Paleolithic period to the present day using Network software v4.5.0.0 (available at http://www.fluxus-engineering.com). Different mutation weights were applied in accordance with previous papers [58–60], and the point insertions and deletions were excluded from the analysis.

3. Results and discussion

Mitochondrial DNA variability was analyzed in 21 skeletal remains recovered from El Aramo Mine, in the Asturias region (Cantabrian fringe of the Iberian Peninsula). The quantification of the template mtDNA number of each of the samples showed values above 1000 molecules/μl in all the DNA extracts from teeth and values below 1000 molecules/μl in all the DNA extracts from bones (**Table 1**). These results indicate the greater efficiency of the DNA extraction from teeth when compared to that from bones. Furthermore, in order to authenticate the results, 5.26% of the samples analyzed were duplicated, and these results were consistent in all the samples (**Table 1**). Moreover, 24 PCR products were cloned, estimating an average of 7.46 mutations per cloned fragment (~100 bp). These mutations have been interpreted as artifacts produced by the postmortem damage of aDNA.

The mitochondrial variability obtained from the 21 human remains from El Aramo Mine showed 15 different haplotypes (genetic diversity: 0.9608 ± 0.0394). The nine skulls studied presented nine different mitochondrial haplotypes, which allow us to rule out the existence of maternal kinship among these individuals. The 12 postcranial remains analyzed showed 7 different mitochondrial haplotypes, which, compared with the haplotypes of the skulls, lead to reject possible coincidences, since the postcranial remains were not associated with the skulls. Finally, the minimum estimated number of individuals was 15, with 15 different mitochondrial haplotypes described (**Table 1**). The high genetic diversity obtained in El Aramo site allows us to indicate that it is a representative sample of the original population, with no evidence of kinship among these individuals.

The 15 mitochondrial haplotypes obtained from El Aramo Mine were classified into 5 different mitochondrial haplogroups (H, T, J, U5b, and I3), with a genetic diversity of 0.6381 ± 0.1288 and a heterogeneous distribution of their frequency values (60, 13, 13, 7, and 7%, respectively). Haplogroup H is the most frequent one in the population of El Aramo (60%), whose value is close to that shown by the current population of the Asturias region (56%), where El Aramo Mine is located, and much higher than the average value found in European (45%) and Near Eastern (16%) populations [54, 55, 61] (**Figure 1**). In El Aramo, haplogroup H is represented

SAMPLE	SAMPLE ID	Molec/μl	HVS-I*	HVS-II	RFLPs	HG
Skull 1 (bone)	AR13	854.6	rCRS	73A	*Alu7025-*	H
Skull 2 (bone)	AR15	551.4	rCRS	73A-263G-315.1C	*Alu7025-*	H
Skull 3 (tooth)[d]	AR22	89190.2	183C-189C-270T	73G	*DdeI10394-; HaeII9052+; HinfI12308+*	U5b1b
Skull 4 (tooth)	AR21	33668.7	189C	73A	*Alu7025-*	H
Skull 5 (tooth)	AR31	17194.3	rCRS	73A-150T-263-309.1C-315.1C-320C	*Alu7025-*	H
Skull 6 (tooth)	AR32	18706.4	51G	73A	*Alu7025-*	H1
Skull 7 (tooth)[d]	AR42	2078.3	rCRS	73A-153T-263G-315.1C	*Alu7025-*	H
Skull 8 (tooth)[d]	AR41	5847.2	126C-292T-294T-296T	73G	*DdeI10394-; NlaIII4216+*	T2c
Skull 9 (tooth)	AR5	178331.7	rCRS	73A-263G-315.1C	*Alu7025-*	H
Mandible (tooth)	AR11	37374.7	126C-355T-362C	73A	*Alu7025-*	H
Hemimandible (tooth)	AR12	133777.7	69T-126C	73G	*DdeI10394-; NlaIII4216+*	J1c
Right Hemimandible (tooth)	AR7-9	153133.6	86C-129A-223T	73G	*DdeI1715-; Alu10032+*	I3
Left Hemimandible (tooth)	AR6	141554.8	69T-126C-320T-360T	73G	*DdeI10394-; NlaIII4216+*	J1c
Right femur (bone)	ARH10	372.5	126C-163G-187T-189T-294T	73G	*DdeI10394-; NlaIII4216+*	T1
Fibule (bone)	ARH13	312.6	086C-129A	—	*Alu7025-*	H

The number of molecules of endogenous mtDNA (molecules/μl), the polymorphisms of HVS-I, HVS-II, those of the coding region (RFLPs), and the mitochondrial haplogroup to which each of the samples belong are indicated.[d]Indicates that this sample has been duplicated.

*The positions of the polymorphisms of HVS-I must have 16,000 added since it is HVS-I (16,000–16,400 pb).

Table 1. Results of the analysis of mtDNA in 15 individuals of El Aramo mine.

by nine different mitochondrial haplotypes, five of which correspond to haplogroup H-rCRS (33%), which is the most frequent one in the present-day European population (15–30%) and in the current population of Asturias (~23.5%). The rest of the haplogroups detected in El Aramo mine have low frequencies in the extant populations of Europe and the Near East [54, 55, 61]. Haplogroup T has a frequency of 13% in El Aramo, which is close to that of the present-day population of Asturias (11.2%) and higher than that of the populations of Europe (6.8%)

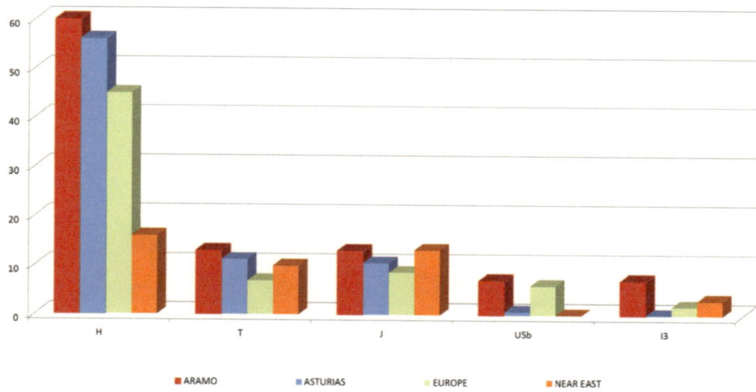

Figure 1. Frequency distribution of mitochondrial haplogroups H, T, J, U5b, and I3 in the sample of El Aramo Mine (Asturias, present study) and the modern populations of Asturias, Europe, and the Near East.

and the Near East (9.91%) (**Figure 1**). Haplogroup J shows similar frequencies in El Aramo and in the extant population of the Near East (13%), and lower frequencies in the present-day populations of Asturias and Europe (10.5 and 8.6%, respectively). Haplogroup U5b in El Aramo Mine has a frequency of 7%, which is close to that observed in the extant population of Europe (6%) and considerably higher than that detected in the current populations of Asturias and the Near East (0.7 and 0.05%, respectively) (**Figure 1**). Lastly, haplogroup I3 shows in El Aramo a value (7%) that is considerably higher than that observed in the current populations, among which the population of the Near East (3%) shows the highest frequency value for this haplogroup, which is absent in the current population of Asturias and very infrequent in Europe (1.8%) (**Figure 1**). To sum up, the main differences in the frequencies of the mitochondrial lineages of El Aramo Mine and the present-day populations lie in haplogroups H, U5b, and I3.

The frequency distribution of the mitochondrial haplogroups of El Aramo Mine was compared with that of other Chalcolithic groups of the Iberian Peninsula and Central Europe [9, 18]. For this analysis, five population groups were defined: (1) El Aramo Mine (Late Chalcolithic-Early Bronze Age) without BBC associated (ARAMO), (2) Chalcolithic from the Cantabrian fringe of the Iberian Peninsula without BBC (CA_Cantabrian), (3) Chalcolithic from Iberia without BBC (CA_Iberian), (4) Chalcolithic from Iberia associated with BBC (BBC_Iberian), and (5) Chalcolithic from Central Europe associated with BBC (BBC_CE) (**Figure 2**). All the populations included in this analysis share the presence of haplogroups H and T, although the distribution of their frequencies is different. The group of El Aramo shows the highest frequency value for haplogroup H (60%), followed by the two Chalcolithic groups of the Iberian Peninsula without BBC, CA_Cantabrian and CA_Iberian (39 and 31.2%, respectively); the lowest frequencies of haplogroup H were found in the BBC-associated groups of the Iberian Peninsula (BBC_Iberian, with 22%) and Central Europe (BBC_CE, with 29%). This frequency distribution of haplogroup H does not support the hypothesis of Brandt et al. [16], who suggest that the BBC was spread from the Iberian Peninsula toward Central Europe by haplogroup H carriers, since the highest frequency values were not found in population associated with the BB culture; moreover, the group of the Iberian Peninsula (BBC_Iberian) has the lowest value (22%) (**Figure 2**).

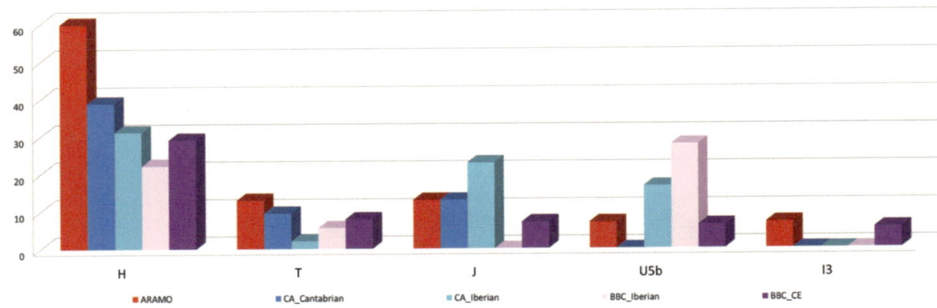

Figure 2. Frequency distribution of mitochondrial haplogroups H, T, J, U5b, and I3 in the sample of El Aramo Mine (Asturias, present study), and in other Chalcolithic groups, both without BB culture (CA_Cantabrian and CA_Iberian) and with BBC associated (BBC_Iberian and BBC_Central Europe).

With respect to haplogroup T, there is also a heterogeneous distribution among the five population groups analyzed. The group of El Aramo shows the highest value for this haplogroup (13%); the Chalcolithic groups associated with BBC (BBC_Iberian and BBC_CE) have frequencies of 5.5 and 7.8%, respectively, which are lower than that of CA_Cantabrian (9.5%) and higher than that of CA_Iberian (2.08%). Given the fact that haplogroup T has been proposed as a marker of the diffusion of the Neolithic culture, the heterogeneity of the frequencies of this haplogroup in the Chalcolithic populations supports the model of random Neolithic cultural diffusion (Hervella et al. [9]). This behavior has also been observed in the MJN (**Figure 3**), where T haplotypes of prehistoric and present-day populations were shown. In MJN main nodes are shared by all the populations compared, both prehistoric and modern. The polymorphisms that define the two T haplotypes of El Aramo Mine are shared with Neolithic and Chalcolithic groups, indicating their relation. Furthermore, the polymorphisms of one of the lineages found in El Aramo Mine are shared with current samples of Europe and the Near East, showing its prevalence to the present time (**Figure 3**).

Haplogroup J shows high-frequency values in the groups that are not associated with BBC (Aramo (13%), CA_Cantabrian (13%), and CA_Iberian (23%)), with the sample of CA_Iberian showing the highest value. The BBC-associated groups have lower frequencies, with 7.8% in the sample of BBC_CE and 0% in BBC_Iberian, showing once again the difference between the Chalcolithic groups with BBC and without BBC. Haplogroup J has also been proposed as a marker of the Neolithic diffusion in Europe. The distribution of frequencies of this haplogroup in the populations analyzed (**Figure 2**) shows a greater Neolithic influence in the non-BBC Chalcolithic groups. This influence of Neolithic diffusion is also observed in the MJN analysis of haplogroup J (**Figure 4**), which shows that the haplotypes of the Chalcolithic samples non- BBC are included in the mitochondrial variability of the Near East. With regard to the BBC-associated populations, the J lineages correspond solely to the BBC_CE population, and not to the BBC_Iberian population (**Figures 2** and **4**), highlighting the differentiation between the two groups with BB culture (BBC_CE and BBC_Iberian). The frequency of haplogroup U5b in El Aramo (7%) indicates the persistence of Paleolithic lineages even after the Neolithic period. The prevalence of this lineage seems to be higher in the Chalcolithic groups of the Iberian Peninsula (16.6% in CA_Iberian and 27.8% in BBC_Iberian) when compared to

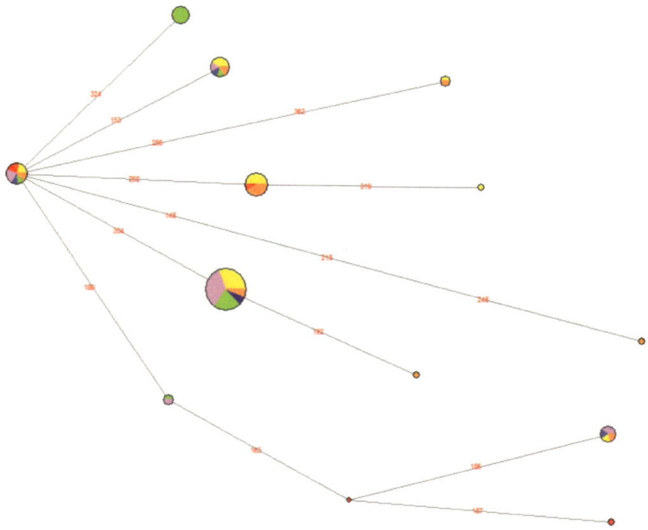

Figure 3. Median Joining Network of mitochondrial haplotypes of haplogroup T. El Aramo (red), Neolithic populations (green), Chalcolithic (blue), BBC (pink), modern Europeans (yellow), and modern Near Easterns (orange).

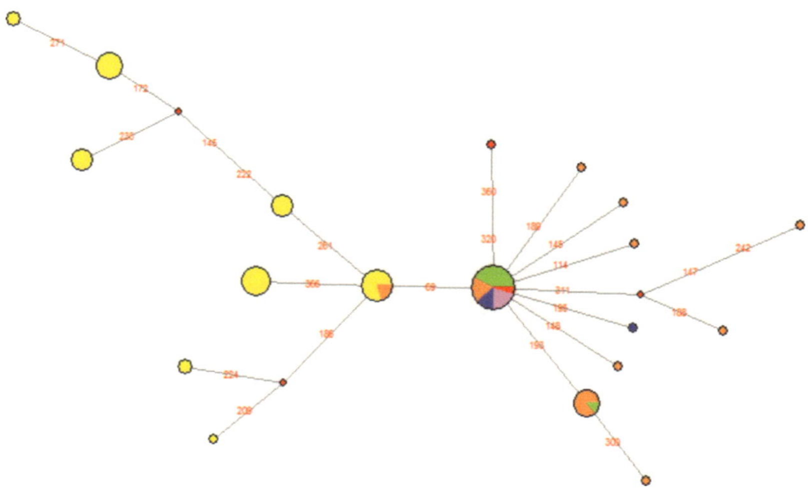

Figure 4. Median Joining Network of mitochondrial haplotypes of haplogroup J. El Aramo (red), Neolithic populations (green), Chalcolithic (blue), BBC (pink), modern Europeans (yellow), and modern Near Easterns (orange).

those of Central Europe (6.3%) (**Figure 2**). The absence of haplogroup U5b in the Chalcolithic sample of the Cantabrian region (CA_Cantabrian) is due to the lack of differentiation in the U lineages published in this sample [43].

Lastly, haplogroup I3 appears only in the sample of El Aramo (7%) and in the BBC population of Central Europe (5.5%). The origin of this mitochondrial lineage has been thoroughly debated, and the consensus reached is that it began in the recent Neolithic period [1], with very low-frequency values found in the modern populations. In the MJN conducted for haplogroup I3, it was observed that El Aramo shares polymorphisms with Neolithic and Chalcolithic groups and with the current populations of Europe and the Near East, showing a low diversity for this lineage (**Figure 5**).

After the comparative analysis of the frequency distribution of the mitochondrial haplogroups of El Aramo and other prehistoric populations, it is possible to distinguish some general tendencies. On the one hand, there is a clear genetic differentiation between the Chalcolithic groups with BB culture (BBC_CE and BBC_Iberian) and those without BB culture (CA_Iberian, CA_Cantabrian and El Aramo); on the other hand, there is a differentiation between the BBC groups of Central Europe and those of the Iberian Peninsula (**Figure 2**). The population of El Aramo Mine shows a distribution of mitochondrial haplotypes that is closer to that of Chalcolithic populations without BBC than to that of chalcolithic populations with BBC, highlighting the specificity of El Aramo, the high frequency of haplogroup H (60%) and the presence of haplogroup I3, whose frequency is, in addition, one of the highest ones described to the present day.

The mitochondrial variability of the population of El Aramo was analyzed in the context of other prehistoric groups and the modern populations of Europe and the Near East through a Multidimensional Scaling analysis (MDS) (**Figure 6**). The MDS was done through a matrix of F_{ST} distances, calculated by the frequencies of the mitochondrial haplogroups of hunter-gatherer,

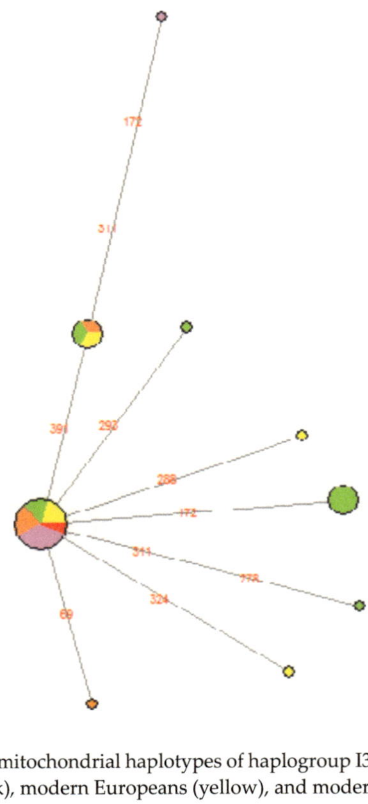

Figure 5. Median Joining Network of mitochondrial haplotypes of haplogroup I3. El Aramo (red), Neolithic populations (green), Chalcolithic (blue), BBC (pink), modern Europeans (yellow), and modern Near Easterns (orange).

http://dx.doi.org/10.5772/intechopen.76438

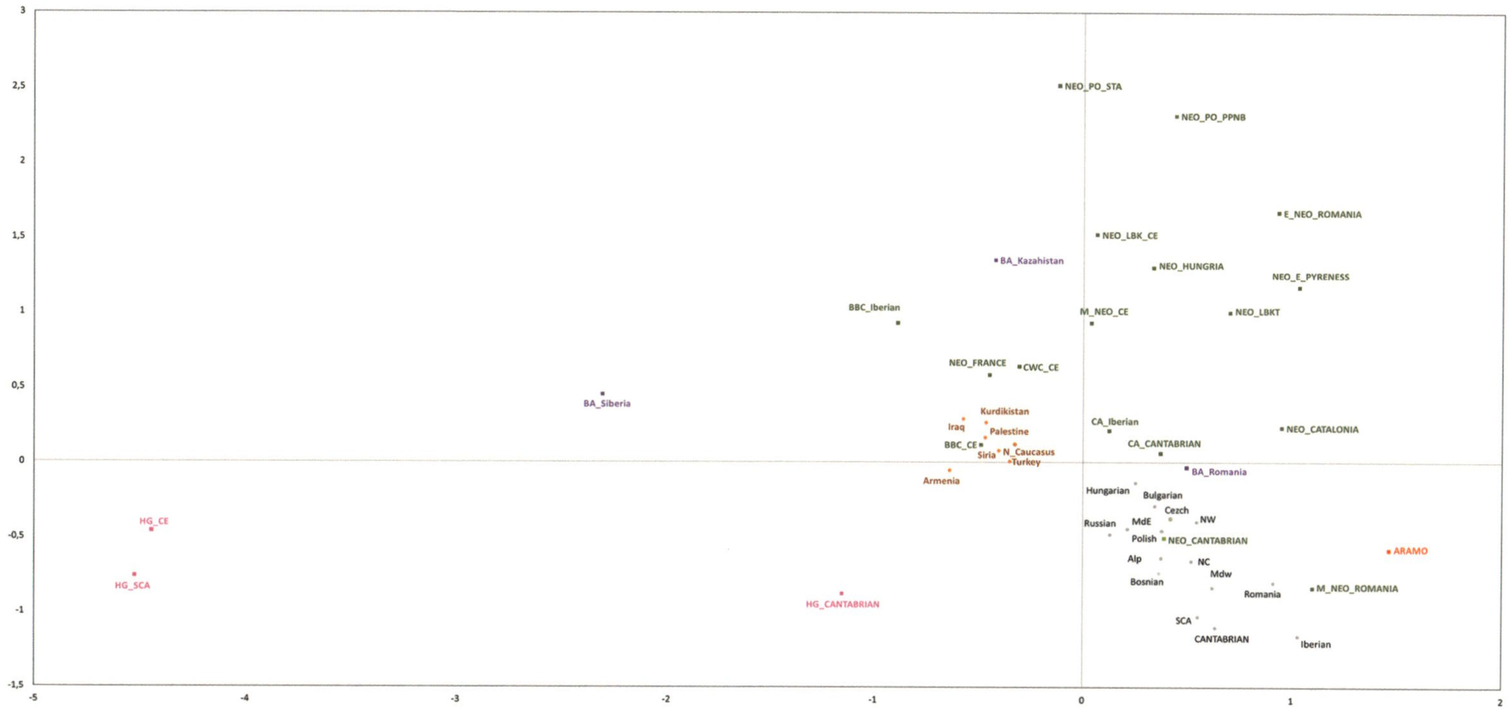

Figure 6. Multidimensional Scaling Analysis performed for haplogroup frequencies of the ancient and present-day European and Near Eastern populations. Hunter-Gatherer groups (pink), Neolithic and Chalcolithic populations (green), Bronze Age groups (purple), El Aramo Mine (red), present-day European populations (grey), and present-day Near Eastern populations (orange). Stress: 0.142 and RSQ: 0.94548. Abbreviations: Hunter-Gatherers (HG), Neolithic (NEO), Bronze Age (BA), present-day populations in Europe: Eastern Mediterranean (MdE), Central Mediterranean (MdC), Western Mediterranean (MdW), Northeast Europe (NE), North-Central Europe (NC), Northwest Europe (NW), Southeast Europe (SE), and Alps (ALP).

farmer, Chalcolithic, Bronze Age, and present-day populations from the Cantabrian fringe, Europe, and the Near East. This analysis shows the differentiation between the two hunter-gatherer populations from Central Europe and Scandinavia (**Figure 6**). It has been proposed that the mtDNA variation of these groups indicates a genetic discontinuity between the hunter-gatherers and later populations in these two geographic regions [13, 14, 50, 51]. However, this suggested discontinuity is not so obvious in the case of the hunter-gatherers from the Cantabrian fringe who separated from those of Central Europe and Scandinavia in this analysis [9, 17] (**Figure 6**).

With regard to the European Neolithic populations, the heterogeneity observed in the mtDNA haplogroup frequency variation is revealed by their position on the two-dimensional plot of the MDS analysis (**Figure 6**). On the one hand, a group of populations (Near East, Central Europe, Hungary, and Eastern Pyrenees) with high-frequency values for haplogroup N is separated from the other Neolithic populations. On the other hand, heterogeneity is also apparent within the Mediterranean area, with a Neolithic population of Southern France being closer to present-day populations in the Near East, due to its high frequency for haplogroups J and U, whereas the Neolithic populations from the Iberian Peninsula (Catalonia and the Cantabrian fringe) show lower frequency for those haplogroups (J and U) (**Figure 6**). The genetic distances observed between the European Neolithic groups suggest a different genetic impact of the Neolithic farmers from the Near East on Central Europe, Mediterranean Europe, and the Cantabrian fringe. These data support a random dispersion model for Neolithic farmers, with different impact on the various geographic regions [9].

With respect to the Chalcolithic prehistoric groups included in the analysis (BBC_CE, BBC_Iberian, CA_Iberian, CA_Cantabrian and Aramo), those with BB culture (BBC_CE and BBC_Iberian) are differentiated from the rest. On the other hand, the distance between the BBC groups of Central Europe and the Iberian Peninsula is due to both the greater persistence of Paleolithic U5 lineages in the BBC_Iberian group and the higher frequency of Neolithic lineages T and J in the BBC_CE group. This differentiation suggests that the relation between these two Chalcolithic groups (BBC_CE and BBC_Iberian) is only cultural but not genetic, supporting the study [18] about the Beaker phenomenon and genomic data from Europe, who reject the hypothesis that the genetic substrate of the BBC_CE groups came from the BBC_Iberian groups [16].

Regarding the Chalcolithic populations without BB culture, CA_Iberian and CA_Cantabrian are genetically close to one another, with El Aramo being further from them due to the high frequencies of haplogroups H and I3. These Chalcolithic groups are not distant from their Neolithic ancestor populations, although they are distant from the present-day populations of these regions (**Figure 6**), which could be attributed to a post-Neolithic population restructuring [20].

In view of the results obtained, it can be inferred that the influence of the Neolithic period on the local groups was complex, and its result could generate the existence of Chalcolithic groups in the Iberian Peninsula with genetic and cultural differences, with the latter being mainly related to the Beaker phenomenon.

The human group of El Aramo Mine, without artifacts associated with BBC, shows some peculiarities. Its chronology expands from the Chalcolithic period to the Early Bronze Age, during which a change in the landscape and the subsistence conditions have been detected in this region [62]. El Aramo consists of males who had a strong relationship with mining, and the burials reflect a ritual related to the exploitation of the mine [63]. Therefore, it is a group with differentiated cultural characteristics within the Chalcolithic groups of the Iberian Peninsula. This cultural differentiation seems to be accompanied by a genetic differentiation, since in the MDS, El Aramo is distant from the rest of the Chalcolithic groups (**Figure 6**). These results indicate the existence of local processes in the Chalcolithic period that could be related to subsistence strategies linked to the characteristics of the environment. In the case of El Aramo (Asturias), these strategies are linked to mining activity, since the region of Asturias is one of the traditional mining areas since the Neolithic period [63].

Acknowledgements

This work was supported by the Basque Government to Research Groups of the Basque University System (IT1138-16) and grant from the Spanish Ministry of Science and Innovation (GCL2016-79093/P). We are grateful to Miguel Angel de Blas Cortina, Director of the archeological intervention in El Aramo Mine, for providing archeological data and fruitful discussion.

Conflict of interest

The authors have declared that no competing interests exist.

Author details

Montserrat Hervella and Concepcion de-la-Rua*

*Address all correspondence to: conchi.delarua@ehu.eus

University of the Basque Country (UPV/EHU), Bizkaia, Spain

References

[1] Revesz PZ. A spatio-temporal analysis of mitochondrial DNA Haplogroup I. MATEC Web Conference. 2016;**76**:04048. DOI: 10.1051/matecconf/2016760

[2] Zvelebil M, Zvelebil KV. Agricultural transition and indo-European dispersal. Antiquity. 1988;**62**:574-583

[3] Ammerman AJ, Cavalli-Sforza LL. The Neolithic Transition and the Genetics of Populations in Europe. Princeton: Princeton University Press; 1984

[4] Haak W, Forster P, Bramanti B, Matsumura S, Brandt G, Tanzer M, Villems R, Renfrew C, Gronenborn D, Alt KW, Burger J. Ancient DNA from the first European farmers in 7500-year-old Neolithic sites. Science. 2005;**310**:1016-1018. DOI: 10.1126/science.1118725

[5] Haak W, Balanovsky O, Sanchez JJ, Koshel S, Zaporozhchenko V, Christina J, Adler C, Der Sarkissian SI, Brandt G, Schwarz C, Nicklisch N, Dresely V, Fritsch B, Balanovska E, Villems R, Meller H, Alt K, Cooper A. Genographic consortium. Ancient DNA from European early Neolithic farmers reveals their near eastern affinities. PLoS One Biology. 2010;**8**:e1000536. DOI: 10.1371/journal.pbio.1000536

[6] Sampietro ML, Lao O, Caramelli DL, Pou R, Marti M, Bertranpetit J, Lalueza-Fox C. Palaeogenetic evidence supports a dual model of Neolithic spreading into Europe. Philosophical Transactions of the Royal Society B: Biological Sciences. 2007;**274**:2161-2167. DOI: 10.1098/rspb.2007.0465

[7] Lacan M, Keyser C, Ricaut FX, Brucato N, Duranthon F, Duranthon F, Guilaine J, Eric Crubézy E, Ludes B. Ancient DNA reveals male diffusion through the Neolithic Mediterranean route. Proceedings of the National Academy of Science of the USA. 2011;**108**:9788-9791. DOI: 10.1073/pnas.1100723108

[8] Deguilloux MF, Soler L, Pemonge MH, Scarre C, Joussaume R, Laporte L. News from the west: Ancient DNA from a French megalithic burial chamber. American Journal of Physical Anthropology. 2011;**144**:108-118. DOI: 10.1002/ajpa.21376

[9] Hervella M, Izagirre N, Alonso S, Fregel R, Alonso A, Cabrera VM, de-la-Rua C. Ancient DNA from hunter-gatherer and farmer groups from northern Spain supports a random dispersion model for the Neolithic expansion into Europe. PLoS One. 2012;**7**:e34417. DOI: 10.1371/journal.pone.0034417

[10] Hervella M, Rotea M, Izagirre N, Constantinescu M, Alonso S, Ioana M, Lazar C, Ridichi F, Soficaru AD, Netea MG, de-la-Rua C. Ancient DNA from south-East Europe reveals different events during early and middle Neolithic influencing the European genetic heritage. PLoS One. 2015;**10**:e0128810. DOI: 10.1371/journal.pone.0128810

[11] Gamba C, Fernández E, Tirado M, Deguilloux MF, Pemonge MH, Utrilla P, Edo M, Molist M, Rasteiro R, Chikhi L, Arroyo-Pardo E. Ancient DNA from an early Neolithic Iberian population supports a pioneer colonization by first farmers. Molecular Ecology. 2012;**21**:45-56. DOI: 10.1111/j.1365-294X.2011.05361.x

[12] Gamba C, Jones ER, Teasdale MD, McLaughlin RL, Gonzalez-Fortes G, Mattiangeli V, Domboróczki L, Kővári I, Pap I, Anders A, Whittle A, János D, Raczky P, Higham TFG, Hofreiter M, Bradley DG, Pinhasi R. Genome flux and stasis in a five millennium transect of European prehistory. Nature Communications. 2014;**5**:5257. DOI: 10.1038/ncomms6257

[13] Skoglund P, Malmström H, Raghavan M, Stora J, Hall P, Willerslev E, Gilbert MT, Götherström A, Jakobsson M. Origins and genetic legacy of Neolithic farmers and hunter-gatherers in Europe. Science. 2012;**336**:466-469. DOI: 10.1126/science.1216304

[14] Skoglund P, Malmström H, Omrak A, Raghavan M, Valdiosera V, Günther T, Hall P, Tambets K, Parik J, Stören KG, Apel J, Hall P, Willerslev E, Stora J, Götherström A, Jakobsson M. Genomic diversity and admixture differs for stone-age Scandinavian foragers and farmers. Science. 2014;**344**:747-750. DOI: 10.1126/science.1253448

[15] Fernández E, Pérez-Pérez A, Gamba C, Prats E, Cuesta P, Cuesta P, Anfruns J, Molist M, Arroyo-Pardo E, Turbón D. Ancient DNA analysis of 8000 B.C. near eastern farmers supports an early Neolithic Pioneer maritime colonization of mainland Europe through Cyprus and the Aegean Islands. PLoS Genetics. 2014;**10**:e1004401. DOI: 10.1371/journal.pgen.1004401

[16] Brandt G, Haak W, Adler CJ, Roth C, Szécsényi-Nagy A, Karimnia S, Möller-Rieker S, Meller H, Ganslmeier R, Friederich S, Dresely V, Nicklisch N, Pickrell JK, Sirocko F, Reich D, Cooper A, Alt KW, Genographic Consortium. Ancient DNA reveals key stages in the formation of central European mitochondrial genetic diversity. Science. 2013;**342**:257-261. DOI: 10.1126/science.1241844

[17] de-la-Rua C, Izagirre N, Alonso S, Hervella M. Ancient DNA in the Cantabrian fringe populations: A mtDNA study from prehistory to late antiquity. Quaternary International. 2015;**364**:306-311. DOI: 10.1016/j.quaint.2015.01.035

[18] Olalde I, Brace S, Allentoft ME, Armit I, Kristiansen K, Booth T, Rohland N, Mallick S, Szécsényi-Nagy A, Mittnik A, Altena E, Lipson M, Lazaridis I, Harper TK, Patterson N, Broomandkhoshbacht N, Diekmann Y, Faltyskova Z, Fernandes D, Ferry M, Harney E, de Knijff P, Michel M, Oppenheimer J, Stewardson K, Barclay A, Alt KW, Liesau C, Ríos P, Blasco C, Miguel JV, García RM, Fernández AA, Bánffy E, Bernabò-Brea M, Billoin D, Bonsall C, Bonsall L, Allen T, Büster L, Carver S, Navarro LC, Craig OE, Cook GT, Cunliffe B, Denaire A, Dinwiddy KE, Dodwell N, Ernée M, Evans C, Kuchařík M, Farré JF, Fowler C, Gazenbeek M, Pena RG, Haber-Uriarte M, Haduch E, Hey G, Jowett N, Knowles T, Massy K, Pfrengle S, Lefranc P, Lemercier O, Lefebvre A, Martínez CH, Olmo VG, Ramírez AB, Maurandi JL, Majó T, JI MK, Mc Sweeney K, Mende BG, Mod A, Kulcsár G, Kiss V, Czene A, Patay R, Endrődi A, Köhler K, Hajdu T, Szeniczey T, Dani J, Bernert Z, Hoole M, Cheronet O, Keating D, Velemínský P, Dobeš M, Candilio F, Brown F, Fernández RF, Herrero-Corral AM, Tusa S, Carnieri E, Lentini L, Valenti A, Zanini A, Waddington C, Delibes G, Guerra-Doce E, Neil B, Brittain M, Luke M, Mortimer R, Desideri J, Besse M, Brücken G, Furmanek M, Hałuszko A, Mackiewicz M, Rapiński A, Leach S, Soriano I, Lillios KT, Cardoso JL, Pearson MP, Włodarczak P, Price TD, Prieto P, Rey PJ, Risch R, Rojo Guerra MA, Schmitt A, Serralongue J, Silva AM, Smrčka V, Vergnaud L, Zilhão J, Caramelli D, Higham T, Thomas MG, Kennett DJ, Fokkens H, Heyd V, Sheridan A, Sjögren KG, Stockhammer PW, Krause J, Pinhasi R, Haak W, Barnes I, Lalueza-Fox C, Reich D. The beaker phenomenon and the genomic transformation of Northwest Europe. Nature. 2018;**555**:190-196. DOI: 10.1038/nature25738

[19] Hervella M, Plantinga TS, Alonso S, Ferwerda B, Izagirre N, Fontecha L, Fregel R, van de Meer JWM, de-la-Rua C, Netea MG. The loss of functional Caspase-12 in Europe is a pre-Neolithic event. PLoS One. 2012;**7**:e37022. DOI: 10.1371/journal.pone.0037022

[20] Alzualde A, Izagirre N, Alonso S, Alonso A, de-la-Rua C. Temporal mitochondrial DNA variation in the Basque Country: Influence of post-Neolithic events. Annals of Human Genetics. 2005;**69**:665-679

[21] Alzualde A, Izagirre N, Alonso S, Alonso A, Albarrán C, Azcarate A, de-la-Rúa C. Insights into the "isolation" of the Basques: mtDNA lineages from the historical site of Aldaieta (6th-7th centuries AD). American Journal Physical Anthropology. 2006;**130**:394-404. DOI: 10.1002/ajpa.20375

[22] Alzualde A, Izagirre N, Alonso S, Alonso A, Albarrán C, Azcarate A, de-la-Rua C. Influence of the European kingdoms of late antiquity on the Basque Country: An ancient DNA study. Current Anthropology. 2007;**48**:155-163. DOI: 10.1086/510464

[23] Fu Q, Posth C, Hajdinjak M, Petr M, Mallick S, Fernandes D, Furtwängler A, Haak W, Meyer M, Mittnik A, Nickel B, Peltzer A, Rohland N, Slon V, Talamo S, Lazaridis I, Lipson M, Mathieson I, Schiffels S, Skoglund P, Derevianko AP, Drozdov N, Slavinsky V, Tsybankov A, Cremonesi RG, Mallegni F, Gély B, Vacca E, Morales MR, Straus LG, Neugebauer-Maresch C, Teschler-Nicola M, Constantin S, Moldovan OT, Benazzi S, Peresani M, Coppola D, Lari M, Ricci S, Ronchitelli A, Valentin F, Thevenet C, Wehrberger K, Grigorescu D, Rougier H, Crevecoeur I, Flas D, Semal P, Mannino MA, Cupillard C, Bocherens H, Conard NJ, Harvati K, Moiseyev V, Drucker DG, Svoboda J, Richards MP, Caramelli D, Pinhasi R, Kelso J, Patterson N, Krause J, Pääbo S, Reich D. The genetic history of Ice Age Europe. Nature. 2016;**534**:200-205. DOI: 10.1038/nature17993

[24] Lazaridis I, Nadel D, Rollefson G, Merrett DC, Rohland N, Mallick S, Fernandes D, Novak M, Gamarra B, Sirak K, Connell S, Stewardson K, Harney E, Fu Q, Gonzalez-Fortes G, Jones ER, Roodenberg SA, Lengyel G, Bocquentin F, Gasparian B, Monge JM, Gregg M, Eshed V, Mizrahi AS, Meiklejohn C, Gerritsen F, Bejenaru L, Blüher M, Campbell A, Cavalleri G, Comas D, Froguel P, Gilbert E, Kerr SM, Kovacs P, Krause J, McGettigan D, Merrigan M, Merriwether DA, O'Reilly S, Richards MB, Semino O, Shamoon-Pour M, Stefanescu G, Stumvoll M, Tönjes A, Torroni A, Wilson JF, Yengo L, Hovhannisyan NA, Patterson N, Pinhasi R, Reich D. Genomic insights into the origin of farming in the ancient Near East. Nature. 2016;**536**:419-424. DOI: 10.1038/nature19310

[25] Green RE, Krause J, Ptak SE, Briggs AW, Ronan MT, Simons JF, Du L, Egholm M, Rothberg JM, Paunovic M, Pääbo S. Analysis of one million base pairs of Neanderthal DNA. Nature. 2006;**444**:330-336. DOI: 10.1038/nature05336

[26] Green RE, Krause J, Briggs AW, Maricic T, Stenzel U, Kircher M, Patterson N, Li H, Zhai W, Fritz MH, Hansen NF, Durand EY, Malaspinas AS, Jensen JD, Marques-Bonet T, Alkan C, Prüfer K, Meyer M, Burbano HA, Good JM, Schultz R, Aximu-Petri A, Butthof A, Höber B, Höffner B, Siegemund M, Weihmann A, Nusbaum C, Lander ES, Russ C, Novod N, Affourtit J, Egholm M, Verna C, Rudan P, Brajkovic D, Kucan Ž, Gušic I, Doronichev VB, Golovanova LV, Lalueza-Fox C, de la Rasilla M, Fortea J, Rosas A, Schmitz RW, Johnson PLF, Eichler EE, Falush D, Birney E, Mullikin JC, Slatkin M, Nielsen R, Kelso J, Lachmann M, Reich D, Pääbo S. A draft sequence of the Neandertal genome. Science. 2010;**328**:710-722. DOI: 10.1126/science.1188021

[27] Noonan JP, Coop G, Kudaravalli S, Smith D, Krause J, Alessi J, Chen F, Platt D, Pääbo S, Pritchard JK, Rubin EM. Sequencing and analysis of Neanderthal genomic DNA. Science. 2006;**314**:1113-1118. DOI: 10.1126/science.1131412

[28] Prüfer K, Racimo F, Patterson N, Jay F, Sankararaman S, Sawyer S, Heinze A, Renaud G, Sudmant PH, de Filippo C, Li H, Mallick S, Dannemann M, Fu Q, Kircher M, Kuhlwilm M, Lachmann M, Meyer M, Ongyerth M, Siebauer M, Theunert C, Tandon A, Moorjani P, Pickrell J, Mullikin JC, Vohr SH, Green RE, Hellmann I, Johnson PL, Blanche H, Cann H, Kitzman JO, Shendure J, Eichler EE, Lein ES, Bakken TE, Golovanova LV, Doronichev VB, Shunkov MV, Derevianko AP, Viola B, Slatkin M, Reich D, Kelso J, Pääbo S. The complete genome sequence of a Neanderthal from the Altai Mountains. Nature. 2014;**505**:43-49. DOI: 10.1038/nature12886

[29] Reich D, Green RE, Kircher M, Krause J, Patterson N, Durand EY, Viola B, Briggs AW, Stenzel U, Johnson PL, Maricic T, Good JM, Marques-Bonet T, Alkan C, Fu Q, Mallick S, Li H, Meyer M, Eichler EE, Stoneking M, Richards M, Talamo S, Shunkov MV, Derevianko AP, Hublin JJ, Kelso J, Slatkin M, Pääbo S. Genetic history of an archaic hominin group from Denisova Cave in Siberia. Nature. 2010;**468**:1053-1060. DOI: 10.1038/nature09710

[30] Meyer M, Kircher M, Gansauge MT, Li H, Racimo F, Mallick S, Schraiber JG, Jay F, Prüfer K, de Filippo C, Sudmant PH, Alkan C, Fu Q, Do R, Rohland N, Tandon A, Siebauer M, Green RE, Bryc K, Briggs AW, Stenzel U, Dabney J, Shendure J, Kitzman J, Hammer MF, Shunkov MV, Derevianko AP, Patterson N, Andrés AM, Eichler EE, Slatkin M, Reich D, Kelso J, Pääbo S. A high-coverage genome sequence from an archaic Denisovan individual. Science. 2012;**338**:222-226. DOI: 10.1126/science.1224344

[31] Meyer M, Fu Q, Aximu-Petri A, Glocke I, Nickel B, Arsuaga JL, Martínez I, Gracia A, Bermúdez de Castro JM, Carbonell E, Pääbo S. A mitochondrial genome sequence of a hominin from Sima de los Huesos. Nature. 2014;**505**:403-406. DOI: 10.1038/nature12788

[32] Keller A, Graefen A, Ball M, Matzas M, Boisguerin V, Maixner F, Leidinger P, Backes C, Khairat R, Forster M, Stade B, Franke A, Mayer J, Spangler J, McLaughlin S, Shah M, Lee C, Harkins TT, Sartori A, Moreno-Estrada A, Henn B, Sikora M, Semino O, Chiaroni J, Rootsi S, Myres NM, Cabrera VM, Underhill PA, Bustamante CD, Vigl EE, Samadelli M, Cipollini G, Haas J, Katus H, O'Connor BD, Carlson MR, Meder B, Blin N, Meese E, Pusch CM, Zink A. New insights into the Tyrolean Iceman's origin and phenotype as inferred by whole-genome sequencing. Nature Communications. 2012;**3**:698. DOI: 10.1038/ncomms1701

[33] Sanchez-Quinto F, Schroeder H, Ramirez O, Avila-Arcos MC, Pybus M, Olalde I, Velazquez AM, Marcos ME, Encinas JM, Bertranpetit J, Orlando L, Gilbert MT, Lalueza-Fox C. Genomic affinities of two 7,000-year-old Iberian hunter-gatherers. Current Biology. 2012;**22**:1494-1499. DOI: 10.1016/j.cub.2012.06.005

[34] Brotherton P, Haak W, Templeton J, Brandt G, Soubrier J, Jane Adler C, Richards SM, Der Sarkissian C, Ganslmeier R, Friederich S, Dresely V, van Oven M, Kenyon R, Van der Hoek MB, Korlach J, Luong K, Ho SYW, Quintana-Murci L, Behar DM, Meller H,

Alt KW, Cooper A, Genographic Consortium. Neolithic mitochondrial haplogroup H genomes and the genetic origins of Europeans. Nature Communications. 2013;**4**:1764. DOI: 10.1038/ncomms2656

[35] Benazzi S, Slon V, Talamo S, Negrino F, Peresani M, Bailey SE, Sawyer S, Panetta D, Vicino G, Starnini E, Mannino MA, Salvadori PA, Meyer M, Pääbo S, Hublin JJ. Archaeology. The makers of the Protoaurignacian and implications for Neandertal extinction. Science. 2015;**348**:793-796. DOI: 10.1126/science.aaa2773

[36] Lazaridis I, Patterson N, Mittnik A, Renaud G, Mallick S, Kirsanow K, Sudmant PH, Schraiber JG, Castellano S, Lipson M, Berger B, Economou C, Bollongino R, Fu Q, Bos KI, Nordenfelt S, Li H, de Filippo C, Prüfer K, Sawyer S, Posth C, Haak W, Hallgren F, Fornander E, Rohland N, Delsate D, Francken M, Guinet JM, Wahl J, Ayodo G, Babiker HA, Bailliet G, Balanovska E, Balanovsky O, Barrantes R, Bedoya G, Ben-Ami H, Bene J, Berrada F, Bravi CM, Brisighelli F, Busby GB, Cali F, Churnosov M, Cole DE, Corach D, Damba L, van Driem G, Dryomov S, Dugoujon JM, Fedorova SA, Gallego Romero I, Gubina M, Hammer M, Henn BM, Hervig T, Hodoglugil U, Jha AR, Karachanak-Yankova S, Khusainova R, Khusnutdinova E, Kittles R, Kivisild T, Klitz W, Kučinskas V, Kushniarevich A, Laredj L, Litvinov S, Loukidis T, Mahley RW, Melegh B, Metspalu E, Molina J, Mountain J, Näkkäläjärvi K, Nesheva D, Nyambo T, Osipova L, Parik J, Platonov F, Posukh O, Romano V, Rothhammer F, Rudan I, Ruizbakiev R, Sahakyan H, Sajantila A, Salas A, Starikovskaya EB, Tarekegn A, Toncheva D, Turdikulova S, Uktveryte I, Utevska O, Vasquez R, Villena M, Voevoda M, Winkler CA, Yepiskoposyan L, Zalloua P, Zemunik T, Cooper A, Capelli C, Thomas MG, Ruiz-Linares A, Tishkoff SA, Singh L, Thangaraj K, Villems R, Comas D, Sukernik R, Metspalu M, Meyer M, Eichler EE, Burger J, Slatkin M, Pääbo S, Kelso J, Reich D, Krause J. Ancient human genomes suggest three ancestral populations for present-day Europeans. Nature. 2014;**513**:409-413. DOI: 10.1038/nature13673

[37] Sikora M, Carpenter ML, Moreno-Estrada A, Henn BM, Underhill PA, Sánchez-Quinto F, Zara I, Pitzalis M, Sidore C, Busonero F, Maschio A, Angius A, Jones C, Mendoza-Revilla J, Nekhrizov G, Dimitrova D, Theodossiev N, Harkins TT, Keller A, Maixner F, Zink A, Abecasis G, Sanna S, Cucca F, Bustamante CD. Population genomic analysis of ancient and modern genomesyields new insights into the genetic ancestry of the Tyrolean Iceman and the genetic structure of Europe. PLoS Genetics. 2014;**10**:e1004353. DOI: 10.1371/journal.pgen.1004353

[38] Sikora M, Seguin-Orlando A, Sousa VC, Albrechtsen A, Korneliussen T, Ko A, Rasmussen S, Dupanloup I, Nigst PR, Bosch MD, Renaud G, Allentoft ME, Margaryan A, Vasilyev SV, Veselovskaya EV, Borutskaya SB, Deviese T, Comeskey D, Higham T, Manica A, Foley R, Meltzer DJ, Nielsen R, Excoffier L, Mirazon Lahr M, Orlando L, Willerslev E. Ancient genomes show social and reproductive behavior of early Upper Paleolithic foragers. Science. 2017;**358**:659-662. DOI: 10.1126/science.aao1807

[39] Günther T, Valdiosera C, Malmström H, Ureña I, Rodriguez-Varela R, Sverrisdóttir ÓO, Daskalaki EA, Skoglund P, Naidoo T, Svensson EM, Bermúdez de Castro JM,

Carbonell E, Dunn M, Storå J, Iriarte E, Arsuaga JL, Carretero JM, Götherström A, Jakobsson M. Ancient genomes link early farmers from Atapuerca in Spain to modern-day Basques. Proceedings of the National Academy of Sciences of the United States of America. 2015;**112**:11917-11922. DOI: 10.1073/pnas.1509851112

[40] Gómez-Sánchez D, Olalde I, Pierini F, Matas-Lalueza L, Gigli E, Lari M, Civit S, Lozano M, Vergès JM, Caramelli D, Ramírez O, Lalueza-Fox C. Mitochondrial DNA from El Mirador cave (Atapuerca, Spain) reveals the heterogeneity of Chalcolithic populations. PLoS One. 2014;**9**:e105105. DOI: 10.1371/journal.pone.0105105

[41] de Blas Cortina MA. Producción e intercambio de metal: la singularidad de las minas de cobre prehistóricas del Aramo y El Milagro (Asturias). Studia Archaeologica. 1998;**88**: 71-103

[42] Ginther C, Issel-Tarver L, King MC. Identifying individuals by sequencing mitochondrial DNA from teeth. Nature Genetics. 1992;**2**:135-138. DOI: 10.1038/ng1092-135

[43] Izagirre N, de-la-Rua C. An mtDNA analysis in ancient Basque populations: Implications for haplogroup V as a marker for a major Paleolithic expansion from southwestern Europe. American Journal of Human Genetics. 1999;**65**:199-207. DOI: 10.1086/302442

[44] Andrews RM, Kubacka I, Chinnery PF, Lightowlers RN, Turnbull DM, Howell N. Reanalysis and revision of the Cambridge reference sequence for human mitochondrial DNA. Nature Genetics. 1999;**23**:147. DOI: 10.1038/13779

[45] Alonso A, Martin P, Albarran C, García P, García O, de Simón LF, García-Hirschfel J, Sancho M, de-la-Rúa C, Fernández-Piqueras J. Multiplex-PCR of short amplicons for mtDNA sequencing from ancient DNA. International Congress Series. 2003;**1239**:585-588

[46] Torroni A, Huoponen K, Francalacci P, Petrozzi M, Morelli L, Scozzari R, Obinu D, Savontaus ML. Classification of European mtDNAs from an analysis of three European populations. Genetics. 1996;**144**:1835-1850

[47] Pääbo S, Poinar H, Serre D, Jaenicke-Despres V, Hebler J, Rohland N, Kuch M, Krause J, Vigilant L, Hofreiter M. Genetic analyses from ancient DNA. Annual Reviews in Genetics. 2004;**38**:645-679. DOI: 10.1146/annurev.genet.37.110801.143214

[48] Gilbert MT, Willerslev E. Authenticity in ancient DNA studies. Medicina Nei Scoli. 2006;**18**:701-723

[49] Handt O, Krings M, Ward RH, Pääbo S. The retrieval of ancient human DNA sequences. American Journal of Human Genetics. 1996;**59**:368-376

[50] Malmström H, Gilbert MT, Thomas MG, Brandstrom M, Stora J, Molnar P, Andersen PK, Bendixen C, Holmlund G, Gotherstrom A, Willerslev E. Ancient DNA reveals lack of continuity between Neolithic hunter-gatherers and contemporary Scandinavians. Current Biology. 2009;**19**:1758-1762. DOI: 10.1016/j.cub.2009.09.017

[51] Bramanti B, Thomas MG, Haak W, Unterlaender M, Jores P, Tambets K, Antanaitis-Jacobs I, Haidle MN, Jankauskas R, Kind CJ, Lueth F, Terberger T, Hiller J, Matsumura

S, Forster P, Burger J. Genetic discontinuity between local hunter-gatherers and Central Europe's first farmers. Science. 2009;**326**:137-140. DOI: 0.1126/science.1176869

[52] Haak W, Lazaridis I, Patterson N, Rohland N, Mallick S, Llamas B, Brandt G, Nordenfelt S, Harney E, Stewardson K, Fu Q, Mittnik A, Bánffy E, Economou C, Francken M, Friederich S, Pena RG, Hallgren F, Khartanovich V, Khokhlov A, Kunst M, Kuznetsov P, Meller H, Mochalov O, Moiseyev V, Nicklisch N, Pichler SL, Risch R, Rojo Guerra MA, Roth C, Szécsényi-Nagy A, Wahl J, Meyer M, Krause J, Brown D, Anthony D, Cooper A, Alt KW, Reich D. Massive migration from the steppe was a source for indo-European languages in Europe. Nature. 2015;**522**:207-211. DOI: 10.1038/nature14317

[53] Keyser C, Bouakaze C, Crubézy E, Nikolaev VG, Montagnon D, Reis T, Ludes B. Ancient DNA provides new insights into the history of south Siberian kurgan people. Human Genetics. 2009;**126**:395-410. DOI: 10.1007/s00439-009-0683-0

[54] Lalueza-Fox C, Sampietro ML, Gilbert MT, Castri L, Facchini F, Pettener D, Bertranpetit J. Unravelling migrations in the steppe: Mitochondrial DNA sequences from ancient central Asians. Proceedings of the Biological Sciences. 2004;**271**:941-947. DOI: 10.1098/rspb.2004.2698

[55] Pardiñas AF, Roca A, García-Vazquez E, López B. Assessing the genetic influence of ancient sociopolitical structure: micro-differentiation patterns in the population of Asturias (Northern Spain). PLoS One. 2012;**7**:e50206. DOI: 10.1371/journal.pone.0050206

[56] Pardiñas AF, Martínez JL, Roca A, García-Vazquez E, López B. Over the sands and far away: interpreting an Iberian mitochondrial lineage with ancient Western African origins. American Journal Human Biology. 2014;**26**:777-783. DOI: 10.1002/ajhb.22601

[57] Schneider S, Excoffier L. Estimation of past demographic parameters from the distribution of pairwise differences when the mutation rates vary among sites: Application to human mitochondrial DNA. Genetics. 1999;**152**:1079-1089

[58] Meyer S, Weiss G, von Haeseler A. Pattern of nucleotide substitution and rate heterogeneity in the hypervariable regions I and II of human mtDNA. Genetics. 1999;**152**:1103-1110

[59] Allard MW, Miller K, Wilson M, Monson K, Budowle B. Characterization of the Caucasian haplogroups present in the SWGDAM forensic mtDNA dataset for 1771 human control region sequences. Scientific Working Group on DNA Analysis Methods. Journal of Forensic Sciences. 2002;**47**:1215-1223

[60] Santos C, Montiel R, Sierra B, Bettencourt C, Fernandez E, Alvarez L, Lima M, Abade A, Aluja MP. Understanding differences between phylogenetic and pedigree-derived mtDNA mutation rate: A model using families from the Azores Islands (Portugal). Molecular Biology and Evolution. 2005;**22**:1490-1505. DOI: 10.1093/molbev/msi141

[61] van Oven M, Kayser M. Updated comprehensive phylogenetic tree of global human mitochondrial DNA variation. Human Mutation. 2009;**30**:386-394. DOI: 10.1002/humu.20921

[62] Hervella M, Fernandez-Crespo T, Schulting RJ, Izagirre N, de Blas MA, de-la-Rua C. Anthropological, genetic and isotopic analysis of human remains recovered from the copper mine of the Aramo mountains (Asturias). Actas del VI Congreso del Neolítico en la Península Ibérica; Granada; 2018, in press

[63] de Blas Cortina MA. La mina como ámbito infraterreno y el cadáver como ofrenda ritual. A propósito de los esqueletos humanos hallados en las explotaciones cupríferas del Aramo. In: Fernández Manzano J, Herrán Martínez JI, editors. Mineros y fundidores en el inicio de la Edad de los Metales. El Midí francés y el Norte de la Península Ibérica. León: Caja España y Fundación Las Médulas; 2003. pp. 32-48

Chapter 7

Phylogenetic Evolution and Phylogeography of Tibetan Sheep Based on mtDNA D-Loop Sequences

Jianbin Liu, Xuezhi Ding, Yufeng Zeng, Xian Guo,
Xiaoping Sun and Chao Yuan

Additional information is available at the end of the chapter

http://dx.doi.org/10.5772/intechopen.76583

Abstract

The molecular and population genetic evidence of the phylogenetic status of the Tibetan sheep (*Ovis aries*) is not well understood, and little is known about this species' genetic diversity. Phylogenetic relationship and phylogeography of 636 individual Tibetan sheep which were collected from the Qinghai-Tibetan Plateau area in China and were assessed using 642 complete sequences of the mitochondrial DNA D-loop. Reference data were obtained from the six reference breed sequences available in GenBank. Phylogeography analysis showed that all four previously defined haplogroups were found in the 15 Tibetan sheep populations but that only one haplogroup was found in Linzhou sheep. Furthermore, clustering analysis divided the 636 individual Tibetan sheep into at least two clusters. The estimated genetic distance and genetic differentiation associate with altitude, suggesting geographic and adaptive effects in Tibetan sheep. These results contribute to the knowledge of Tibetan sheep populations and will help inform future conservation programs about the Tibetan sheep native to the Qinghai-Tibetan Plateau in China.

Keywords: Tibetan sheep, mtDNA D-loop, phylogeography, maternal lineage

1. Introduction

In China, Tibetan sheep (*Ovis aries*) play an important role in agriculture, economy, culture and religion in Qinghai-Tibetan Plateau areas, and provide meat, wool, and pelts for local populations [1]. Due to the rich Tibetan sheep genetic resources, there are approximately 17 indigenous sheep populations in the Qinghai-Tibetan Plateau area. All indigenous Tibetan sheep adapted to the local environment [2]. Moreover, they are considered as critical genetic resources, so they are one of the most important components in agro-animal husbandry societies. However, in reality, most indigenous Tibetan sheep suffer a serious situation because of the low numbers of each population, which decline steadily since 30 years [3]. Qinghai-Tibetan Plateau areas have special climate and landforms in geography, which provide a different livelihood for Tibetan nomads because of high altitude and cold mountains [4]. Besides, Tibetan sheep bind up with their herders in culture, religion, and social life. The fossil remains indicate that the domestic Tibetan sheep date their wild ancestors from the Pleistocene period [5]. Archeological evidences indicate that domestication of the yak is likely to have been performed approximately 5000 YBP (years before present) by the ancient Qiang people in Northern Tibet [6]. According to the temporal scale, indigenous animals are considered as an ideal model for cold and hypoxia environment adaption studies, on account of their adaptions for high-altitude hypoxia. In addition, Tibetan sheep are isolated from other local sheep in China, due to the unavailable traffic to other parts of China or external countries (Nepal, India, Pakistan, etc.). The severe changes of the ecological environment, value of Tibetan sheep in illegal commerce, and deficiency of animal conservation may result in extinction [7]. So far, the genetic diversity, phylogenetic relationship, and maternal origin of the Qinghai-Tibetan Plateau populations remain uncertain and controversial.

The study of mitochondrial DNA (mtDNA) polymorphisms has been useful for describing the molecular phylogeny and diversity of this sheep [8–11], due to the extremely low rate of recombination of mtDNA, its maternal lineage heredity and its relatively fast substitution rate as compared to nuclear DNA [12]. In particular, the CR (the D-loop) is the main noncoding regulatory region for the transcription and replication of mtDNA [13]. Based on mtDNA sequence analysis, we investigate the history and phylogenic relationships of modern domestic Tibetan sheep populations [14].

It is possible to describe the genetic polymorphisms and maternal origin of Tibetan sheep, according to the variability and structure of the mtDNA control region because mtDNA merely has no recombination and follows simple maternal inheritance [14, 15] and evolves relatively rapidly [16]. The higher substitution rate of CR, compared with the heterogeneity rate in the other parts of mtDNA, can characterize intraspecific and interspecific genetic diversity optimally [17–21]. This high mutation rate is because the CR remains single stranded for long periods during mitochondrial replication and transcription [22–26].

Here, we investigate the mtDNA D-loop variability of Tibetan sheep indigenous to the Qinghai-Tibetan Plateau areas. We increase the number of Tibetan sheep samples by including six available reference genomes from GenBank for our population genetic and phylogenetic analysis of the 15 Tibetan sheep populations, based on completion of the mtDNA control region. Our results provide insight into the phylogenetic evolution and maternal origin of Tibetan sheep and improve the management of sheep genetic resources and conservation of their genetic diversity.

2. Materials and methods

2.1. Sample collection

We selected 15 Chinese local Tibetan sheep populations for investigation in this study. For analysis, 10 mL blood samples were collected from the jugular vein of each animal. From the 10 mL samples, 2 mL samples were quickly frozen in liquid nitrogen and stored at −80°C for genomic DNA extraction, as described previously [27]. The total DNA was extracted from the blood using the saturated salt method [28], quantified spectrophotometrically, and adjusted to 50 ng/μL. Blood samples were collected from 636 sheep from 15 populations, living in the Qinghai-Tibetan Plateau areas in China. The genetic characteristics for these Tibetan sheep populations were analyzed in order to ascertain the phylogenetic evolution and phylogeography for the populations. The investigated populations included the following numbers and corresponding population types: 39 Guide Black Fur sheep (GD), 44 Qilian White Tibetan sheep (QL), 64 Tianjun White Tibetan sheep (TJ), 44 Qinghai Oula sheep (QH), 67 Minxian Black Fur sheep (MX), 58 Ganjia Tibetan sheep (GJ), 71 Qiaoke Tibetan sheep (QK), 52 Gannan Oula sheep (GN), 10 Langkazi Tibetan sheep (LKZ), 46 Jiangzi Tibetan sheep (JZ), 85 Gangba Tibetan sheep (GB), 34 Huoba Tibetan sheep (HB), 8 Duoma Tibetan sheep (DM), 5 Awang Tibetan sheep (AW), and 9 Linzhou Tibetan sheep (LZ) raised in China. The sampling information (population code, sample number, altitude, longitude and latitude, accession number, sampling location, and geographical location) for the 15 indigenous Tibetan sheep populations is shown by Liu et al. [29].

2.2. Data collection

To achieve good coverage of the tested populations, a dataset of six referenced breeds was completed using the six submitted sequences containing the *Ovis aries*, *Ovis vignei*, and *Ovis ammon* mtDNA D-loops for the six individuals in GenBank [29, 30].

Primers flanking sequences of the complete mtDNA D-loop was designed by an available genome sequence using the Primer Premier 5.0 software [31] and synthesized by BGI Shenzhen Technology Co., Ltd. (Shenzhen, China). The nucleotide sequence of reverse primer was 5′-GAACAACCAACCTCCCTAAG-3′, and the nucleotide sequence of forward primer was 5′-GGCTGGGACCAAACCTAT-3′. Polymerase chain reaction system (PCRs) took place in a 30 μL reaction system containing 2 μL genomic DNA (10 ng/μL) template, 2 μL dNTP (2.5 mM), 3 μL (3 pM) each primer, 3 μL 10× Ex Taq reaction buffer, 0.2 μL Taq DNA polymerase (5 μL/U) (TaKaRa, China), and 16.8 μL ddH_2O approximately. The PCR conditions were as follows: initial denaturation for 5 min at 94°C, 36 cycles of denaturation at 94°C for 30 s, annealing at 56°C for 30 s, and extension at 72°C for 1.5 min. The final extension step was followed by a 10 min extension at 72°C. The PCR amplification products were subsequently stored at 12°C until use.

The amplified D-loop fragment was purified using a PCR gel extraction kit from Sangon Biotech Co., Ltd. (Shenzhen, China) and sequenced directly using a BigDye Terminator v3.1 cycle sequencing ready reaction kit (Applied Biosystems, Darmstadt, Germany) in an automatic sequencer (ABI-PRISM 3730 genetic analyzer, Applied Biosystems, Foster City, California, United states of America). PCR for the sequencing was performed in an automatic sequencer with a total reaction volume of approximately 5 μL containing 3 μL genomic DNA (10 ng/μL), 1 μL (3 pM) of each sequencing primer, 0.5 μL BigDye, and 0.5 μL ddH_2O. The sequencing conditions were as follows: initial denaturation for 2 min at 95°C, 25 cycles of denaturation at 95°C for 10 s, and annealing at 51°C for 10 s. The final extension step was followed by a 190 s extension at 60°C. The PCR sequencing products were subsequently stored at 12°C until use.

2.3. Data analysis

The sequences were arranged for multiple comparisons using Clustal Omega [32] and were aligned using ClustalW and BLAST [33]. These results were compared with other sequences obtained from GenBank. The reference sequences for tree construction were taken from the maternal lineages of each tree: haplogroup A (AF039578), haplogroup B (AF039577, AY582801, and AY091487), haplogroup E (AY091490, AJ238300). The diversity parameters, including the haplotype diversity, nucleotide diversity and average number of nucleotide differences, were estimated using DnaSP (Sequence Polymorphism Software) 5.10.01 [34]. G_{ST}, F_{ST}, N_m, AMOVA test, and neutrality tests were estimated using Arlequin version 3.5.1.2 [35]. To identify differences between the geographic regions using the AMOVA program, four groups were established. The phylogenetic and molecular evolutionary relationships, D_{xy}, D_a, ME phylogenetic haplotype and clustering tree, and genetic distance were assessed using MEGA version 6.0 [36]. We sketched the network and mismatched distribution graphs using the median-joining method implemented in the NETWORK version 4.6.1.2 software to assess the haplotype relationships [37].

3. Results

3.1. Polymorphic site and sequencing analysis of the complete control region

Based on the reference sequences from GenBank accession numbers (AY091487, AY091490, AJ238300, AF039578, AF039577, AY582801), all of the sequences were aligned with 1274 comparative sites, and 350 haplotypes were obtained from the 642 sequenced individuals. The length of the sequences obtained from the 636 individuals varied considerably, between 1031 and 1259 bp, although the majority were between 1180 and 1183 bp [29]. A total of 196 variable sites were obtained from the sequences, including 63 singleton variable sites and 133 parsimony-informative variable sites. There were 158 transitions and 38 transversions within the 196 variable sites, among which 15 sites had both transitions and transversions. Transition mutations were caused by observed substitutions. The variability of the number of 75 bp tandem repeat motifs [38] caused the observed variation in the length of the mtDNA D-loop sequences of the Tibetan sheep, with the exception of the insertion or deletion of several nucleotide sites.

Whole haplotypes' nucleotide composition was 32.96% A, 29.71% T, 22.89% C, 14.44% G, 62.67% A+T, and 37.33% G+C, and the A+T were more common than the G+C haplotype substantially, showing an AT bias [29]. The largest haplogroup A consisted of 490 individuals and 259 haplotypes; the next largest haplogroup B and haplogroup C consisted of 145 individuals and 43 haplotypes. The smallest haplogroup D consisted of 1 individual and 1 haplotype. The number of haplotypes, individuals, and frequency detected in each Tibetan sheep population of haplotype group varied from 1 to 49, from 0 to 62, and from 0 to 0.88, respectively. The haplotype diversity and nucleotide diversity were calculated separately for each Tibetan sheep population and were estimated to be 0.99 ± 0.01 and 0.02 ± 0.00, respectively. The values of haplotype diversity and nucleotide diversity ranged from 0.90 ± 0.16 to 1.00 ± 0.05 and from 0.01 ± 0.00 to 0.03 ± 0.00, respectively, thus demonstrating the high level of genetic diversity in the 15 Tibetan sheep populations. The nucleotide diversity value of the LZ and JZ populations was higher than that of the remaining 13 Tibetan sheep populations, indicating a relatively high level of diversity. Similarly, the haplotype diversity values were highest in LKZ and LZ populations and the lowest in the AW population.

3.2. Genetic distance and average number of nucleotide differences

The study presents the genetic distance and average number of nucleotide differences between and within the 15 Tibetan sheep populations. The genetic distance values ranged from 0.01 to 0.04 within the population diagonals, and the genetic distance values ranged from 0.01 to 0.04 among populations in Liu et al. [29]. Among the Tibetan sheep populations, the genetic distance within populations reached a maximum value in LZ and a minimum value in AW. Similarly, the genetic distance between the populations had a maximum value for LZ and JZ and a minimum value for AW and TJ. The average number of nucleotide differences values ranged from 10.00 to 29.81 within populations along the digital diagonal, and the average number of nucleotide difference values ranged from 10.73 to 30.99 between the populations below the diagonals. Among the Tibetan sheep populations, the average number of nucleotide differences within the populations reached its value maximum in LZ and its minimum value in AW. Similarly, the average number of nucleotide differences between populations reached a value maximum in LZ and JZ and a minimum value in AW and TJ populations [29].

3.3. Genetic distances and altitude

We test whether genetic distances between populations can be explained by absolute differences between altitudes for the 15 Tibetan sheep populations. Graphically, for the focal population of LZ, **Figure 1** plots the genetic distance between population LZ and each of the remaining populations as a function of the absolute difference in altitudes. Genetic distance tends to decrease with absolute difference in altitudes, as estimated by the Pearson correlation coefficient ($r = -0.4136$, two tailed $P = 0.063$, square root of 0.1711 indicated in **Figure 1**). This tendency is observed in 10 among the 15 sheep populations, but is never statistically significant at $P < 0.05$ (see **Table 1**). It is strongest (most negative) for high altitude populations and weakest (most positive) for populations living at low altitudes. This association between altitude and Pearson correlation coefficients obtained between genetic distances and absolute differences in altitudes (**Table 1**) has itself $r = -0.65$, one tailed $P = 0.0044$.

3.4. Genetic differentiation

To examine the genetic differentiation between the 15 Tibetan sheep populations, we calculated F_{ST} and G_{ST}. We also calculated N_m, D_{xy}, and D_a among the 15 studied Tibetan sheep

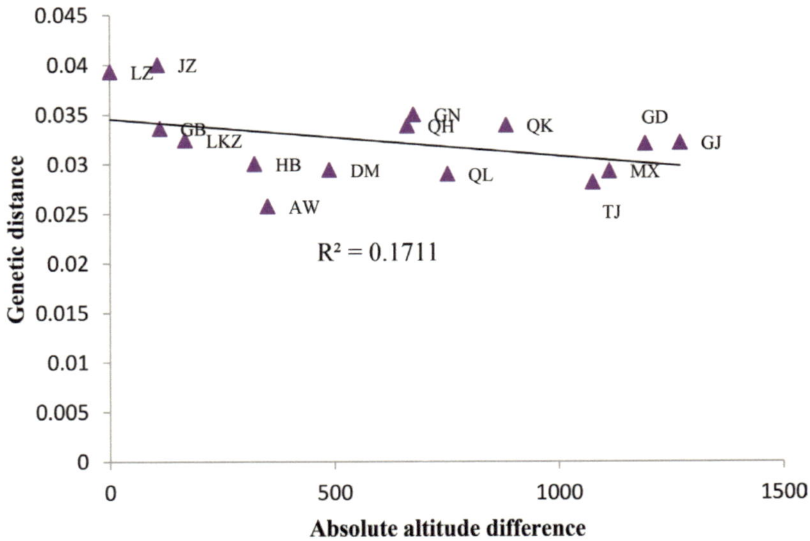

Figure 1. Genetic distance and absolute difference between altitudes for population LZ.

populations [29]. The estimated pairwise F_{ST} values are from Liu et al. [29]. The F_{ST} values ranged from −0.05 to 0.24. DM and LKZ had the closest pairwise F_{ST} value among the 15 Tibetan sheep populations and AW were more distantly related to JZ, compared with other

Population	Altitude, m	Genetic dist, r	Genetic diff, r
GD	3100	0.07	0.43
QL	3540	−0.13	0.53
TJ	3217	0.06	0.54
QH	3630	−0.21	0.58
MX	3180	0.08	0.56
GJ	3022	0.06	0.42
QK	3410	0.01	0.53
GN	3616	−0.13	0.60
LKZ	4459	−0.29	0.09
JZ	4398	−0.41	−0.17
GB	4403	−0.36	−0.51
HB	4614	−0.12	−0.46
DM	4780	−0.11	0.34
AW	4643	−0.05	−0.01
LZ	4292	−0.42	−0.11

Table 1. Altitude and Pearson correlation coefficients between absolute differences in altitude and each genetic distance and genetic differentiation between 15 Tibetan sheep populations.

Tibetan sheep populations. No F_{ST} values were larger than 0.25 [39], indicating that there was no significant genetic differentiation among the whole Tibetan sheep populations. The decreasing sequence of F_{ST} values among Tibetan sheep were 14 MX, 13 GD and JZ, 12 QK, 10 GB and GN and TJ, 9 GJ and HB and QH, 7 QL, 4 LKZ and LZ, 3 DM, and 1 AW.

The distribution of the 15 Tibetan sheep populations varied according to their F_{ST} values ($P < 0.05$, or $P < 0.01$). The G_{ST} values ranged from 0.01 to 0.05 in Liu et al. [29]. The G_{ST} value between the LKZ and LZ was the smallest, and the G_{ST} value was the largest (JZ and AW, MX and AW, respectively). The mean G_{ST} was 0.02, which indicates that most of the genetic diversity occurred within populations and that 1.76% of the total population differentiation came from inter-population comparisons, whereas the remaining 98.24% came from differences among individuals within each population. Thus, the gene divergence between the populations was very low. Variation observed among and within the 15 Tibetan sheep populations indicate lack of differentiation among geographic populations.

Liu et al. present the 15 Tibetan sheep populations' N_m of the sequence values and haplotype values [29]. The N_m of sequences ranged from −731.04 to 495.66, demonstrating that gene exchange was either extremely frequent or extremely rare. The sequence value between GN and QK was the smallest, and MX and QL was the largest. The mean N_m of the sequences was −9.40, implying a relationship with distance relatively. The N_m of the haplotype values ranged from 5.04 to 177.66. Notably, the value between QL and GJ was 35.24 times greater than the N_m between JZ and AW. The N_m of the haplotype values between JZ and AW was the smallest, and the N_m of the haplotype values between GJ and QL was the greatest. The mean haplotype N_m was 22.59, failed to indicate that gene flow occurred between the populations in the past time.

Liu et al. provided the data of the D_{xy} and D_a values among the 15 Tibetan sheep populations [29]. The D_{xy} value between JZ and AW was the largest, and the D_{xy} value between LKZ and LZ was the smallest. The D_a values were from 0.01 to 0.03. The mean D_a was 0.02. Similarly, the number of net nucleotide substitutions per site between populations of the 15 Tibetan sheep populations was highest JZ and LZ and lowest TJ and AW.

3.5. Genetic differentiation and altitude

We test whether genetic differentiation between populations can be explained by altitude. Graphically, for the focal population of GD, **Figure 2** plots genetic differentiation between GZ and each of the remaining populations as a function of the absolute value of the difference between their altitudes. Genetic differentiation tends to increase with altitude (r = 0.4315, one-tailed P = 0.062) (square root of 0.1862 indicated in **Figure 2**). Analyses similar to those in **Figure 2** showed that genetic differentiation increases with absolute differences in altitude, specifically for nine populations ((significance at P < 0.05 indicated by *) QL*, TJ*, QH*, MX*, GJ, QK*, GN*, DM, and LKZ) and decreases for the remaining five populations (GB,HB, JZ, LZ, and AW), mainly GB* and HB* (**Table 1**).

This association between genetic differentiation and absolute difference between altitudes is most positive for populations at high altitudes and most negative for those at low altitudes. This association between altitude and Pearson correlation coefficients obtained between genetic differentiations and absolute differences in altitudes (**Table 1**) has itself r = −0.75, one-tailed P = 0.0011.

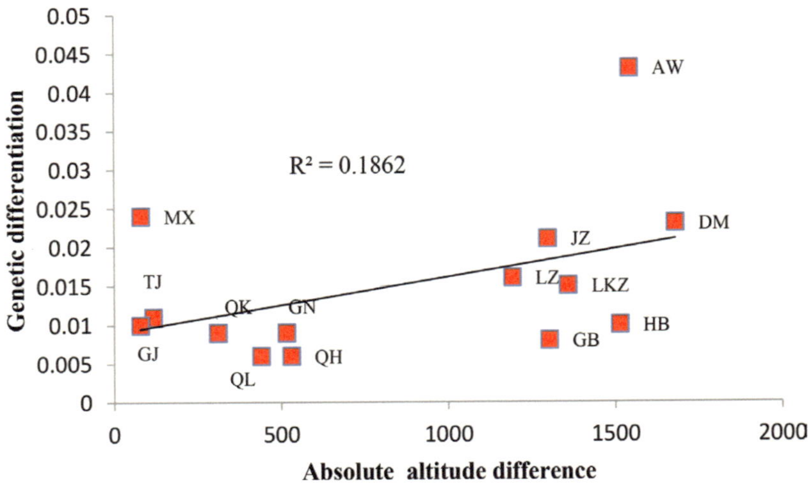

Figure 2. Genetic differentiation and absolute difference between altitudes for population GD.

3.6. Phylogenetic relationships

To extend our knowledge of the phylogenetic relationship of the 15 Tibetan sheep populations, a phylogenetic tree was constructed using ME based on the complete mtDNA D-loop sequences of 642 individuals and 350 haplotypes from 15 Tibetan sheep populations and six reference breeds [29]. We determined four distinct cluster haplogroups: A, B, C and D. Of the 350 haplotypes, there was no common haplotype identified in all of the Tibetan sheep populations; 98 haplotypes were shared, and 252 haplotypes were singletons, which including 38 in GB, 33 in GJ, 28 in TJ, and 24 in QH. The leading haplotype (Hap 39) was found in 39 individuals. The next most common haplotype was Hap 42, composed of 19 individuals, and the remaining nine haplotypes were composed of 7–10 individuals. Haplotype 42 was composed of JZ, MX, QL and TJ. Haplotype 4 was composed of 14 of the Tibetan sheep populations, but excluding LKZ, indicating close clustering. The majorities of the 490 individuals were grouped in haplogroup A, followed by haplogroups B and C; however, only one animal from the LZ belonged to haplogroup D. The DM was composed of two haplogroups, the AW was composed of one haplogroup and the remaining 13 Tibetan sheep populations were composed of three haplogroups [29]. Moreover, the maximum composite likelihood method was used to analyze the genetic distance between populations, which were in the units of the number of base substitutions per site. More specifically, the neighbor-joining phylogenetic tree of the 642 sequences of the mtDNA D-loop, based on units of the number of base substitutions per site divided the 15 Tibetan sheep populations and six reference breeds into four groups effectively. *O. ammon* and *O. vignei* were genetically distinct and separated initially. The 15 Tibetan sheep populations and four reference breeds were then divided into three sub-clusters. The first cluster included JZ, QL, QH, GN, QK, MX and GD. The second cluster included *OasiaA*, AW, TJ, GJ, LKZ, DM, GB, HB and LZ. The third cluster included *Omexic*, *Oeuro*reB and *Omusimon*. The AMOVA was conducted, and the results are shown in Liu et al. [29]. The AMOVA revealed a variation of 4.46% among the populations and of 95.54% within the populations significantly ($P < 0.05$). The F_{ST} was 0.05, which indicated that 4.50% of the total genetic variation was due to differences between populations, and the remaining 95.50% came from differences among individuals within each population.

3.7. Population expansions

The sample size for most of the populations was more than 30, so the detection of population expansion was performed at the individual population level (data not shown) and in all haplotype sequences. Liu et al. showed the mismatch distribution analysis of the complete dataset (lineages A, B, C, D and 15 Tibetan sheep populations of mtDNA D-loop) [29]. Neutrality tests (Ewens-Watterson test, Chakraborty's test, Tajima's D test, Fu's FS test) were used to detect population expansion [29]. The charts of the mismatch distribution for the samples of the 15 Tibetan sheep populations and the total samples were multimodal. However, the mismatch distribution for LZ was a unimodal function. The mismatch distribution of the complete dataset showed that there were two major peaks, with maximum values at 4 and 27 pairwise differences and two smaller peaks at 45 and 51 pairwise differences [29]. These results suggest that at least two expansion events occurred during the population demographic history of the Tibetan sheep population. The mismatch distribution analysis revealed a unimodal bell-shaped distribution of pairwise sequence differences in lineages A, B and C, but that of the lineage D was a sampling function duo to small sample effects. The complete dataset of 15 Tibetan sheep populations did not produce a significantly negative Ewens-Watterson test, whereas Chakraborty's neutrality test of JZ was significant (12.63, $p = 0.03$), and Tajima's D neutrality of TJ test was also significant (−0.47, $p = 0.02$). Fu's F_S value was −7.48 for the 15 Tibetan sheep populations, of which GN, QK, HB, GB, GJ, QH, QL and TJ were highly significant ($p < 0.01$ or $p < 0.001$). This finding suggests the occurrence of two expansion events in the demographic history of the 15 Tibetan sheep populations. This result is consistent with a demographic model showing two large and sudden expansions, as inferred from the mismatch distribution.

4. Discussion

4.1. High mtDNA D-loop diversity of Tibetan sheep populations

The 15 Tibetan sheep populations in our study showed a high level of genetic diversity. This finding is consistent with archeological data and other genetic diversity studies [21, 40–43], while in this study, the haplotype diversity was higher than that found in a previous study [44], and the nucleotide diversity was lower compared with the data in a previous study [7]. The genetic diversity among the 15 Tibetan sheep populations was relatively higher compared with other sheep populations [1, 44]. For instance, the haplotype diversity values of Turkish sheep breeds distributed in a Turkish population were 0.95 ± 0.01 [44]. However, according to Walsh's work, based on the required sample size for the diagnosis of conservation units [45], a sample of 59 individuals fails necessary to support the hypothesis that individuals with unstamped ("hidden") character states exist in the population size. Thus, the sample size necessary to reject a hidden state frequency of 0.05 is 56 when sampling from a finite population of 500 individuals. Therefore, because of the large sample size, genetic diversity estimation reflects precisely Tibetan sheep. For the LZ, LKZ, HB, QH, GD, TJ, GJ, QK, GB and GN with broad distribution, a high genetic diversity could only be observed within the studies containing large sample size or wide collection areas. However, if more samples were involved in the study, a higher diversity could be found, suggesting further investigation of the genetic diversity of these 15 Tibetan sheep populations. These Tibetan sheep populations had been experiencing a genetic bottleneck during the twentieth century and were classified as the rarest sheep populations [46]. In addition, among the 15 Tibetan sheep populations, the positive Ewens-Watterson and Chakraborty's values were significantly different, suggesting a previous decline in the population size of the mtDNA D-loop diversity. This finding was consistent with the results of a previous study [46]. Such genetic diversity may be caused by an increased mutation rate in the mtDNA D-loop, the maternal effects of multiple wild ancestors, overlapping generations, the mixing of populations from different geographical locations, natural selection favoring heterozygosis or subdivision accompanied by genetic drift [42, 43].

4.2. Maternal origins of the Tibetan sheep populations

The sequence motifs from the 1180 bp to the 1183 bp region of the mtDNA D-loop form the basis for the four major maternal lineages in the Tibetan sheep mtDNA haplotypes. Maternal lineage D was the rarest. The Tibetan sheep haplotypes belonged to all four major maternal lineages, although only 0.16% belonged to maternal lineages D. This finding demonstrated that populations of Tibetan sheep possess abundant mtDNA diversity, and therefore, there is a widespread origin of their maternal lineages. Furthermore, the thoroughbred Tibetan sheep has been proposed to be shared in the maternal lineages A, and the contribution of Asian sheep breeds to this population has also been reported in Liu et al. [29]. In this study, maternal lineages B and C were found in common among the overall sequences of all 15 Tibetan sheep populations, including the 14 Tibetan sheep populations respectively other than DM and AW. It is generally acknowledged that domestic sheep have two maternal lineages (A and B), based on the earlier mtDNA analysis [7, 13, 16, 47]. Recently, a new maternal lineage (C) was found in Chinese domestic sheep [40, 42, 43]. The ME phylogenetic tree median-joining analyses, revealed the presence of four maternal lineages in the Tibetan sheep populations. Of these groups, the maternal lineage A was predominant, and the maternal lineage B and C were the second most common. The proportion of maternal lineage D was 0.16%, further demonstrating that lineage D is the rarest among mtDNA sheep lineages [29]. Our findings coincided with previous studies and supported the results on domestic sheep breeds in China [48, 49]. Three mtDNA of maternal lineages were identified in both China [39, 42, 43, 49] and other countries [50–52]. The four mtDNA maternal lineages found in the Tibetan sheep populations in the Qinghai-Tibetan plateau areas further supported the hypothesis of multiple maternal origins in Chinese domestic sheep.

4.3. Genetic differentiation of Tibetan sheep populations

In this study, the AMOVA analysis revealed the distinct population of Qinghai-Tibetan Plateau areas among other Tibetan sheep populations, with a significant positive variance in the meanwhile. Gene flow (N_m), also known as gene migration, refers to the transfer of alleles from one population to another. Poor gene exchange is indicated when N_m haplotype values are >1 and N_m sequences <1, a, which means that genetic drift results in substantial local differentiation [53, 54].

The low G_{ST} value, combined with the low N_m of sequences used in this study, indicates that the great differentiation mainly resulted from the independent evolution of each isolated population and substantial local differentiation caused by genetic drift [55]. The lower effective population sizes may contribute too, as the GN, QK, GJ and QL live in canyons and valleys, so lower population sizes were not available for migration compared with other Tibetan sheep. As the effective population size declines, the nucleotide substitutions might reach fixation [48, 56]. Overall, the study showed that the 15 Tibetan sheep populations from the Qinghai-Tibetan Plateau divide into two phylogeography lineages: 5 Tibetan populations (GB, HB, JZ, LZ and AW) represent the phylogenetic clusterings of the phylogeography lineages in Tibet Autonomous Region, 9 Tibetan populations (QL, TJ, QH, MX, GJ, QK, GN, DM and LKZ) represent the phylogenetic clusterings of the phylogeography lineages in Gansu and Qinghai Province. Associations between genetic differentiation and absolute differences between altitudes are positive for eight populations and negative for seven populations. These two groups separated by the direction of the association between genetic differentiation and (absolute difference between) altitudes correspond for 12 among 15 populations to the two main phyletic clusters found for these populations using neighbor-joining (Liu et al., 2016, therein **Figure 2**). This association is statistically significant according to Fisher's exact test (an one-tailed $P = 0.032$). The exceptions to this association with phylogeny are populations GJ, TJ and JZ. These results on associations between genetic differentiation and altitude suggest that part of the genetic differentiation between populations might be adaptive in relation to altitude and/or climate.

4.4. Genetic relationships among the Tibetan sheep populations

The study showed that the 15 Tibetan sheep populations from the Qinghai-Tibetan Plateau divide into four maternal lineages: 490 Tibetan sheep represent the maternal origin of the maternal lineage A, 64 Tibetan sheep represent the maternal origin of the maternal lineage B, 81 Tibetan sheep represent the maternal origin of the maternal lineage C, and 1 Tibetan sheep represents the maternal origin of the maternal lineage D. This genetic relationship displayed a high consistency with traditional classification schemes and the results of previous studies [40, 57–61]. Fifteen Tibetan sheep populations derived from four maternal lineages. On the one hand, Tibetan sheep show a great value as portable food and wool resource; on the other hand, the commercial trade and extensive transport of sheep, along with human migratory paths, might promote the observed genetic exchange. Other study methods such as genetic approaches, including the degree method and the phylogenetic relationship clustering method, also indicated that indigenous sheep were the maternal lineages A, B, C, and D [58, 60].

The study presents the Pearson correlation coefficient of genetic differentiation with the corresponding altitude difference between the 15 Tibetan sheep populations. The study showed that the correlation between altitude and genetic differentiation increases with altitude, specifically for 10 populations (GJ, GD, TJ, MX, QK, QL, QH, GN, DM and LKZ), with r ranging from 0.089 to 0.584, and decreases for the remaining five populations (GB, HB, JZ, LZ and AW), with r from −0.512 to −0.011. This evidence based on the large-scale mtDNA D-loop sequences analysis of 15 Tibetan sheep populations indicates effects associated to climate or isolation of phylogeography on genetic differentiation. These results indicate an adaptive effect associated with altitude or geography, which coincides with previous studies [29, 42, 43, 62].

4.5. Population expansion of Tibetan sheep populations

The mismatch distribution analysis of the complete dataset, maternal lineages A, B, C, D, and 15 Tibetan sheep populations of the mtDNA D-loop, is presented [29]. Neutrality tests (Ewens-Watterson test, Chakraborty's test, Tajima's D test, Fu's FS test) were used to detect population expansion [29]. The complete dataset of all Tibetan sheep populations had a significantly large negative Tajima's D value and F_S value. This result shows two large and sudden expansions, consistent with a demographic model, as inferred from the mismatch distribution. The mismatch distribution of the complete dataset suggested that there were two major peaks with maximum values at 4 and 27 pairwise differences and two smaller peaks at 45 and 51 differences. Based on the results, it could be implied that there are at least two expansion events occurred in the population demographic history of the Tibetan sheep, which live on the Qinghai-Tibetan Plateau. The mismatch distribution analysis revealed a unimodal bell-shaped distribution of the pairwise sequence differences in maternal lineages A, B and C. However, the distribution of maternal lineage D was a sambong function, duo to the geographic distribution patterns of species diversity. Mismatch analysis of maternal lineages A, B, and C suggested that it happened in the demographic history of Tibetan sheep populations that single population expansion events occurred before. Similar results were found in previous reports [42, 43].

4.6. Phylogenetic analysis of the Tibetan sheep populations

Phylogenetic analyses of complete mitogenomes showed a high resolution among wild sheep as well as among the major lineages of domestic sheep [62]. The complete mitogenomes of *O. orientalis* and *O. musimon* formed a monophyletic group that was incorporated within lineage B of domestic sheep. However, the analysis of full control region and D-loop fragments showed that *O. orientalis* is also closely related to other lineages of *O. aries*. This difference could be ascribed to the small number of *O. musimon* and *O. orientalis* complete mitogenomes available in this study.

Full control region from the complete mitogenomes produced similar phylogenies with fully resolved phylogenetic relationships of wild sheep, but they failed to define the phylogenetic relationships among the major lineages of domestic sheep. Our results suggest that partial fragments of the complete mitogenomes would be problematic when making phylogenetic inferences about domestic sheep. This problem arises due to diagnostic substitutions located elsewhere in the mitogenome [62]. Thus, the diagnostic substitutions for species and lineages presented [62] here can serve as an important resource for maternal genetic differentiation between domestic and wild sheep as well as between the lineages within domestic sheep. Also, they might be helpful for addressing certain conflicts described above in future.

5. Conclusion

High mtDNA genetic diversity in the sheep from the Qinghai-Tibetan Plateau areas is a rich resource for China. The evidences indicate the high diversity of four maternal lineages by doing the large-scale mtDNA D-loop sequences analysis of 15 Tibetan sheep populations. Although the maternal lineage D was only found in a single LZ, phylogenetic analysis showed that four maternal lineages (A, B, C and D), previously defined, could be identified in the 636 tested individuals of the 15 Tibetan sheep populations. The estimation of demographic parameters from the mismatch analyses shows that maternal lineages A, B and C had at least one demographic expansion in the Tibetan sheep of the Qinghai-Tibetan Plateau areas.

Acknowledgements

The authors appreciated constructive comments from the editor Hervé Seligmann. This work was supported by the special fund from the Major International (Regional) Joint Research Project (NSFC-CGIAR 31461143020), and Gansu Provincial Agricultural biotechnology research and application projects (GNSW-2014-21, GNSW-2016-13), and the Central Level, Scientific Research Institutes for Basic R & D Special Fund Business (1610322016016).

Conflict of interest

This study did not involve endangered or protected Tibetan sheep populations. All experimental and sampling procedures were approved by the Institutional Animal Care and Use Committee, Lanzhou Institute of Husbandry and Pharmaceutical Sciences, Peoples Republic of China.

Author contributions

Conceived and designed the experiments: LJB DXZ ZYF GX SXP. Performed the experiments: LJB DXZ ZYF GX SXP. Analyzed the data: GX SXP YC. Wrote the paper: LJB DXZ ZYF GX YC.

Author details

Jianbin Liu[1,2†‡*], Xuezhi Ding[1†‡], Yufeng Zeng[1†‡], Xian Guo[1†‡], Xiaoping Sun[1,2†‡] and Chao Yuan[1,2†‡]

*Address all correspondence to: liujianbin@caas.cn

1 Lanzhou Institute of Husbandry and Pharmaceutical Sciences of the Chinese Academy of Agricultural Sciences, Lanzhou, China

2 Sheep Breeding Engineering Technology Research Center of Chinese Academy of Agricultural Sciences, Lanzhou, China

†These authors contributed equally to this work

‡These authors are co-first authors on this work

References

[1] Zhao Y, Zhao E, Zhang N, Duan C. Mitochondrial DNA diversity, origin, and phylogenic relationships of three Chinese large-fat-tailed sheep breeds. Tropical Animal Health and Production. 2011;**43**:1405-1410. DOI: 10.1007/s11250-011-9869-2

[2] China National Commission of Animal Genetic Resources. Animal Genetic Resources in China (Sheep and Goats). 1st ed. Beijing: China Agricultural Press; 2011

[3] Zeng XC, Chen HY, Hui WQ, Jia B, Du YC, Tian YZ. Genetic diversity measures of 8 local sheep breeds in northwest of China for genetic resource conservation. Asian-Australasian Journal of Animal Sciences. 2010;**23**:1552-1556. DOI: 10.5713/ajas.2010.10132

[4] Ding XZ, Guo X, Yan P, Liang CN, Bao PJ, Chu M. Seasonal and nutrients intake regulation of lipoprotein lipase (LPL) activity in grazing yak (*Bos grunniens*) in the Alpine Regions around Qinghai Lake. Livestock Science. 2012;**143**:29-34. DOI: 10.1016/j.livsci.2011.08.004

[5] Wiener G, Han JL, Long RJ. The Yak. 2nd ed. Bangkok, Thailand: Regional Office for Asia and the Pacific Food and Agriculture Organization of the United Nations; 2003

[6] Zhang RC. China Yak. Lanzhou: Gansu Scientific and Technology Press, China; 1989

[7] Zhao E, Yu Q, Zhang N, Kong D, Zhao Y. Mitochondrial DNA diversity and the origin of Chinese indigenous sheep. Tropical Animal Health and Production. 2013;**45**:1715-1722. DOI: 10.1007/s11250-013-0420-5

[8] Smith DG, McDonough J. Mitochondrial DNA variation in Chinese and Indian rhesus macaques (*Macaca mulatta*). American Journal of Primatology. 2005;**65**:1-25 PMID: 15645455

[9] Xu S, Luosang J, Hua S, He J, Ciren A, Wang W, Tong X, Liang Y, Wang J, Zheng X. High altitude adaptation and phylogenetic analysis of Tibetan horse based on the mitochondrial genome. Journal of Genetics and Genomics. 2007;**34**:720-729. DOI: 10.1016/S1673-8527(07)60081-2

[10] Peng R, Zeng B, Meng X, Yue B, Zhang Z, Zou F. The complete mitochondrial genome and phylogenetic analysis of the giant panda (*Ailuropoda melanoleuca*). Gene. 2007;**397**:76-83. DOI: 10.1016/j.gene.2007.04.009

[11] He L, Dai B, Zeng B, Zhang X, Chen B, Yue B, Li J. The complete mitochondrial genome of the Sichuan Hill Partridge (*Arborophila rufipectus*) and a phylogenetic analysis with related species. Gene. 2009;**435**:23-28. DOI: 10.1016/j.gene.2009.01.001

[12] Brown JR, Beckenbach AT, Smith MJ. Mitochondrial DNA length variation and heteroplasmy in populations of white sturgeon (*Acipenser transmontanus*). Genetics. 1992;**132**: 221-228. PMID: 1398055

[13] Hiendleder S, Mainz K, Plante Y, Lewalski H. Analysis of mitochondrial DNA indicates that domestic sheep are derived from two different ancestral maternal sources: No evidence for contributions from Urial and Argali sheep. The Journal of Heredity. 1998;**89**: 113-120. DOI: 10.1093/jhered/89.2.113

[14] Fritsch ES, Chabbert CD, Klaus B, Steinmetz LM. A genome-wide map of mitochondrial DNA recombination in yeast. Genetics. 2014;**198**(2):755-771. PMCID: PMC4196626

[15] Leducq JB, Henault M, Charron G, Nielly-Thibault L, Terrat Y, Fiumera HL, Shapiro BJ, Landry CR. Mitochondrial recombination and introgression during speciation by hybridization. Molecular Biology and Evolution. 2017;**34**(8):1947-1959. DOI: 10.1093/molbev/msx139

[16] Hiendleder S, Lewalski H, Wassmuth R, Janke A. The complete mitochondrial DNA sequence of the domestic sheep (*Ovis aries*) and comparison with the other major ovine haplotype. Journal of Molecular Evolution. 1998;**47**:441-448. DOI: 10.1007/PL00006401

[17] Loehr J, Worley K, Grapputo A, Carey J, Veitch A, Coltman DW. Evidence for cryptic glacial refugia from north American mountain sheep mitochondrial DNA. Journal of Evolutionary Biology. 2005;**19**:419-430. DOI: 10.1111/j.1420-9101.2005.01027.x

[18] Castro AL, Stewart BS, Wilson SG, Hueter RE, Meekan MG, Motta PJ. Population genetic structure of Earth's largest fish, the whale shark (*Rhincodon typus*). Molecular Ecology. 2007;**16**:5183-5192. DOI: 10.1111/j.1365-294X.2007.03597.x

[19] Jia S, Chen H, Zhang G, Wang Z, Lei C, Yao R. Genetic variation of mitochondrial D-loop region and evolution analysis in some Chinese cattle breeds. Journal of Genetics and Genomics. 2007;**34**:510-518. DOI: 10.1016/S1673-8527(07)60056-3

[20] Li D, Fan L, Ran J, Yin H, Wang H, Wu S, et al. Mitochondrial DNA. Mitochondrial DNA. 2008;**19**:446-452. PMID: 19489138

[21] Hassan AA, El Nahas SM, Kumar S, Godithala PS, Roushdy K. Mitochondrial D-loop nucleotide sequences of Egyptian river buffalo: Variation and phylogeny studies. Livestock Science. 2009;**125**:37-42. DOI: 10.1016/j.livsci.2009.03.001

[22] Seligmann H, Krishnan NM, Rao BJ. Mitochondrial tRNA sequences as unusual replication origins: Pathogenic implications for Homo sapiens. Journal of Theoretical Biology. 2006;**243**:375-385. DOI: 10.1016/j.jtbi.2006.06.028

[23] Seligmann H. Mutation patterns due to converging mitochondrial replication and transcription increase lifespan, and cause growth rate-longevity tradeoffs. In: Seligmann H, editor. DNA Replication-Current Advances. InTech; 2011. pp. 151-80 (book chapter 6)

[24] Seligmann H. Coding constraints modulate chemically spontaneous mutational replication gradients in mitochondrial genomes. Current Genomics. 2012;**13**:37-54. DOI: 10.2174/138920212799034802

[25] Reyes A, Gissi C, Pesole G, Saccone C. Asymmetrical directional mutation pressure in the mitochondrial genome of mammals. Molecular Biology and Evolution. 1998;**15**(8):957-966. DOI: 10.1093/oxfordjournals.molbev.a026011

[26] Chong RA, Mueller RL. Evolution along the mutation gradient in the dynamic mitochondrial genome of salamanders. Genome Biology and Evolution. 2013;**5**(9):1652-1660. DOI: 10.1093/gbe/evt119

[27] D'Angelo F, Ciani E, Sevi A, Albenzio M, Ciampolini R, Cianci D. The genetic variability of the Podolica cattle breeds from the Gargano area. Preliminary results. Italian Journal of Animal Science. 2006;**5**:79-85. DOI: 10.4081/ijas.2006.79

[28] Sambrook J, Russell DW. Molecular Cloning: A Laboratory Manual. 3rd ed. New York: Cold Spring Harbor Laboratory Press; 2001

[29] Liu J, Ding X, Zeng Y, Yue Y, Guo X, Guo T, Chu M, Wang F, Han J, Feng R, Sun X, Niu C, Yang B, Guo J, Yuan C. Genetic diversity and phylogenetic evolution of Tibetan sheep based on mtDNA D-loop sequences. PLoS One. 2016;**11**(7):e0159308. DOI: 10.1371/journal.pone.0159308

[30] Wu C, Zhang Y, Bunch T, Wang S, Wang W. Molecular classification of subspecies of *Ovis ammon* inferred from mitochondrial control region sequences. Mammalia. 2006;**67**: 109-118

[31] Singh VK, Mangalam AK, Dwivedi S, Naik S. Primer premier: Program for design of degenerate primers from a protein sequence. BioTechniques. 1998;**24**:318-319. PMID:9494736

[32] Sievers F, Wilm A, Dineen D, Gibson TJ, Karplus K, Li W. Fast, scalable generation of high-quality protein multiple sequence alignments using Clustal Omega. Molecular Systems Biology. 2011;**7**:539. DOI: 10.1038/msb.2011.75

[33] Hall TA. BioEdit: A user-friendly biological sequence alignment editor and analysis program for Windows 95/98/NT. Nucleic Acids Symposium Series. 1999;**41**:95-98

[34] Librado P, Rozas J. DnaSP v5: A software for comprehensive analysis of DNA polymorphism data. Bioinformatics. 2009;**25**:1451-1452. DOI: 10.1093/bioinformatics/btp187

[35] Excoffier L, Lischer HEL. Arlequin suite ver 3.5: A new series of programs to perform population genetics analyses under Linux and Windows. Molecular Ecology Resources. 2010;**10**:564-567. DOI: 10.1111/j.1755-0998.2010.02847.x

[36] Tamura K, Stecher G, Peterson D, Filipski A, Kumar S. MEGA6: Molecular evolutionary genetics analysis version 6.0. Molecular Biology and Evolution. 2013;**30**:2725-2729. PMID: 24132122

[37] Bandelt HJ, Forster P, Rohl A. Median-joining networks for inferring intraspecific phylogenies. Molecular Biology and Evolution. 1999;**16**:37-48. PMID: 10331250

[38] Lopez-Oceja A, Gamarra D, Cardoso S, Palencia-Madrid L, Juste RA, De Pancorbo MM. Two ovine mitochondrial DNAs harboring a fifth 75/76 bp repeat motif without altered gene expression in Northern Spain. Electrophoresis. 2017;**38**(6):869-875. DOI: 10.1002/elps.201600308

[39] Chen SY, Duan ZY, Sha T, Xiangyu JT, Wu SF, Zhang YP. Origin, genetic diversity, and population structure of Chinese domestic sheep. Gene. 2006;**376**:216-223. DOI: 10.1016/j.gene.2006.03.009

[40] Luo YZ, Cheng SR, Batsuuri L, Badamdorj D, Olivier H, Han JL. Origin and genetic diversity of Mongolian and Chinese sheep using mitochondrial DNA D-loop sequences. Journal of Genetics and Genomics. 2005;**32**(12):1256-1265. PMID:16459654

[41] Lei X, Xu T, Chen Y, Chen H, Yuan Z. Microsatellite markers on genetic relationships of six Chinese indigenous sheep breeds. Chinese Journal of Biochemistry and Molecular Biology. 2006;**22**:81-85. DOI: 10.3969/j.issn.1007-7626.2006.01.014

[42] Wang X, Ma YH, Chen H, Guan WJ. Genetic and phylogenetic studies of Chinese native sheep breeds (*Ovis aries*) based on mtDNA D-loop sequences. Small Ruminant Research. 2007;**72**:232-236. DOI: 10.1016/j.smallrumres.2006.10.016

[43] Liu J, Ding X, Guo T, Yue Y, Zeng Y, Guo X, Chu M, Han J, Feng R, Sun X, Niu C, Yang B, Guo J, Yuan C. The complete mitochondrial genome sequence of the wild Huoba Tibetan sheep of the Qinghai-Tibetan Plateau in China. Mitochondrial DNA. 2015;**6**:4689-4690. DOI: 10.3109/19401736.2015.1106504

[44] Oner Y, Calvo JH, Elmaci C. Investigation of the genetic diversity among native Turkish sheep breeds using mtDNA polymorphisms. Tropical Animal Health and Production. 2013;**45**:947-951. DOI: 10.1007/Js11250-012-0313-z

[45] Walsh PD. Sample size for the diagnosis of conservation units. Conservation Biology. 2000;**14**:1533-1537. DOI: 10.1046/j.1523-1739.2000.98149.x

[46] Tapio M, Ozerov M, Tapio I, Toro MA, Marzanov N, Cinkulov M, Gomcharenko G, Kiselyova T, Murawski M, Kantanen J. Microsatellite-based genetic diversity and population structure of domestic sheep in northern Eurasia. BMC Genetics. 2010;**11**:76. DOI: biomedcentral.com/1471-2156/11/76

[47] Hiendleder S. Molecular characterization of the sheep mitochondrial genome. Journal of Animal Breeding and Genetics. 1996;**113**:293-302. DOI: 10.1111/j.1439-0388.1996.tb00619.x

[48] Gong Y, Li X, Liu Z, Wu J, Zhang Y. mtDNA cytochrome B gene polymorphisms on some Chinese indigenous sheep breeds. Chinese Journal of Veterinary Science. 2006;**26**:213-215

[49] Meadows JRS, Cemal I, Karaca O, Gootwine E, Kijas JW. Five ovine mitochondrial lineages identified from sheep breeds of the near east. Genetics. 2007;**175**:1371-1379. DOI: 10.1534/genetics.106.068353

[50] Tapio M, Marzanov N, Ozerov M, Cinkulov M, Gonzarenko G, Kiselyova T, Murawski M, Viinalass H, Kantanen J. Sheep mitochondrial DNA variation in European, Caucasian, and Central Asian areas. Molecular Biology and Evolution. 2006;**23**(9):1776-1783. PMID: 16782761

[51] Pedrosa S, Arranz JJ, Brito N, Molina A, Primitivo FS, Bayon Y. Mitochondrial diversity and the origin of Iberian sheep. Genetics, Selection, Evolution. 2007;**39**:91-103. DOI: 10.1051/gse:2006034

[52] San Primitivo F, Pedrosa S, Arranz JJ, Brito NV, Molina A, Bayon Y. Mitochondrial DNA variability in Spanish sheep breeds. Archivos de Zootecnia. 2007;**56**:455-460. DOI: 10.1051/gse:2006034

[53] Millar C, Libby W. Strategies for conserving clinal, Ccotypic, and disjunct population diversity in widespread species. In: Falk DA, Holsinger KE, editors. Genetics and Conservation of Rare Plants. New York: Oxford University Press; 1991. pp. 140-170

[54] Liu W, Yao YF, Yu Q, Ni QY, Zhang MW, Yang JD, Mei MM, Xu HL. Genetic variation and phylogenetic relationship between three serow species of the genus Capricornis based on the complete mitochondrial DNA control region sequences. Molecular Biology Reports. 2013;**40**:6793-6802. DOI: 10.1007/S11033-013-2796-8

[55] Bossart JL, Prowell DP. Genetic estimates of population structure and gene flow: Limitations, lessons and new directions. Trends in Ecology & Evolution. 1998;**13**:202-206. DOI: 10.1016/S0169-5347(97)01284-6

[56] Kimura M. On the probability of fixation of mutant genes in a population. Genetics. 1962;**47**:713-719. PMID:14456043

[57] Nei M, Maruyama T, Chakraborty R. The bottleneck effect and genetic variability in populations. Evolution. 1975;**29**(1):1-10. DOI: 10.2307/2407137

[58] Lei X, Chen Y, Chen H, Yuan Z, Xu T, Guo M. Microsatellite markers on the genetic relationships of 6 Chinese indigenous sheep breeds. Animal Biotechnology Bulletin. 2004;**9**(1):1-7. DOI: 10.1051/gse:2002032

[59] Cai D-W, Han L, Zhang X-L, Zhou H, Zhu H. DNA analysis of archaeological sheep remains from China. Journal of Archaeological Science. 2007;**34**:1347-1355. DOI: 10.1038/srep07170

[60] Sun W, Chang H, Yang Z, Geng R, Tsunoda K, Ren Z, Chen C, Hussein H. Analysis on the origin and phylogenetic status of Tong sheep using 12 blood protein and nonprotein markers. Journal of Genetics and Genomics. 2007;**34**(12):1097-1105. DOI: 10.1016/S1673-8527(07)60125-8

[61] Zhong T, Han JL, Guo J, Zhao QJ, Fu BL, He XH, Jeond JT, Guana WJ, Ma YH. Genetic diversity of Chinese indigenous sheep breeds inferred from microsatellite markers. Small Ruminant Research. 2010;**90**:88-94. DOI: 10.1016/j.smallrumres.2010.02.001

[62] Lv FH, Peng WF, Yang J, Zhao YX, Li WR, Liu MJ, Ma YH, Zhao QJ, Yang GL, Wang F, Li JQ, Liu YG, Shen ZQ, Zhao SG, Hehua EE, Gorkhali NA, Vahidi MF, Muladno M, Naqvi AN, Tabell J, Iso-Touru T, Bruford MW, Kantanen Han JL, Li MH. Mitogenomic meta-analysis identifies two phases of migration in the history of eastern Eurasian sheep. Molecular Biology and Evolution. 2015;**32**(10):2515-2533. DOI: 10.1093/molbev/msv139

Section 3

The Human Mitogenome in Health and Disease

Chapter 8

Mitochondrial Aging and Metabolism: The Importance of a Good Relationship in the Central Nervous System

Genaro Gabriel Ortiz, Mario A Mireles-Ramírez,
Héctor González-Usigli, Miguel A Macías-Islas,
Oscar K Bitzer-Quintero,
Erandis Dheni Torres-Sánchez,
Angélica L Sánchez-López, Javier Ramírez-Jirano,
Mónica Ríos-Silva and Blanca Torres-Mendoza

Additional information is available at the end of the chapter

http://dx.doi.org/10.5772/intechopen.76652

Abstract

The mitochondrial theory of aging suggests that mitochondria have a decrease in production capacity of adenosine triphosphate (ATP). The question may seem trivial, but it becomes more complex when considering that dysfunctional mitochondria can be eliminated by lysosomal digestion and that cell with dysfunctional mitochondria can undergo the process of apoptosis. In organs with regenerative capacity, like the liver, cell proliferation can almost completely hide mitochondrial dysfunction. However, evidence indicates selective damage in mitochondria during aging, and so the mitochondrial aging theory is gaining recognition and respect. There is solid evidence that accumulated DNA damage in mitochondria is a cause directly related to metabolic disorders such as diabetes and degenerative disorders such as Alzheimer's disease. The central nervous system is particularly susceptible to oxidative damage due to several factors, among which are its high oxygen consumption, its dependence on aerobic carbohydrate metabolism, and its complex composition of membrane lipids. Free radicals are generated at many cell sites, and the mitochondrial respiratory chain is one of the main sources. While many studies have been conducted in experimental animal models, the results are relevant because at least some of their interventions suggest a directing aim at reducing the effects of aging.

Keywords: mitochondria, aging, nervous system, regulation, oxidative stress

1. Mitochondria and DNA

Mitochondria are double-membrane organelles that are found in the cytoplasm of most eukaryotic cells, and they are essential for the functioning of tissues that are highly dependent on aerobic metabolism, like the brain and heart, since they produce more than 90% of the energy needed for cellular functions [1]. The human mitochondrial genome (mtDNA) is a double circular molecule of 16,571 pairs of nucleotides (16.5 Kb) which contains 37 genes that code for 22 transfer RNAs, 2 ribosomal RNAs, and 13 subunits that encode mitochondrial DNA. These 13 subunits are key in the respiratory chain and in the oxidative phosphorylation system which contains 7 subunits of complex I, 1 subunit of complex III, 3 subunits of complex IV or cytochrome oxidase, and 2 subunits of complex V or ATP synthase (ATPase6 and ATPase8) (**Figure 1**) [1–3].

1.1. Specific characteristics of mitochondrial genetics

The type of inheritance of the mitochondrial genetic system, its location in a cytoplasmic organelle, and the continuous arrangement of genes with almost no intermediate nucleotides or introns and polyplasmy (high number of copies in each cell) provide genetic characteristics that clearly differentiate them from those of nuclear DNA. Each cell contains between 1000 and 10,000 copies of mtDNA depending on the tissue, surpassing a few hundred in the sperm and up to 100,000 in the oocyte [4]. Each mitochondrion contains between 2 and 10 molecules. The mtDNA is primarily maternally inherited by a vertical non-Mendelian pattern. Very small amounts of parental mtDNA have been detected; for example, a case of a 28-year-old male with mitochondrial myopathy was reported due to a new 2 bp deletion in the mtDNA of the ND2 gene (also known as MTND2), which encodes a subunit of the complex I enzyme of the mitochondrial respiratory chain. In this study, it was determined that

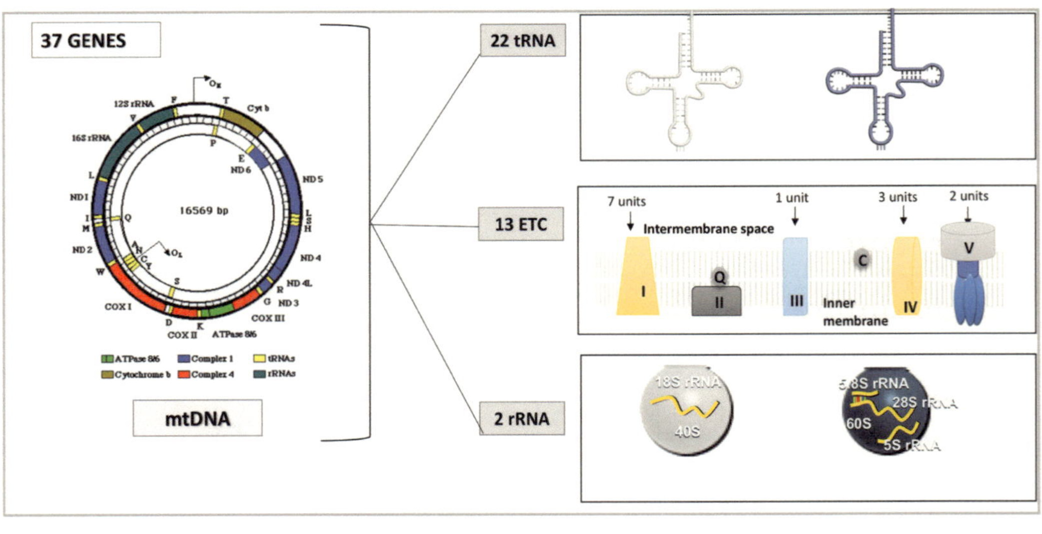

Figure 1. The mitochondrial genome. Mitochondrial DNA (mtDNA) contains essential genes for normal mitochondrial function, including protein production and electron transport chain (ETC) assembly. This image is a modification of QIAGEN's original [Sánchez-Lopez AL].

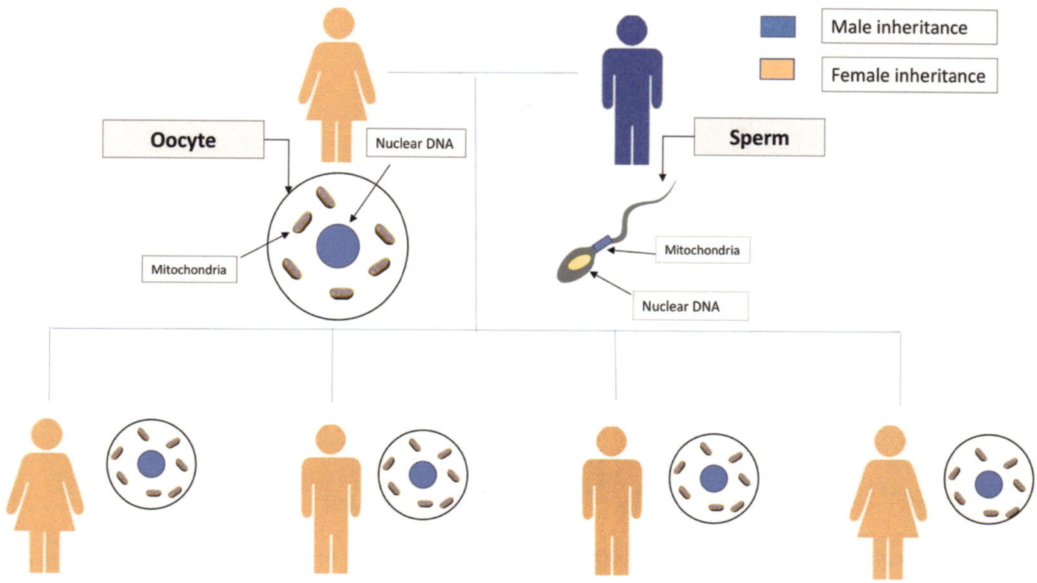

Figure 2. Inheritance pattern of mitochondrial DNA. mtDNA is transferred along material lineage; sperm-derived paternal mitochondria enter the oocyte cytoplasm after fertilization but are eliminated from the cytoplasm of gametes. Mitochondrial disease is always related in the maternal line.

the mtDNA harboring the mutation was of paternal origin and was calculated to be present in 90% of the mtDNA of the patient's muscle [5].

The general pattern is that mothers transmit their mitochondrial genome to all of their offspring, but only daughters will pass it on to all of the members of the next generation. This is due to the high number of mtDNA molecules that exist in the ovules (between 100,000 and 200,000 copies) compared to a few hundred in the sperm. In addition, paternal mitochondria that enter the fertilized ovum are eliminated by an active process (**Figure 2**) [6, 7].

1.2. Mitotic segregation

The phenotype of a cell line can vary during cell division because the mitochondria are randomly distributed among daughter cells; so, if in a cell two populations of mtDNA coexist, one normal and one mutated (heteroplasmy), throughout divisions three different genotypes may originate: homoplasmic for normal mitochondrial DNA, homoplasmic for mutated mitochondrial DNA, and heteroplasmic DNA. Therefore, the phenotype of a cell with heteroplasmy will depend on the percentage of mutated DNA it contains. If the number of damaged mtDNA molecules is relatively low, complementation with normal DNA molecules occurs, and the genetic defect will not manifest [8]. When the mutated DNA exceeds a certain threshold, a pathogenic phenotype will develop according to a threshold effect: if ATP production is below the minimum necessary for the functioning of the tissues, due to defective proteins encoded in the mtDNA, illness might develop [7, 9, 10]. The number of DNA molecules is different in each organ and tissue depending on the required energy amounts for functioning. Therefore, the most affected organs and systems are vision, the central nervous system, skeletal muscle, heart, pancreatic islets, kidney, and liver (**Figure 3**) [6, 11, 12].

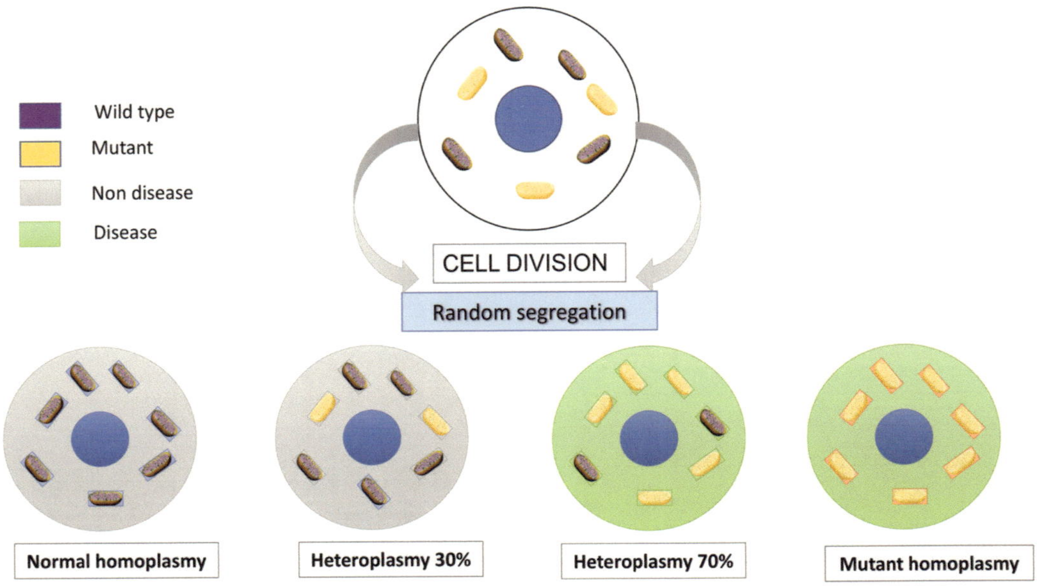

Figure 3. Mitochondrial homoplasmy and heteroplasmy. The expression of mitochondrial diseases is variable; a single cell may receive a uniform collection of mtDNA (homoplasmy) or a mixture of mutant and wild-type mtDNA (heteroplasmy). The proportion of mutant mtDNA molecules determines the penetrance and severity of expression.

1.3. High mutation speed

The mtDNA has a spontaneous mutation rate 10 times higher than that of nuclear DNA. Continuous mitochondrial production of oxygen radicals by the final oxidation of carbon compounds probably damages the unprotected mtDNA (e.g., mtDNA reminds bacterial genomes as it lacks histones). Therefore, the within-species individual sequence variation is large, up to about 70 nucleotides. Within single individuals, low heterogeneity levels in the mtDNA will be generated throughout life. It has been proposed that the decrease in respiratory capacity of the tissues, which takes place during aging, may be due to an accumulation of such mitochondrial damages. This theory was first evidenced in a study by the Attardi Group, who documented that the mitochondria deteriorate with age as a result of the accumulation of mutations [13]. Mitochondrial dysfunction is characterized by a deficient production of energy, a failure in calcium homeostasis, an activation of proteases and phospholipases, activation of nitric oxide synthase, and an abundant generation of free radicals [14–16]. Mitochondria, besides being the main source of free radicals, are also very susceptible to oxidative stress, which is made evident by a massive induction of lipid peroxidation, protein oxidation, and mutations in mtDNA. Oxidative stress also induces apoptotic death, and the mitochondria play a central role in this phenomenon since there is cytochrome c release to the cytoplasm and opening of the permeability transition pore [16].

1.4. Metabolic regulation and the central nervous system: the central role of mitochondria

Mitochondria provide the energy required for neuron function because they transform the potential chemical energy stored in covalent bonds of glucose or fatty acids into chemical energy stored in the covalent bonds between ATP phosphates. This last form of potential chemical energy is easily usable by the cell and has been selected throughout evolution as the mechanism by means of which all cellular processes that require the use of energy readily dispose of it [10, 17]. The body must maintain a balance between the needs of cells and the availability of fuel, which is called metabolic homeostasis. The constant availability of fuel in the blood is called caloric homeostasis, whereby the blood level of fuel (in ATP equivalents) does not decrease below certain limits regardless of whether the individual is in a state of good nutrition or fasting. The maintenance of metabolic homeostasis is achieved through the integration of three main factors: (1) the concentration of nutrients in the blood, which affects the speed with which these are used and stored in different tissues, (2) hormone levels in blood (first messengers) that transmit information to specific tissues on the state of the organism and the contribution or demand of nutrients, and (3) the central nervous system (CNS) that by way of neural signals controls the metabolism directly or through the release of hormones [9, 18]. Despite its essential role in the energy metabolism of the brain and other tissues, the amount of circulating glucose is limited. To ensure its continued provision, the body stores metabolic fuels to provide glucose or energy in case of need. Within the homeostatic mechanisms that allow regulation of the availability of combustible molecules, hormonal control is one of the most important. Insulin and glucagon are the main hormones that regulate the storage and use of fuels. Insulin is an anabolic hormone that promotes the storage, while glucagon is the hormone that stimulates the mobilization of the combustible molecules [17, 18]. Other hormones, such as adrenaline, are released as a CNS response to hypoglycemia, exercise, and other types of physiological stress. Along with other stress hormones (glucocorticoids), adrenaline increases the availability of fuels. One of the requirements to maintain and perpetuate life is the preservation of homeostasis, that is, the constancy of the internal environment (blood levels of ions, lipids, and carbohydrates) within narrow limits. These conditions must be maintained even in varied situations such as rest, exercise, satiety, or fasting. How is our body harmonized to survive in different metabolic situations? In mammals, the coordination of metabolism is achieved through the neuroendocrine system. The main hormones involved in the regulation of intermediate metabolism are insulin, glucagon, catecholamines, and cortisol [19–21].

The brain must generate large amounts of ATP to maintain the membrane potential, which is essential for the transmission of nerve impulses. Under normal conditions the brain only uses glucose as fuel, oxidizing it through aerobic glycolysis. It does not use fatty acids. In fact, 60% of the total glucose consumed by the body is used by the brain. The metabolism of the brain is totally aerobic, consuming 20% of the total oxygen consumed by the body. It does not have appreciable reserves of glycogen or other fuels so it requires the constant supply of oxygen and glucose that cross the blood–brain barrier with ease [19, 22].

Practically, until adulthood, we are well protected against damage to mitochondria since the body is able to produce antioxidant systems that defend us from it [23]. But as we get older, changes occur inside our cells that determine the progressive destruction of mitochondria and, therefore, bring about aging and disease [24].

The sequence variations existing between different individuals have been very useful for anthropological, ethnological, and forensic studies and are the basis for the hypothesis that all existing humans descend from a woman who lived in Africa about 250,000 years ago (**Figure 4**) [25–27].

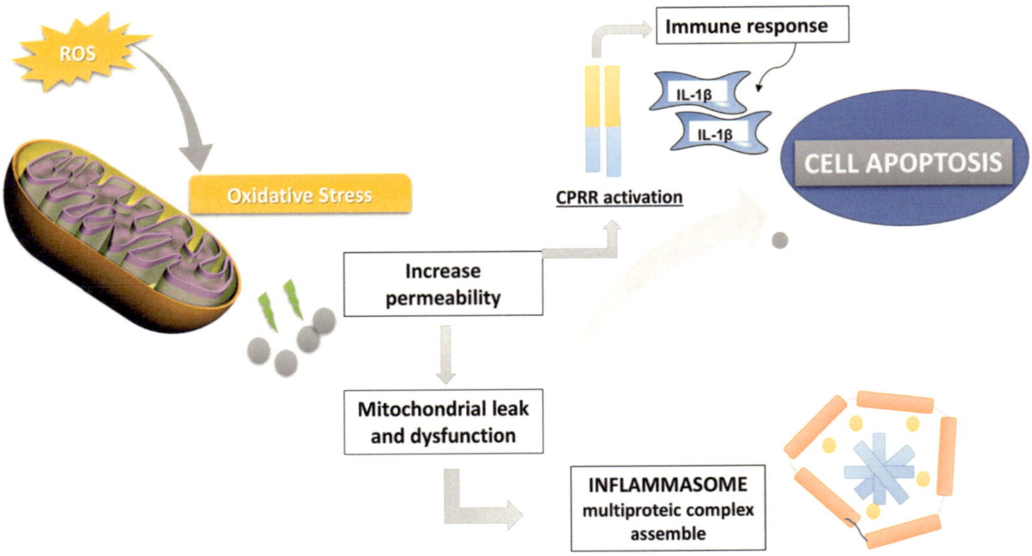

Figure 4. Mitochondrial aging theory. The production of intracellular free radicals, and its effects on cellular components, is a determinant of lifespan. Mitochondria is the prime target for oxidative damage; accumulation of reactive oxygen species (ROS) leads to changes of the inner membrane permeability causing release of intramitochondrial content and activating a cytoplasmic immune response leading to apoptotic cell death.

Mitochondria in the elderly are, for the most part, dysfunctional, unlike young individuals in whom little mitochondrial damage is observed: with the passage of time, devastating changes occur inside our cells that lead to the destruction of mitochondria and consequently trigger aging and disease [15, 28]. Production rates of superoxide anions and hydrogen peroxide (free radicals) increase significantly, specifically deteriorating the mitochondria. At the same time, the levels of endogenous antioxidants (which would contribute to diminishing the harmful effects of free radicals) decrease. There is also a significant reduction of molecules capable of capturing free radicals before they can attack other molecules. Both factors decrease mitochondrial defenses which then become more vulnerable [29, 30]. Oxidative damage accumulated in mitochondrial DNA and other components of the mitochondria (as well as in the cell as a whole) leads to the deterioration of mitochondria, and as a consequence of that deterioration, more free radicals are produced [24].

According to the mitochondrial theory of aging, this growing spiral of deterioration is a process of aging in itself; the number and functional state of the mitochondria determine, in a very specific way, the biologically determined lifespan of individuals. The recent research identifies this mitochondrial aberration associated with age as one of the main mechanisms in chronic inflammation [Ref]. Specifically, mitochondrial dysfunction acts as a mechanism of inflammation in the following manner [31, 32]:

a. The accumulation of free radicals induces a greater permeability in the membrane of the mitochondria.

b. The molecular components normally contained within the mitochondria pass into the cell cytoplasm.

c. The cytoplasmic pattern recognition receptors (CPRRs), which detect and initiate the immune response against intracellular pathogens, recognize the molecules of the mitochondrial discharge as potential threats.

d. After detecting potential threat, the CPRRs form a complex called inflammasome that captures the inflammatory cytokine interleukin-1β, which then recruits components of the immune system to destroy the altered cell.

These four steps represent a simplified diagram of mitochondrial dysfunction that leads to cell destruction; however, free radicals are not the only inducers of cell death by inflammation [33, 34].

Circulating carbohydrates, mainly glucose and fructose, also participate in aging processes. When these blood sugars come into contact with proteins and lipids, a harmful reaction occurs that forms compounds called advanced glycation end products (AGEs). The AGEs bind to a receptor on the surface of the cells called the PFG receptor (receptor for advanced glycation end products (RAGE)). After activation, the RAGEs induce the movement of the nuclear mediator factor kappa-B (NF-kB) to the nucleus where numerous inflammatory genes are activated. AGEs are formed mainly in vivo, and glycation is exacerbated by elevated blood glucose levels. Dietary AGE also contributes to inflammation [17, 18, 35].

Hence, molecules that protect and revitalize mitochondria could recreate a "juvenile" state of protection against free radicals (**Figure 5**) [36].

Mitochondria in the elderly are, for the most part, are dysfunctional, unlike young individuals in whom no mitochondrial damage is observed. So much so is the mitochondrial dysfunction caused by oxidative damage due to free radicals that are already a marker of aging and pathologies associated with age [37].

The mitochondrial theory, which proposes that mitochondrial defects associated with age are controlled by the accumulation of mutations in mitochondrial DNA. There is, however, a growing body of contradictory evidence that has raised questions about the validity of this theory. It has been suggested that the mitochondrial defects associated with age are not controlled by the accumulation of mutations in mitochondrial DNA but by another form of genetic regulation. Contrary to the mitochondrial theory of aging, the epigenetic regulation of respiration controls defects associated with age [37].

Damage to mitochondrial DNA causes changes or mutations in the DNA sequence. The accumulation of these changes is associated with a reduced life expectancy and the early onset of characteristics related to aging such as weight and hair loss, the curvature of the spine, and osteoporosis [38]. There is, however, a growing body of contradictory evidence that has raised questions about the validity of this theory. Tsukuba's team, in particular, has made a compelling research that has led them to propose that the mitochondrial defects associated with age are not controlled by the accumulation of mitochondrial DNA mutations but by another form of genetic regulation [2, 39, 40]. The researchers compared mitochondrial respiration and the amount of DNA damage in the mitochondria, expecting that respiration would decrease and DNA damage would increase in the cells of the elderly group. The elderly group had lower respiration as the accepted theory indicates; however, there was no difference in amounts of

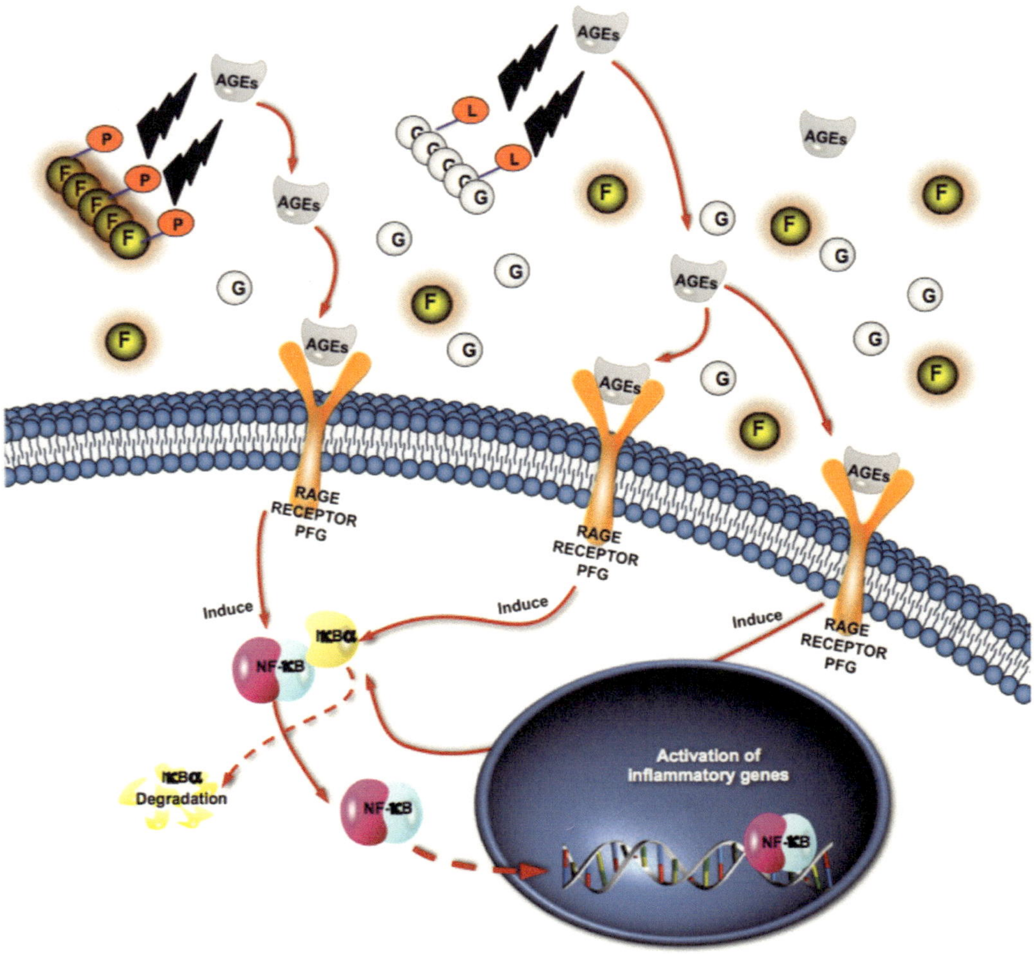

Figure 5. AGEs. The activation of inflammatory genes is triggered by the formation of AGEs. AGEs activate NF-kB through a cascade of reactions. This image is a modification of QIAGEN's original [Torres-Sánchez ED].

DNA damage. This epigenetic regulation may be responsible for the effects associated with age that is seen in mitochondria [7, 41, 42].

To test this theory, a research reprogrammed human fibroblast cell lines derived from the young and from the old to a state similar to that of embryonic stem cells. Then, they returned these cells back to their fibroblast form, and their mitochondrial respiratory function was examined; the researchers looked for genes that could be controlled epigenetically causing these mitochondrial defects associated with age and found two that regulate the production of glycine in the mitochondria, CGAT, and SHMT2 and showed that by changing the regulation of these genes, they can produce defects or restore mitochondrial function in fibroblast cell lines. The addition of glycine for 10 days in the culture medium of the fibroblast cell line of the 97-year-old people restored its respiratory function. This suggests that glycine treatment can reverse the breathing defects associated with aging in elderly human fibroblasts.

Incredibly, the defects associated with age had reversed: all fibroblasts had respiration rates comparable to those of the fetal fibroblast cell line, regardless of whether they were derived from the young or the elderly. This indicates that the aging process in the mitochondria is controlled by epigenetic regulation, not by mutations [37].

2. Oxidative stress and aging

Mitochondria are the easiest target for damage by free radicals due to two reasons:

1. They are exactly where free radicals are produced.
2. They lack the antioxidant defenses that are present in other parts of the cell [43, 44].

There is strong evidence that the accumulated DNA damage of mitochondria is directly related to aging metabolic disorders and diseases [45]. The difference between mitochondria and other intracellular compartments is that the mitochondria have their own DNA. The production of free radicals (including superoxide anions and hydrogen peroxide) in mitochondria is a corollary to energy production (**Figure 6**). The accumulation of these by-products inside mitochondria damages their structure and their DNA. This damage is similar to that produced by ionizing radiation, and today there is an important scientific consensus that considers it as one of the main factors of aging [46]; so much so, that mitochondrial dysfunction caused by oxidative damage due to free radicals is already a marker of aging and the pathologies associated with aging, like in Alzheimer's disease, Parkinson's disease, and cancer [47–49].

The energy metabolism intrinsic to the maintenance of the organism and environmental factors (pollution, smoking) determine the continuous generation of oxygen radicals. These radicals produce oxidative damage to lipids, proteins, and DNA, and damaged molecules accumulate during aging [44, 46]. The deterioration secondary to aging is observed more clearly in postmitotic cells, which, when damaged, cannot be replaced by new cells, as is the case of the neuron. Although it has not been possible to demonstrate with certainty what is the role of this damage in senescence, oxidative stress would be one of the mechanisms possibly involved in neurodegenerative diseases [50].

Oxidative stress can increase with aging, both due to increased generation of oxygen radicals and by the decrease in the ability to eliminate these radicals (antioxidant mechanisms) [51]. There is still discussion regarding the apparent decrease in antioxidant mechanisms during aging [51, 52]. However, the available evidence, with respect to the maximum lifespan of individuals, suggests that the mechanisms of defense against oxidation would not be very relevant [52, 53]. The levels of antioxidant enzymes and the low molecular weight antioxidants show an inverse correlation with the maximum longevity of the animals, which indicates that pro-oxidative activity as such is the most relevant one [54]. Nor has it been found that supplementation with antioxidants (or the opposite effect, the elimination of antioxidant mechanisms) significantly modifies the maximum lifespan of an animal. In contrast, studies

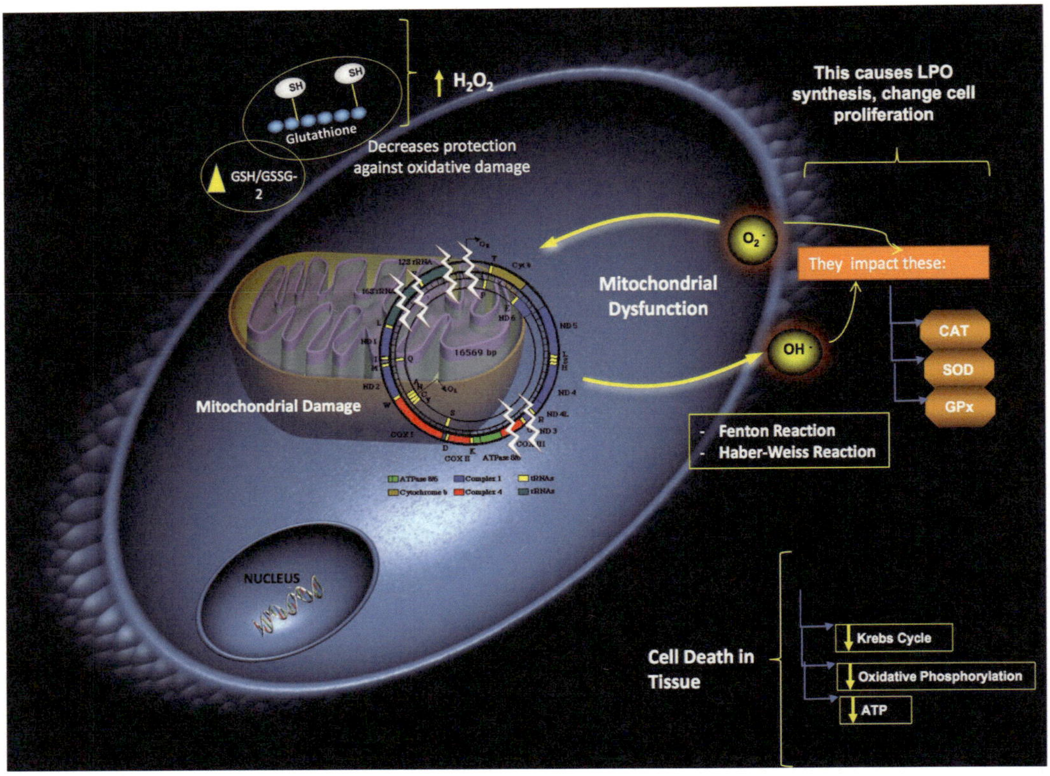

Figure 6. Mitochondrial dysfunction. The mitochondria are the main endogenous generator of free radicals. This production acts in a vicious circle that damages the mitochondria and therefore the mitochondrial primordial functions as shown in the figure. This image is a modification of QIAGEN's original [Torres-Sánchez ED].

of average survival suggest that in animals treated with antioxidant therapy these can effectively, nonspecifically protect against various causes of early mortality [55, 56]. These protective effects can have great importance for the human population given that due to their living conditions humans live in an adverse environment and are subjected, for example, to radiation and toxic compounds, so they are exposed to damage by oxidative stress of exogenous origin [57–59].

The animals would have regulatory mechanisms active during development that would monitor mitochondrial activity and, in response, establish the rates of respiration, behavior, and aging that persist during adult life [15, 60]. Although many of these studies have been carried out in experimental models, the results are relevant since they suggest that at least some of the interventions aimed at reducing the effects of aging should be considered in the early stages and not during the adult life of the individual [61]. Also, mitochondria that have suffered oxidative damage also contribute to the aging process [62–64]. Based on the studies that associate the increase of oxidative stress with aging, a line of research has been strengthened which proposes that the decrease in caloric intake is associated with an increase in the resistance of the central nervous system to suffer the neurodegenerative disorders of aging (**Figure 7**) [65]. The neuroprotective effect would depend on the decrease in the generation of oxygen radicals and an increase in the production of neurotrophic factors and protein chaperones [66, 67].

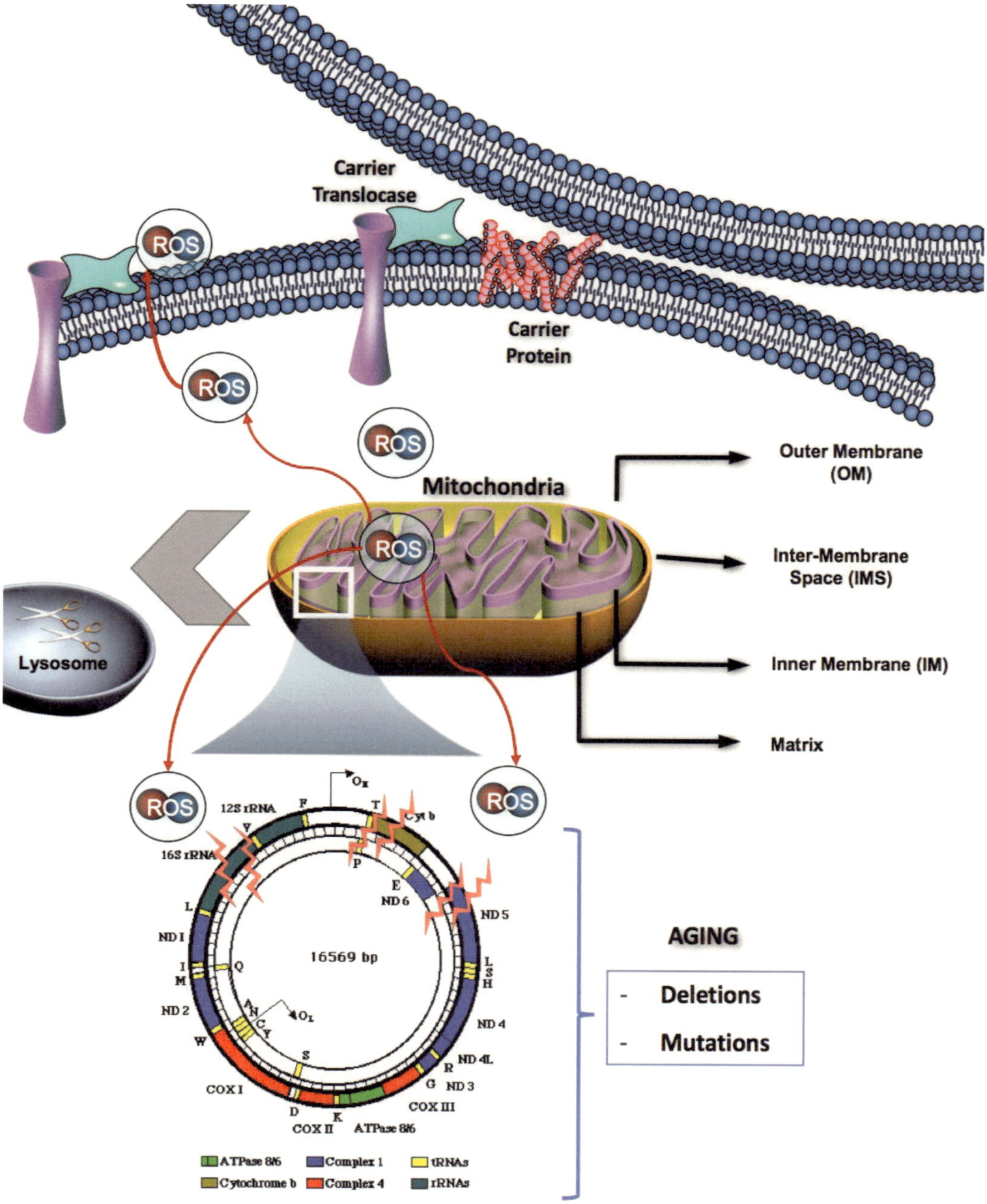

Figure 7. Aging and mitochondrial DNA. DNA damage is important for aging; reactive oxygen species (ROS) generated damage mtDNA and therefor mutations and other alterations. This image is a modification of QIAGEN's original [Torres-Sánchez ED].

3. DNA mitochondria and disease

Mitochondrial diseases are a group of disorders whose common feature is a defect in the production of ATP. However, this term is frequently applied to disorders caused by damage to the oxidative phosphorylation (OXPHOS) system because for many years only mutations in mtDNA related to these diseases had been detected. But, identification of nuclear genes encoding proteins of the OXPHOS system complexes, or responsible for their assembly, has been described [68].

Mitochondrial disease can associate with any symptom, in any organ, at any age, but some symptoms and signs are actually more suggestive of a mitochondrial disorder than others. These "warning signs" warrant the onset of a diagnostic assessment of mitochondrial diseases. In contrast, numerous nonspecific symptoms occur frequently in infants and children with mitochondrial disease, but they have a broad differential diagnosis and lead more often to other diagnoses [68]. For example, pigmentary retinopathy in a preadolescent child may be a trait of mitochondrial disease but should suggest the possibility of juvenile neuronal ceroid lipofuscinosis or another genetic syndrome. Thus, nonspecific symptoms, especially isolated ones, do not indicate per se a mitochondrial problem. However, when combined, the likelihood of mitochondrial disorder increases, especially if the nonspecific aspects affect different organ systems, which leads to the initiation of appropriate initial diagnostic investigations [53, 69].

The defects of the respiratory chain of Mendelian inheritance are included in four groups:

1. Mutations in genes that code for subunits of the respiratory chain
2. Mutations in genes that code for anchor proteins
3. Defects in intergenomic communication
4. Defects that affect the constituent lipids of the inner mitochondrial membrane where CR is embedded

4. Diseases caused by mutations in genes that encode subunits of the respiratory chain

The most frequent of these diseases are those that code for subunits of complexes I and II and cause Leigh's syndrome, which is a fatal neurodegenerative disease that begins in the first years of life due to a profound defect in the production of ATP in the developing brain. It is defined by the presence of bilateral necrotic lesions in ganglia of the base and brain stem, characterized histologically by cavitated areas, vascular proliferation, neuronal loss, and demyelination. Individuals with Leigh's syndrome can also present variable symptoms that do not fit into any defined syndrome (hypotonia, cardiomyopathy, ataxia, developmental delay, etc.) [70]. The most important genes that code for complex I subunits are NDUFS1, NDUFS2, NDUFS3, NDUFS4, NDUFS6, NDUFS8, NDUFV1, and NDUFV2 [71–73].

4.1. Diseases caused by mutations in genes that code for anchor proteins

This group of diseases includes mutations in genes that code for proteins that, while not part of the mitochondrial respiratory chain, are necessary for the correct assembly of proteins encoded by the nuclear and the mitochondrial genomes. Examples are mutations in the nuclear SURF1, LRPPRC, and NDUFA12L genes, which code for proteins necessary for the assembly of cyclooxygenase (COX) [73, 74].

Primary deficits of coenzyme Q10 (CoQ10) include various disorders caused by defects of their biosynthesis at different levels. The CoQ10 transports electrons from complexes I and II to complex III and receives electrons from the beta-oxidation pathway via electron-transferring-flavoprotein dehydrogenase (ETFDH) [75]. There are at least nine enzymes necessary for the synthesis of CoQ10, and mutations in the genes that encode them are responsible for different cases of encephalomyopathies. There are also disorders due to CoQ10 secondary deficits, including autosomal recessive cases of cerebellar ataxia of unknown cause in children, apraxia syndrome with oculomotor ataxia 2 (AOA2) caused by mutations in the aprataxin gene (APTX), and myopathic form of glutaric aciduria type II (GAII) caused by mutations in the gene that encodes the ETFDH [76, 77]. The importance of knowledge of these disorders is that supplements with CoQ10 improve the symptoms in these patients. Defects have also been described in proteins involved in the assembly of complex III (BCS1L) and complex V (ATPAF2) [3, 74].

4.2. Diseases secondary to defects in intergenomic communication

These diseases are due to defects in nuclear factors involved in the replication, maintenance, and translation of mtDNA. The resulting disorders are characterized by quantitative alterations (depletion syndromes) or qualitative alterations (multiple deletions) of mtDNA or by defects in the translation of respiratory chain components encoded in the mtDNA. Thus, many of these disorders are due to alterations in the pool of nucleotides necessary for the synthesis of mtDNA or in the enzymes necessary for the replication of mtDNA itself [78, 79].

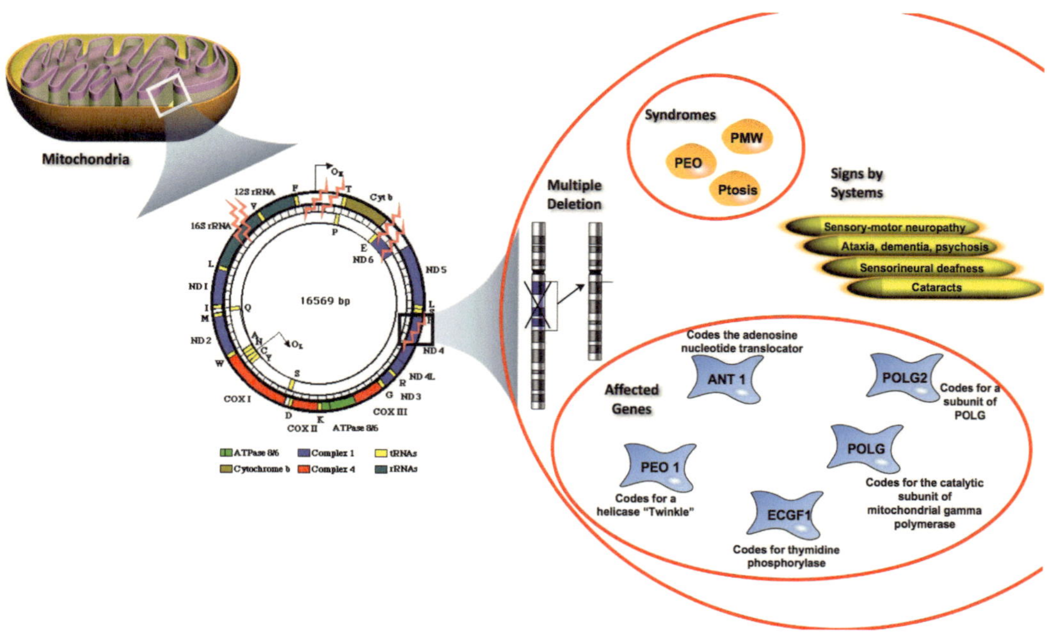

Figure 8. Multiple deletions of mtDNA. Mitochondrial damage is regulated by multiple deletions in the PEO, ANT1, ECGF I, POLG, and OLG2 genes. The deletions will trigger the syndromes and signs that are illustrated in the image. This image is a modification of QIAGEN's original [Torres-Sánchez ED].

4.3. Multiple deletions of mtDNA

From the clinical point of view, the multiple deletion syndromes of mtDNA are characterized by progressive external ophthalmoparesis (PEO), ptosis, and proximal muscle weakness associated with signs of involvement of other systems that include the peripheral nerves (sensory-motor neuropathy), the brain (ataxia, dementia, psychosis), the ear (sensorineural deafness), and the eye (cataracts). Genes involved in the homeostasis of the mitochondrial pool of nucleotides are associated with the presence of PEO and multiple deletions in mtDNA. They include ANT1 (encodes the adenosine nucleotide translocator), PEO1 (codes for a helicase known as Twinkle), ECGF1 (which codes for thymidine phosphorylase or TP), POLG (encodes for the catalytic subunit of mitochondrial gamma polymerase), and POLG2 (which codes for a subunit of POLG) (**Figure 8**) [14, 80, 81].

Mitochondrial neurogastrointestinal encephalomyopathy or MNGIE is a multisystemic disease of autosomal recessive inheritance, of presentation in young adults secondary to mutations in TP (thymidine phosphorylase). It is characterized by PEO, neuropathy, leukoencephalopathy, and severe gastrointestinal dysmotility, leading to profound cachexia and early death. The decrease in thymidine phosphorylase activity leads to a defect in the synthesis of mtDNA, causing not only multiple deletions in the mtDNA but also depletion of same and point mutations that are reflected in the muscle, even though it expresses little TP. The damage, therefore, seems to be mediated by toxins. Thus, thymidine and deoxyuridine are toxic intermediaries that accumulate in the blood of these patients, and their elimination leads to clinical improvement. Different approaches have been carried out to favor the elimination of these toxic intermediaries from the blood, by means of hemodialysis, platelet transfusion, and, finally, allogeneic bone marrow transplantation [35, 80].

Mutations in mitochondrial gamma polymerase (POLG) may occur in the form of PEO at the onset of adulthood and multiple deletions in mtDNA and be accompanied by ataxia, peripheral neuropathy, Parkinsonism, psychiatric symptoms, myoclonic epilepsy, and gastrointestinal symptoms. These disorders can have both dominant and recessive inheritances. An example of a clinical syndrome secondary to mutations in this gene is SANDO (sensory ataxic neuropathy, dysarthria, ophthalmoparesis). Mutations in POLG are also responsible for the Alpers syndrome in children, a recessively inherited disorder characterized by encephalopathy and severe hepatopathy and associated with mtDNA depletion [80].

4.4. Depletion of mtDNA

Some mutations in POLG are responsible for a fatal hepatocerebral syndrome in children (Alpers syndrome) characterized by a profound depletion of mtDNA. Mutations in proteins that affect the control of the pool of nucleotides in mitochondria also produce depletion of mtDNA, highlighting two syndromes:

- Hepatocerebral syndrome caused by mutations in POLG or in DGUOK (encodes the enzyme deoxyguanosine kinase (dGK))
- Myopathic syndrome caused by mutations in TK2 (which codes for the mitochondrial form of thymidine kinase), in SUCLA2 (beta subunit of succinyl-CoA synthetase), or in RRM2B (p-53 inducible ribonucleotide reductase) [80, 82]

4.5. Defects in mtDNA translation

In the translation of the 13 subunits of the respiratory chain encoded in the mtDNA, the participation of many nuclear coding factors such as polymerases, ribosomal proteins, RNA-modifying enzymes and initiation, elongation, and termination factors, among others, is necessary. These defects result in deep combined deficits of all the respiratory chain complexes. Clinically, they manifest as necrotizing leukoencephalopathies, cardiomyopathies, and hepatocerebral syndromes among others. Genes involved include GFM1 (encodes a ribosomal elongation factor), MRPS16 (encodes the 16 subunit of the mitochondrial ribosomal protein), TSFM (encodes the mitochondrial elongation factor EFTs), and TUFM (encodes the elongation factor Tu) [80, 82, 83].

4.6. Mitochondrial secondary disease

Even when a sophisticated biochemical analysis confirms mitochondrial dysfunction, it can be challenging to distinguish whether the cause of this dysfunction is a gene that directly affects the electron transport or is secondary to an unrelated genetic or environmental cause. Thus, the definitive diagnosis of mitochondrial disease cannot be based solely on biochemical findings, since the in vitro activity of the electron transport chain enzyme in a sample of patient tissue may be diminished as a consequence of other metabolic diseases or issues related to the handling of samples. Mitochondrial dysfunction that may or may not be clinically relevant is observed when the main defect lies in another metabolic pathway related to energy, such as the oxidation of fatty acids or the metabolism of amino acids. In addition, alteration of OXPHOS has been observed with decreased in vitro activity of the electron transport chain enzyme in up to 50% in tissue samples from patients with other metabolic diseases [84]. Of course, other diagnoses that have finally been confirmed in individuals with suspected mitochondrial disease and biochemical samples of mitochondrial dysfunction in vitro include disorders of copper metabolism (Menkes disease and Wilson's disease), lysosomal disorders (neuronal ceroid lipofuscinosis and Fabry disease), peroxisomal disorders, neurodegeneration associated with pantothenate kinase, holocarboxylase synthetase deficiency, molybdenum cofactor deficiency, and neonatal hemochromatosis [85]. It is increasingly accepted that the alteration of OXPHOS may contribute to the pathology in some genetic alterations that are not typically classified as mitochondrial or metabolic disorders, such as Rett syndrome, Aicardi-Goutières syndrome, various neuromuscular disorders, and Duchenne muscular dystrophy. In addition, the activities of the electron transport complexes in skeletal muscle can decrease in malnourished children, correcting to normal values after improvement of nutrition [41, 74, 86].

Medications and toxins can also significantly alter mitochondrial function. Sodium valproate can alter mitochondrial function by inducing carnitine deficiency, depression of intramitochondrial oxidation of fatty acids, and/or inhibition of OXPHOS, which should suggest the use of an alternative anticonvulsant in mitochondrial disease, especially in patients with POLG1 mutations. Other important examples of drugs that can induce mitochondrial dysfunction are retroviral nucleoside analogs in HIV infection, as well as salicylates that can alter the hepatic mitochondria in Reye syndrome. Since there are so many nonspecific clinical features that can raise the suspicion of mitochondrial diseases, the differential diagnosis can be very broad. The clinical presentation of mitochondrial disease in children can mimic other multisystem disorders, such as congenital disorders of glycosylation or Marinesco-Sjögren syndrome, or even be confused with a syndrome of vascular or immunological stroke. Although the clinical

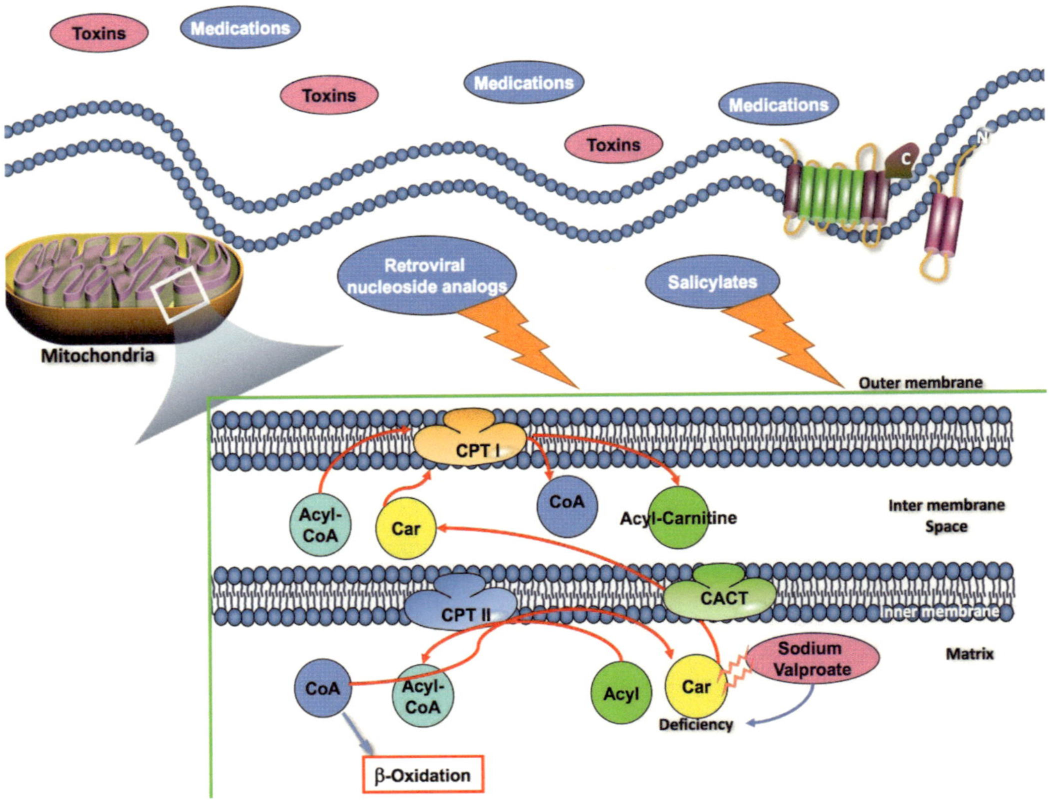

Figure 9. Medications and toxin in mitochondria: Alteration of mitochondrial function by exogenous metabolites; the main damage affects cell respiration, but also damage in the oxidation of fatty acids is observed. This image is a modification of QIAGEN's original [Torres-Sánchez ED].

and neuroimaging features of Leigh's syndrome often clearly suggest a mitochondrial disorder, other alterations may give rise to striatal necrosis, which should be taken into account. Similarly, clinical and neuroimaging findings may sometimes suggest other leukoencephalopathies or degenerative disorders (**Figure 9**) [85, 86].

5. Assessment and diagnostic process

The main challenge to correctly establish mitochondrial dysfunction as the cause of the presentation of a specific patient is the absence of a definitive biomarker that characterizes mitochondrial disease in all patients. Thus, the diagnostic assessment is necessarily broad and of many levels, with a focus on integrated training from many sources: complete medical and family history, clinical findings that may suggest a mitochondrial disease, abnormalities of the biochemical laboratory such as lactic acidosis (which, as we analyzed earlier, is not sensitive or specific as an isolated biomarker in many mitochondrial disorders), tissue biopsy tests of the abnormal activity of the electron transport chain enzyme or an alteration of the respiratory capacity, and, if possible, the identification of a pathogenic mutation of mtDNA or nDNA. This process usually involves sophisticated tests that request invasive procedures, such as muscle or liver biopsy to obtain the tissue for assessment in specialized laboratories. These investigations may offer intermediate or ambiguous results, and the decrease in the activities of the enzymes of the electron transport chain may be secondary to non-respiratory chain disorders. To assist in the interpretation, two diagnostic schemes have been proposed for infants and children to classify the probability of a specific patient's mitochondrial disease as clear, probable, possible, or improbable. Recently, guidelines were proposed for the diagnosis and treatment of mitochondrial disorders in infants and children; however, these complex and sophisticated diagnostic algorithms are aimed for the metabolic specialist and have a limited clinical utility for the family physician who contemplates the start of the diagnostic evaluation of a specific patient [20, 21, 87].

The diagnostic evaluation typically begins with the general clinical assessment and goes through the systematic, imaging, and metabolic screening tests up to the most specific biochemical and genetic determinations. This starts with the less invasive evaluations and moves on to the biopsy-based, more invasive analyses, as needed. Obviously, the complete diagnostic process can be complicated and including the early intervention of a local specialist in metabolism can be very useful. Recommendation to a metabolic specialist should occur whenever the symptoms and signs clearly suggest a mitochondrial disease, patients are potentially unstable with the classic features of metabolic disease, there is lactic acidosis in the blood or the cerebrospinal fluid (CSF), a pattern of maternal inheritance is observed, or anomalies are identified in the initial diagnostic assessment. Referral by a primary care physician is also prudent when a more elaborate study is necessary, such as a provocation test or a muscle biopsy with the study of the enzymes of the electron transport chain [79, 88]. If a biochemical diagnosis has been established but its molecular basis remains unknown, further study and genetic counseling should be coordinated by a specialist. Mitochondrial disease is clearly not a single entity but rather a heterogeneous disorder of energy dysfunction caused by hundreds of different mutations, deletions, duplications, and other defects of nuclear and mitochondrial genes. Thus, at present, there is no accepted and gene-based diagnostic algorithm that is useful for all patients or used by all metabolic specialists. The study of nDNA mutations can be performed on any tissue, including blood. However, most of the diagnostic study of nDNA genes should not be done a priori but guided by the clinical picture, the specific headlines, and the biochemical findings in a given patient. On the contrary, the most informative study of mtDNA mutations is performed in a muscle biopsy sample, although urinary sediment and buccal cells may also be useful.

It is important to recognize that dietary advice should always be offered in a specialized setting. In addition, although there are only a few viable therapeutic options for mitochondrial disease, it is best to be offered by clinicians with experience in these disorders [89].

What was once considered a few rare diseases to be described in clinical sessions or in the form of clinical cases in journals are today disorders that are commonly known and observed in a wide range of consultations.

Author details

Genaro Gabriel Ortiz[1]*, Mario A Mireles-Ramírez[2], Héctor González-Usigli[2], Miguel A Macías-Islas[3], Oscar K Bitzer-Quintero[4], Erandis Dheni Torres-Sánchez[5], Angélica L Sánchez-López[6], Javier Ramírez-Jirano[4], Mónica Ríos-Silva[7] and Blanca Torres-Mendoza[8]

*Address all correspondence to: genarogabriel@yahoo.com

1 Desarrollo-Envejecimiento, Enfermedades Neurodegenerativas, División de Neurociencias, Centro de Investigación Biomédica de Occidente, Instituto Mexicano del Seguro Social, Guadalajara, Jalisco, Mexico

2 Departamento de Neurología, Unidad Médica de Alta Especialidad, Hospital de Especialidades, Centro Médico de Nacional de Occidente, Instituto Mexicano del Seguro Social, Guadalajara, Jalisco, Mexico

3 Departamento de Farmacología, Centro Universitario de Ciencias de la Salud, Universidad de Guadalajara, Guadalajara, Jalisco, Mexico

4 Neuroinmunomodulación, División de Neurociencias, Centro de Investigación Biomédica de Occidente, Instituto Mexicano del Seguro Social, Guadalajara, Jalisco, Mexico

5 Centro Universitario de la Ciénega, Universidad de Guadalajara, Guadalajara, Jalisco, Mexico

6 Departamento de Bioingeniería, Instituto Tecnológico de Monterrey-Campus Guadalajara, Guadalajara, Jalisco, Mexico

7 Centro Universitario de Investigaciones Biomédicas, Universidad de Colima, Colima, Colima, Mexico

8 División de Neurociencias, Centro de Investigación Biomédica de Occidente, Instituto Mexicano del Seguro Social, Guadalajara, Jalisco, Mexico

References

[1] Malik AN, Czajka A. Is mitochondrial DNA content a potential biomarker of mitochondrial dysfunction? Mitochondrion. 2013;**13**(5):481-492

[2] Carelli V, Chan DC. Mitochondrial DNA: Impacting central and peripheral nervous systems. Neuron. 2014;**84**(6):1126-1142

[3] Ojaimi J et al. Mitochondrial respiratory chain activity in the human brain as a function of age. Mechanisms of Ageing and Development. 1999;**111**(1):39-47

[4] Reynier P et al. Mitochondrial DNA content affects the fertilizability of human oocytes. Molecular Human Reproduction. 2001;**7**(5):425-429

[5] Schwartz M, Vissing J. Paternal inheritance of mitochondrial DNA. The New England Journal of Medicine. 2002;**347**(8):576-580

[6] Chinnery PF et al. Point mutations of the mtDNA control region in normal and neurodegenerative human brains. American Journal of Human Genetics. 2001;**68**(2):529-532

[7] Tin A et al. Association between mitochondrial DNA copy number in peripheral blood and incident CKD in the atherosclerosis risk in communities study. Journal of the American Society of Nephrology. 2016;**27**(8):2467-2473

[8] Song J et al. Peripheral blood mitochondrial DNA content is related to insulin sensitivity in offspring of type 2 diabetic patients. Diabetes Care. 2001;**24**(5):865-869

[9] Kakiuchi C et al. Quantitative analysis of mitochondrial DNA deletions in the brains of patients with bipolar disorder and schizophrenia. The International Journal of Neuropsychopharmacology. 2005;**8**(4):515-522

[10] Kennedy ED, Maechler P, Wollheim CB. Effects of depletion of mitochondrial DNA in metabolism secretion coupling in INS-1 cells. Diabetes. 1998;**47**(3):374-380

[11] Krishnan KJ et al. Mitochondrial DNA deletions cause the biochemical defect observed in Alzheimer's disease. Neurobiology of Aging. 2012;**33**(9):2210-2214

[12] Lin MT et al. High aggregate burden of somatic mtDNA point mutations in aging and Alzheimer's disease brain. Human Molecular Genetics. 2002;**11**(2):133-145

[13] Michikawa Y et al. Aging-dependent large accumulation of point mutations in the human mtDNA control region for replication. Science. 1999;**286**(5440):774-779

[14] Chang SW et al. The frequency of point mutations in mitochondrial DNA is elevated in the Alzheimer's brain. Biochemical and Biophysical Research Communications. 2000;**273**(1):203-208

[15] Mecocci P et al. Oxidative damage to mitochondrial DNA shows marked age-dependent increases in human brain. Annals of Neurology. 1993;**34**(4):609-616

[16] Qiu X, Chen Y, Zhou M. Two point mutations in mitochondrial DNA of cytochrome c oxidase coexist with normal mtDNA in a patient with Alzheimer's disease. Brain Research. 2001;**893**(1-2):261-263

[17] Park KS et al. Depletion of mitochondrial DNA alters glucose metabolism in SK-Hep1 cells. American Journal of Physiology, Endocrinology and Metabolism. 2001;**280**(6):E1007-E1014

[18] Lehnhardt FG et al. Altered cerebral glucose metabolism in a family with clinical features resembling mitochondrial neurogastrointestinal encephalomyopathy syndrome in association with multiple mitochondrial DNA deletions. Archives of Neurology. 2008;**65**(3):407-411

[19] Blanchard BJ et al. A mitochondrial DNA deletion in normally aging and in Alzheimer brain tissue. NeuroReport. 1993;**4**(6):799-802

[20] Brierley EJ et al. Role of mitochondrial DNA mutations in human aging: Implications for the central nervous system and muscle. Annals of Neurology. 1998;**43**(2):217-223

[21] Corral-Debrinski M et al. Mitochondrial DNA deletions in human brain: Regional variability and increase with advanced age. Nature Genetics. 1992;**2**(4):324-329

[22] Abramov AY et al. Mechanism of neurodegeneration of neurons with mitochondrial DNA mutations. Brain: A Journal of Neurology. 2010;**133**(Pt 3):797-807

[23] Lowes DA et al. Antioxidants that protect mitochondria reduce interleukin-6 and oxidative stress, improve mitochondrial function, and reduce biochemical markers of organ dysfunction in a rat model of acute sepsis. British Journal of Anaesthesia. 2013;**110**(3):472-480

[24] Balaban RS, Nemoto S, Finkel T. Mitochondria, oxidants, and aging. Cell. 2005;**120**(4): 483-495

[25] de la Monte SM et al. Mitochondrial DNA damage as a mechanism of cell loss in Alzheimer's disease. Laboratory Investigation. 2000;**80**(8):1323-1335

[26] Tanaka N et al. Mitochondrial DNA variants in a Japanese population of patients with Alzheimer's disease. Mitochondrion. 2010;**10**(1):32-37

[27] Tranah GJ et al. Mitochondrial DNA sequence associations with dementia and amyloid-beta in elderly African Americans. Neurobiology of Aging. 2014;**35**(2):442 e1-442 e8

[28] Williams SL et al. Somatic mtDNA mutation spectra in the aging human putamen. PLoS Genetics. 2013;**9**(12):e1003990

[29] Gadaleta MN et al. Mitochondrial DNA copy number and mitochondrial DNA deletion in adult and senescent rats. Mutation Research. 1992;**275**(3-6):181-193

[30] Pandya JD et al. Age- and brain region-specific differences in mitochondrial bioenergetics in Brown Norway rats. Neurobiology of Aging. 2016;**42**:25-34

[31] Swerdlow RH, Khan SM. A "mitochondrial cascade hypothesis" for sporadic Alzheimer's disease. Medical Hypotheses. 2004;**63**(1):8-20

[32] Theurey P, Pizzo P. The aging mitochondria. Genes. 2018;**9**(1):1-13

[33] Cui H, Kong Y, Zhang H. Oxidative stress, mitochondrial dysfunction, and aging. Journal of Signal Transduction. 2012;**2012**:646354

[34] Mammucari C, Rizzuto R. Signaling pathways in mitochondrial dysfunction and aging. Mechanisms of Ageing and Development. 2010;**131**(7-8):536-543

[35] Kang CM, Kristal BS, Yu BP. Age-related mitochondrial DNA deletions: Effect of dietary restriction. Free Radical Biology & Medicine. 1998;**24**(1):148-154

[36] Valko M et al. Free radicals, metals and antioxidants in oxidative stress-induced cancer. Chemico-Biological Interactions. 2006;**160**(1):1-40

[37] Hashizume O et al. Epigenetic regulation of the nuclear-coded GCAT and SHMT2 genes confers human age-associated mitochondrial respiration defects. Scientific Reports. 2015;**5**:10434

[38] Taylor RW, Turnbull DM. Mitochondrial DNA mutations in human disease. Nature Reviews. Genetics. 2005;**6**(5):389-402

[39] Mancuso M et al. Is there a primary role of the mitochondrial genome in Alzheimer's disease? Journal of Bioenergetics and Biomembranes. 2009;**41**(5):411-416

[40] Phillips NR, Simpkins JW, Roby RK. Mitochondrial DNA deletions in Alzheimer's brains: A review. Alzheimer's & Dementia: The Journal of the Alzheimer's Association. 2014;**10**(3):393-400

[41] Szczepanowska K, Trifunovic A. Different faces of mitochondrial DNA mutators. Biochimica et Biophysica Acta. 2015;**1847**(11):1362-1372

[42] Zheng LD et al. Mitochondrial epigenetic changes link to increased diabetes risk and early-stage prediabetes indicator. Oxidative Medicine and Cellular Longevity. 2016;**2016**:5290638

[43] Lenaz G et al. Role of mitochondria in oxidative stress and aging. Annals of the New York Academy of Sciences. 2002;**959**:199-213

[44] Sastre J et al. Mitochondria, oxidative stress and aging. Free Radical Research. 2000;**32**(3):189-198

[45] Picca A et al. Aging and calorie restriction oppositely affect mitochondrial biogenesis through TFAM binding at both origins of mitochondrial DNA replication in rat liver. PLoS One. 2013;**8**(9):e74644

[46] Barja G. Free radicals and aging. Trends in Neurosciences. 2004;**27**(10):595-600

[47] Gredilla R. DNA damage and base excision repair in mitochondria and their role in aging. Journal of Aging Research. 2010;**2011**:257093

[48] Richter C. Oxidative damage to mitochondrial DNA and its relationship to ageing. The International Journal of Biochemistry & Cell Biology. 1995;**27**(7):647-653

[49] Srivastava S. The mitochondrial basis of aging and age-related disorders. Genes. 2017; **8**(12):1-23

[50] Filburn CR et al. Mitochondrial electron transport chain activities and DNA deletions in regions of the rat brain. Mechanisms of Ageing and Development. 1996;**87**(1):35-46

[51] Kujoth GC et al. Mitochondrial DNA mutations, oxidative stress, and apoptosis in mammalian aging. Science. 2005;**309**(5733):481-484

[52] Cadenas E, Davies KJ. Mitochondrial free radical generation, oxidative stress, and aging. Free Radical Biology & Medicine. 2000;**29**(3-4):222-230

[53] Wei YH, Kao SH, Lee HC. Simultaneous increase of mitochondrial DNA deletions and lipid peroxidation in human aging. Annals of the New York Academy of Sciences. 1996;**786**:24-43

[54] Barja G. Rate of generation of oxidative stress-related damage and animal longevity. Free Radical Biology & Medicine. 2002;**33**(9):1167-1172

[55] Barnham KJ, Masters CL, Bush AI. Neurodegenerative diseases and oxidative stress. Nature Reviews. Drug Discovery. 2004;**3**(3):205-214

[56] Pham-Huy LA, He H, Pham-Huy C. Free radicals, antioxidants in disease and health. International Journal of Biomedical Sciences. 2008;**4**(2):89-96

[57] McInerny SC, Brown AL, Smith DW. Region-specific changes in mitochondrial D-loop in aged rat CNS. Mechanisms of Ageing and Development. 2009;**130**(5):343-349

[58] Takasaki S. Mitochondrial haplogroups associated with Japanese centenarians, Alzheimer's patients, Parkinson's patients, type 2 diabetic patients and healthy non-obese young males. Journal of Genetics and Genomics = Yi Chuan Xue Bao. 2009;**36**(7): 425-434

[59] Trifunovic A et al. Premature ageing in mice expressing defective mitochondrial DNA polymerase. Nature. 2004;**429**(6990):417-423

[60] Trifunovic A et al. Somatic mtDNA mutations cause aging phenotypes without affecting reactive oxygen species production. Proceedings of the National Academy of Sciences of the United States of America. 2005;**102**(50):17993-17998

[61] Borland MK et al. Chronic, low-dose rotenone reproduces Lewy neurites found in early stages of Parkinson's disease, reduces mitochondrial movement and slowly kills differentiated SH-SY5Y neural cells. Molecular Neurodegeneration. 2008;**3**:21

[62] Chomyn A, Attardi G. MtDNA mutations in aging and apoptosis. Biochemical and Biophysical Research Communications. 2003;**304**(3):519-529

[63] Kauppila JH, Stewart JB. Mitochondrial DNA: Radically free of free-radical driven mutations. Biochimica et Biophysica Acta. 2015;**1847**(11):1354-1361

[64] Kujoth GC et al. The role of mitochondrial DNA mutations in mammalian aging. PLoS Genetics. 2007;**3**(2):e24

[65] Luchsinger JA et al. Caloric intake and the risk of Alzheimer disease. Archives of Neurology. 2002;**59**(8):1258-1263

[66] Muftuoglu M, Mori MP, de Souza-Pinto NC. Formation and repair of oxidative damage in the mitochondrial DNA. Mitochondrion. 2014;**17**:164-181

[67] Spina Purrello V et al. Effect of growth factors on nuclear and mitochondrial ADP-ribosylation processes during astroglial cell development and aging in culture. Mechanisms of Ageing and Development. 2002;**123**(5):511-520

[68] DiMauro S. Mitochondrial diseases. Biochimica et Biophysica Acta. 2004;**1658**(1-2): 80-88

[69] Skuratovskaia DA et al. The association of the mitochondrial DNA oriB variants with metabolic syndrome. Biomeditsinskaia Khimiia. 2017;**63**(6):533-538

[70] Quintana A et al. Complex I deficiency due to loss of Ndufs4 in the brain results in progressive encephalopathy resembling Leigh syndrome. Proceedings of the National Academy of Sciences of the United States of America. 2010;**107**(24):10996-11001

[71] Avola R et al. Nuclear and mitochondrial DNA synthesis and energy metabolism in primary rat glial cell cultures. Neurochemical Research. 1986;**11**(6):789-800

[72] de Souza-Pinto NC et al. Mitochondrial DNA, base excision repair and neurodegeneration. DNA Repair. 2008;**7**(7):1098-1109

[73] Keogh MJ, Chinnery PF. Mitochondrial DNA mutations in neurodegeneration. Biochimica et Biophysica Acta. 2015;**1847**(11):1401-1411

[74] Reeve AK, Krishnan KJ, Turnbull D. Mitochondrial DNA mutations in disease, aging, and neurodegeneration. Annals of the New York Academy of Sciences. 2008;**1147**:21-29

[75] Bentinger M, Tekle M, Dallner G. Coenzyme Q—Biosynthesis and functions. Biochemical and Biophysical Research Communications. 2010;**396**(1):74-79

[76] Castellotti B et al. Ataxia with oculomotor apraxia type1 (AOA1): Novel and recurrent aprataxin mutations, coenzyme Q10 analyses, and clinical findings in Italian patients. Neurogenetics. 2011;**12**(3):193-201

[77] Lamperti C et al. Cerebellar ataxia and coenzyme Q10 deficiency. Neurology. 2003;**60**(7):1206-1208

[78] Krishnan KJ et al. Mitochondrial DNA mutations and aging. Annals of the New York Academy of Sciences. 2007;**1100**:227-240

[79] LeDoux SP et al. Mitochondrial DNA repair: A critical player in the response of cells of the CNS to genotoxic insults. Neuroscience. 2007;**145**(4):1249-1259

[80] Dai Y et al. Behavioral and metabolic characterization of heterozygous and homozygous POLG mutator mice. Mitochondrion. 2013;**13**(4):282-291

[81] Kraytsberg Y et al. Mitochondrial DNA deletions are abundant and cause functional impairment in aged human substantia nigra neurons. Nature Genetics. 2006;**38**(5):518-520

[82] Soong NW et al. Mosaicism for a specific somatic mitochondrial DNA mutation in adult human brain. Nature Genetics. 1992;**2**(4):318-323

[83] Kang BY et al. The 5178C/A and 16189T/C polymorphisms of mitochondrial DNA in Korean men and their associations with blood iron metabolism. Molecular Biology Reports. 2010;**37**(8):4051-4057

[84] Saxena R et al. Comprehensive association testing of common mitochondrial DNA variation in metabolic disease. American Journal of Human Genetics. 2006;**79**(1):54-61

[85] Onyango I et al. Mitochondrial genomic contribution to mitochondrial dysfunction in Alzheimer's disease. Journal of Alzheimer's Disease. 2006;**9**(2):183-193

[86] Weng SW et al. Peripheral blood mitochondrial DNA content and dysregulation of glucose metabolism. Diabetes Research and Clinical Practice. 2009;**83**(1):94-99

[87] Mecocci P, MacGarvey U, Beal MF. Oxidative damage to mitochondrial DNA is increased in Alzheimer's disease. Annals of Neurology. 1994;**36**(5):747-751

[88] Pinto M, Moraes CT. Mitochondrial genome changes and neurodegenerative diseases. Biochimica et Biophysica Acta. 2014;**1842**(8):1198-1207

[89] Scarpelli M et al. Strategies for treating mitochondrial disorders: An update. Molecular Genetics and Metabolism. 2014;**113**(4):253-260

Chapter 9

Long Noncoding Mitochondrial RNAs (LncmtRNAs) as Targets for Cancer Therapy

Jaime Villegas Olavarria, Verónica A. Burzio,
Vincenzo Borgna, Lorena Lobos-Gonzalez,
Mariela Araya, Francisca Guevara,
Claudio Villota and Luis O. Burzio

Additional information is available at the end of the chapter

http://dx.doi.org/10.5772/intechopen.75453

Abstract

Mitochondria are traditionally been viewed as the cell's powerhouse, generating most of its ATP. However, besides this fundamental metabolic role, mitochondria are implicated in diverse other processes, including apoptosis, inflammation and metastasis. These functions are exerted in part by the growing class of long noncoding mitochondrial RNAs (lncmtRNAs). We found that normal human proliferating cells express a family of noncoding mitochondrial RNAs (ncmtRNAs), comprised of sense (SncmtRNA) and antisense (ASncmtRNA). However, tumor cells express only sense transcripts, suggesting that ASncmtRNA downregulation as a cancer new hallmark. The few ASncmtRNAs copies in tumor cells seem essential to tumor cell viability: knockdown of these transcripts with antisense oligonucleotides (ASO) causes massive apoptotic death of tumor cells, preceded by cell cycle arrest. Preclinical assays show that systemic administration of ASO delayed tumor growth in melanoma and renal cancer models and, caused total remission in subcutaneous renal cancer tumors. The same treatment, however, does not affect normal tissue, suggesting this approach for the development of an efficient and safe therapeutic strategy for several cancer types.

Keywords: cancer, mitochondria, long noncoding RNAs, antisense oligonucleotides, therapy

1. Introduction

Mitochondria are eukaryotic cell organelles that represent a universal system in higher organisms which generate most of the cellular energy, in the form of ATP, necessary for different cell processes. However, many other functions have been assigned to this tiny organelle, such as apoptosis, reactive oxidative species (ROS) signaling, inflammation and metastasis. Mitochondria play a central role in apoptosis, principally due to the release of proteins from the mitochondrial inter-membrane space [1], linking mitochondria to cell suicide. Mitochondria also represent a major source of DNA-damaging reactive oxygen species (ROS), mainly as by-products of oxidative phosphorylation. In comparison to nuclear DNA, mitochondrial DNA (mtDNA) is more susceptible to DNA damage due to the reduced capacity of the cell to repair mtDNA, potentially promoting cancer [2].

In inflammation, mitochondria mainly serve as a source of various signaling molecules, termed damage-associated molecular patterns or DAMPS, which propagate inflammatory signals and therefore activate inflammation [3].

Cancer death is most often due to secondary tumors or metastasis. This process requires a complex series of events, which include epithelial-to-mesenchymal transition, stromal remodeling, invasion and ultimately migration of cancer cells. In this context, mitochondrial ROS play a key role, leading to angiogenesis and metastasis [4] and promoting the migratory plasticity of cells through activation of two essential factors, Src and protein tyrosine kinase 2 [5]. The basic understanding of the dependence of cancer cells on various mitochondrial roles is already endorsing novel therapeutic approaches in cancer.

Along that line, an expanding group of evidences indicate that the mitochondrial genome is not only responsible for the synthesis of the canonical 13 proteins, 22 tRNAs and two ribosomal RNAs (12S and 16S). Novel and expanding evidence suggest that mtDNA compensates for reduced length by using little known phenomena that potentially increase DNA's protein coding repertoire, such as so called swinger polymerization, that consists of systematic exchanges between nucleotides during DNA or RNA polymerization, producing so-called swinger sequences [6, 7]. These transformations alter gene and mRNA coding properties. Moreover, in human mitochondria systematic deletions of mono- and dinucleotides after each trinucleotide have been reported, producing delRNAs. Recently, an exhaustive analysis of human nanoLc mass spectrometry peptidome data detect numerous tetra- and pentapeptides translated from the human mitogenome, and this peptide subgroup would be the result of the translation of delRNAs. Therefore, non-canonical transcriptions and translations could considerably expand the coding potential of mitochondrial DNA and RNA sequences [8, 9].

Finally, in the field of antisense RNAs and because mitochondrial tRNA mutations are 6.5 times more frequently pathogenic than in other mitochondrial sequences, a potential additional tRNA gene function is that of templating for antisense tRNAs. Most antisense tRNAs probably function routinely in translation and extend the tRNA pool and mutation pathogenicity, probably frequently resulting from a mixture of effects due to sense and antisense tRNA translational activity for many mitochondrial tRNAs [10, 11]. These could link to mitochondrial disorders and cancer.

This small but powerful organelle is also a novel source of noncoding RNAs (ncRNAs), and growing evidence shows that mammalian mitochondria can also import/export ncRNAs, turning this organelle into a pivotal player not only in cellular physiology but also in cancer, representing potential targets for innovative ncRNA-based treatment strategies [12].

In this chapter we discuss the importance of long noncoding mitochondrial RNAs (lncmtRNAs) in diagnostic and pharmaceutical targeting in cancer.

2. Mitochondrial transcripts and noncoding RNAs

Human mitochondrial DNA (mtDNA) is a circular molecule of 16,569 bp in length [13] which encodes a small subset of 13 proteins required for OxPhos, 22 tRNAs and two ribosomal RNAs, 12S rRNA and 16S rRNA, which form part of the small (28S) and large (39S) subunits of the 55S mitoribosome [14]. All other protein components are encoded by nuclear genes and imported into mitochondria from the cytosol.

Replication and transcription of mtDNA is initiated from the D loop, a small noncoding region, and is regulated by nuclear-encoded proteins imported into mitochondria [15]. Mitochondrial RNAs are transcribed as long polycistronic precursors from both strands, termed heavy (H) and light (L) strands [16]. Except for NADH dehydrogenase 6 (ND6), all the 13-mitochondrial proteins are encoded in the H-strand. Additionally, the H-strand encodes 14 of the 22 tRNAs and the 2 rRNAs. The remaining 8 tRNAs are encoded on the L-strand [17]. The precursor transcripts are processed according to the tRNA punctuation model, whereby 22 interspersed tRNAs are excised at their 5′ and 3′ends by RNase P [18] and by RNase Z, elaC homology 2 (ELAC2), respectively, releasing simultaneously individual rRNAs and mRNAs [19]. The RNAs then undergo maturation, involving polyadenilation at the 3′eextremitoess of mRNAs and rRNAs, and specific nucleotide modifications and addition of CCA trinucleotides to the 3′eextremities of tRNAs [20]. The data of several groups indicate that 250–300 nuclear-encoded proteins are dedicated exclusively to serve mitochondrial gene expression. This includes RNA polymerase, endonucleases for RNA processing, translation factors, biogenesis factors for the mitochondrial ribosome, aminoacyl-tRNA synthetases, and other auxiliary factors [21, 22].

However, evidence has accumulated supporting the notion that, besides proteins, many types of RNAs transcribed from the nuclear genome are actively delivered to mitochondria. Among these transcripts are different types of noncoding RNAs, such as tRNAs, 5S rRNA, MRP RNA (RMRP) and RNase P RNA (RPPH1) [23], as well as microRNAs (mitomiRs) [24]. The logical explanation is that, despite their critical function, the handfuls of mitochondrial- and nuclear-encoded proteins are insufficient to maintain mitochondrial structure or activity.

Noncoding RNAs (ncRNAs) are divided in two major groups according to size, as small non-coding RNAs and long noncoding RNAs. Among the small ncRNAs, microRNAs (miRNAs) are the most-studied class in mammals. These RNAs (20–24 nucleotides in length) negatively regulate gene expression through binding with their target mRNA and have been implicated actively in pathogenic processes of many human diseases [24] and, as such, are important regulators of cancer cell metabolism [25]. The observation of association of miRNAs with/inside mitochondria may have important implications in several cellular processes and suggest that the role of mitochondria clearly extends beyond its role in energy metabolism and other cellular processes. The newfound destination of miRNAs indicates novel roles of mitochondria in normal and pathological events [25].

The class of long noncoding RNAs (lncRNAs) has been recently recognized, and is defined as transcripts longer than 200 nucleotides. The size cutoff is arbitrary and many functional lncRNAs are considerably longer than 200 nucleotides, including X-inactive specific transcript (XIST) [26], its antisense form Tsix [27], and Hox transcript antisense intergenic RNA (HOTAIR) [28], which are several kilobases (kb) in length.

LncRNAs are able to interact with DNA, RNA, and proteins. In doing so, they regulate several processes including chromatin dynamics, gene transcription, splicing, and translation [29]. Their involvement in these processes implicates lncRNAs in various aspects of human physiology and disease, which include cancer. Aberrant lncRNA expression has been associated to various cancer types [30]. Moreover, deregulated lncRNA expression patterns can modulate several hallmarks of cancer [31], including sustained growth signaling, repressed growth inhibition, apoptosis evasion, stimulated proliferation, and the promotion of angiogenesis [32].

2.1. Long noncoding RNAs are generated in the mitochondria

Both strands of the mtDNA are entirely transcribed but the light strand carries only genes for seven tRNAs and the ND6 protein. Therefore, large noncoding sequences are thus generated and released upon transcript processing. Three lncRNAs generated from mtDNA transcription have been proposed. Their presence was authenticated by Northern blot and qRT-PCR analysis. These transcripts are complementary to MTND5, MTND6 and MTCYTB genes. These molecules form intermolecular duplexes that resist RNase 1 digestion, suggesting regulation of their complementary coding mRNA. Therefore, pairing of these lncRNAs with their mRNA targets might, for instance, control translation [33].

Recently, a novel mitochondrial long noncoding RNA (mtlncRNA) was identified in the plasma of patients with left ventricular (LV) remodeling post-myocardial infarction. Levels of LIPCAR (long intergenic noncoding RNA predicting cardiac remodeling) decline in early stages after myocardial infarction, but increase in late stages, coinciding with LV remodeling. Therefore, high levels of LIPCAR associate with identified patients with high risk of heart failure, even death, suggesting that this lncmtRNA as a potential biomarker for patients with recent episodes of acute myocardial infarction [34].

In the year 2000, our laboratory described a novel chimeric mitochondrial RNA present in mouse testis and sperm cells. This transcript contained an inverted repeat of 120nt joined to the 5′ end of the 16S mitochondrial rRNA. The presence of this novel mitochondrial RNA in sperm, testis, and somatic tissues was demonstrated by RT-PCR. As to the origin of this novel RNA, one possibility was that it arose from transcription altered mtDNA which contained an insert of 121bp between the tRNAVal and the 16S rRNA genes. However, PCR of sperm, testis, liver, and blood cell mtDNA between these two genes yielded a fragment of 342bp consistent with a normal mtDNA lacking the putative insertion of 121bp. The most surprising result was the localization of this novel RNA in the sperm nucleus. In situ hybridization (ISH) demonstrated that the sequence of the 16S rRNA and that of the inverted repeat were localized in the sperm nucleus [35].

Nuclear localization of this mitochondrial transcript is not specific to mouse since, by ISH, we found that at least the sequence of the 16S rRNA was also localized in the nucleus of human sperm. To determine when during spermatogenesis the mitochondrial RNA is localized in the nucleus, ISH of mouse and human testis was carried out. The nuclei of spermatogonia, spermatocytes and round and elongated spermatids were all positively stained. In human spermatocytes, the nuclear staining pattern was fibrillar, suggesting an association of the mitochondrial transcript with the meiotic chromosomes [36].

These results suggested that the nuclear localization of the 16S mitochondrial rRNA in spermatogenic cells is the result of an intriguing process of translocation of the transcript from the organelle to the nucleus. This hypothesis leads to several important questions; for example, how does the organelle regulate the exit of the 16S mitochondrial rRNA without affecting the number of copies needed to assemble mitoribosomes for normal mitochondrial translation? Or what is the mechanism by which this RNA is exported from mitochondria? At present these questions remain unanswered.

However, the extramitochondrial localization of the 16S mitochondrial rRNA described by us is not unique, since the same transcript has been found consistently in the cytoplasm of Drosophila and Xenopus embryos [37, 38]. Moreover, injection of an anti-16S rRNA ribozyme into cleavage embryos of Drosophila demonstrated that the rRNA is actively involved in the generation of pole cells, progenitors of the germ line [39].

As mentioned above, ISH revealed that this lncRNA is over-expressed in human sperm and precursor cells [36]. These results suggest that human cells might contain a transcript with structural features similar to the mouse RNA. We found that the human RNA is over-expressed in several human proliferating cells but not in resting cells. The structure of this transcript of 2374 nt, which we designated sense noncoding mitochondrial RNA or SncmtRNA, revealed the presence of an inverted repeat (IR) of 815 nt linked to the 5′ end of the 16S mtrRNA. The expression of this transcript can be induced in resting lymphocytes stimulated with phytohaemagglutinin (PHA), together with DNA synthesis and the expression of the proliferation markers proliferating cell nuclear antigen (PCNA), Ki-67 and phosphohistone H3. On the other hand, treatment of DU145 cells with aphidicolin reversibly blocks cell proliferation as well as the expression of the ncmtRNA. These results suggested that the ncmtRNA is a new marker of cell proliferation [40].

Afterwards, we described 2 mitochondrial transcripts (ASncmtRNAs) in human cells containing stem-loop structures similar to that of the previously described SncmtRNA. Regarding expression of the SncmtRNA and the ASncmtRNAs, 3 different phenotypes of human cells can be defined. Normal proliferating cells express both families of transcripts; in striking contrast, tumor cells express the SncmtRNA and down-regulate the ASncmtRNAs. Finally, neither of these transcripts is expressed in nondividing cells. Down-regulation of the ASncmtRNAs was observed in 15 different tumor cell lines and in tumor cells present in 273 cancer biopsies corresponding to 17 different cancer types [41]. SncmtRNA is expressed in all proliferating cells, independently whether we are dealing with a regulated or a dysfunctional cell cycle. The fact that the ASncmtRNAs are always down-regulated in tumor cells suggests that, hypothetically, the ASncmtRNAs might function as a unique mitochondria-encoded tumor suppressor. **Figure 1** shows a panel of ISH for S and ASncmtRNA in non-proliferating tissue (liver), tumor tissue (cervix carcinoma) and normal proliferating tissue (normal cervix epithelium), representing the concept of differential expression mentioned. For in situ hybridization, tissue sections were incubated with hybridization mixture

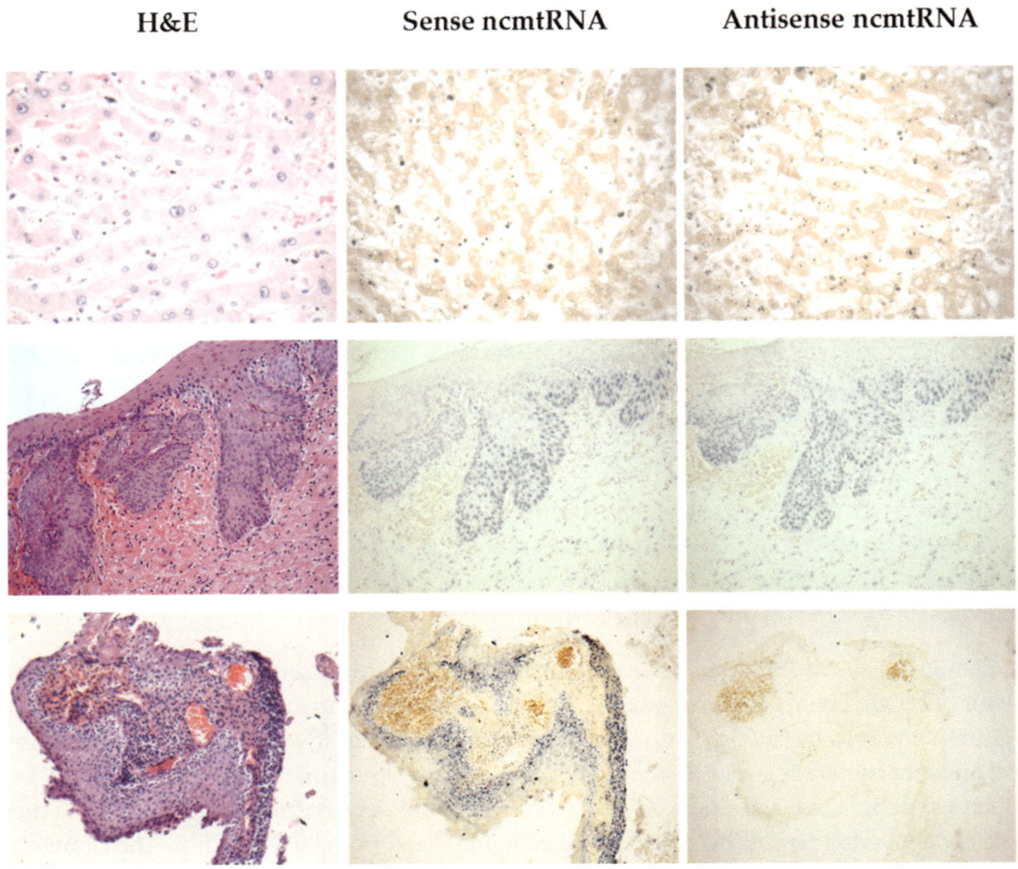

Figure 1. Representative in situ hybridization assay showing the differential expression pattern of lncmtRNAs in tissues according to proliferative status. Upper panel shows absence of signal for both RNAs in non-proliferating tissues such as liver. Middle panel shows presence of strong punctuate signal, corresponding to nuclei in normal proliferating cervix epithelium. Lower panel shows a strong signal corresponding only to SncmtRNA and complete absence of signal corresponding to ASncmtRNA in a tumor tissue, exemplified by cervix carcinoma. H&E, hematoxylin-eosin staining. Magnification in upper panel, ×200. Magnification in cervix tissues, ×100.

containing probes complementary to sense or antisense ncmtRNAs, previously labeled at the 3′ end with digoxigenin-11-dUTP (Boehringer Mannheim, Germany) as described previously [36]. For detection, sections were incubated with a monoclonal anti-digoxigenin antibody conjugated to alkaline phosphatase, and after color development, positive signal correspond to a blue color, representing the expression of the corresponding RNA (see **Figure 1**).

Regarding subcellular localization, we found that in biopsies of normal and cancer tissues, nuclear localization of these transcripts was frequently observed. The extra-mitochondrial localization of these transcripts was confirmed by electron microscopy ISH. In normal cells, SncmtRNA and the ASncmtRNAs were found in the nucleus associated to chromatin. In tumor cells, SncmtRNA shows similar localization plus association with nucleoli, while the ASncmtRNAs are down-regulated. Although the meaning of the nuclear localization in normal proliferating cells of SncmtRNA and the ASncmtRNAs is unclear, the results suggest that these transcripts might play a role in retrograde signaling. Down regulation of the ASncmtRNAs seems to be an important step in neoplastic transformation and cancer progression [42].

The study of RNA and DNA oncogenic viruses has proven valuable in the discovery of key cellular pathways that are rendered dysfunctional during cancer progression. Because of this, we studied human foreskin keratinocytes (HFK) immortalized with HPV in order to gain insight on the role of the lncmtRNAs in cell proliferation. We showed that immortalization of HFK with HPV-16 or 18 causes downregulation of the ASncmtRNAs and induces the expression of a new sense transcript termed SncmtRNA-2.

Transduction of HFK with both E6 and E7 oncoproteins is sufficient to induce expression of SncmtRNA-2. On the other hand, the E2 oncogene is involved in downregulation of the ASncmtRNAs. Knockdown of E2 in immortalized cells reestablishes in a reversible manner the expression of the ASncmtRNAs, suggesting that endogenous cellular factors(s) could play functions analogous to E2 during non-viral-induced oncogenesis [43]. Our results suggest that a fraction of SncmtRNA-1 is processed outside of the organelle, to give rise to SncmtRNA-2 and a 63-nt fragment released from the IR. In silico analysis of this sequence revealed that the 63-nt fragment is highly complementary to hsa-miR-620. Using the TargetScan algorithm (www.targetscan.com), we found >100 predictive targets for hsa-miR-620 [44]. An interesting example is the mRNA of promyelocytic leukemia (PML) protein, which is a core component of PML nuclear bodies found in tumor cells, important structures involved in HPV replication. Several reports indicate that the E6 and E7 oncoproteins are localized in these nuclear structures [45].

2.2. Differential expression of lncmtRNAs as a tool for cancer diagnostics

As mentioned above, the ASncmtRNAs are downregulated in tumor cell lines and cells in tumor biopsies, independently of the tissular origin of the tumor analyzed. Therefore, this differential expression might be used for screening of cancer cells.

Cervical cancer is the fourth most common cancer in women worldwide. In 2012, this disease accounted for 528,000 new cases and 266,000 deaths among females [46]. Cervical cancer is of slow progression and, according to histopathological studies, there are at least three well-defined stages preceding cervical squamous carcinoma, known as cervical intraepithelial neoplasia (CIN). These stages (CIN1, CIN2 and CIN3) correspond to the progressive invasion of the cervical epithelium from the basal cell layer to the surface of the squamous epithelium [47]. Therefore, detection of premalignant lesions is key to preventing disease progression to advanced stages.

Therefore, we performed a study in order to evaluate and quantify the differential expression of non-coding mitochondrial RNAs during the progression of the disease. We found down-regulation of the antisense mitochondrial transcripts at early stages of cervical neoplasia (CIN1). Moreover, differential expression of ASncmtRNA v/s S-ncmtRNA showed significant difference, while, as expected, normal proliferating tissues did not display downregulation of ASncmtRNAs. Moreover, downregulation of ASncmtRNAs correlated with the over-expression of the tumor suppressor protein p16INK-4a [48, 49].

Bladder cancer (BC) is a significant cause of morbidity and mortality with a high recurrence rate. Early detection of bladder cancer is essential in order to remove the tumor, to preserve the organ and to avoid metastasis. The "gold standard" in the detection of BC is cystoscopy. This examination, however, is unpleasant, time consuming, expensive and may result in infections and urethral damage [50]. In a pilot study, we analyzed the differential expression of SncmtRNA and ASncmtRNAs in cells isolated from voided urine from patients with bladder cancer as a noninvasive diagnostic assay. For this purpose, we developed a test based on a multiprobe mixture labeled with different fluorophores, which takes about 1 hour to complete. We examined the expression of these transcripts in cells isolated from urine of 24 patients with BC and 15 healthy donors. The samples from BC patients revealed expression of SncmtRNA and downregulation of the ASncmtRNAs. Exfoliated cells recovered from the urine of healthy donors did not express these mitochondrial transcripts. The differential expression of the SncmtRNA and the ASncmtRNAs in cells isolated from voided urine can be explored as a new non-invasive diagnostic test for bladder cancer [51].

2.3. Targeting antisense noncoding mitochondrial RNA: From bench to clinic

As mentioned before, we postulated that the ASncmtRNAs might function as a unique mitochondria-encoded tumor suppressor. Therefore, we tested whether ASncmtRNA knockdown (ASK for short) induces alteration of cancer cell function. We found, in several tumor cell lines, that knockdown of the low copy number of the ASncmtRNAs with antisense oligonucleotides (ASO) induces massive cancer cell death by apoptosis without affecting the viability of normal cells. Apoptosis is triggered or potentiated by a drastic reduction in levels of survivin, a member of the inhibitor of apoptosis (IAP) family that is overexpressed in virtually all human cancers. Down-regulation of survivin is at the post-transcriptional level and probably mediated by microRNAs generated by Dicer from the ASncmtRNAs after ASO-induced RNase H processing [52]. It is important to highlight that the ASO treatment is efficient in inducing knockdown of the ASncmtRNAs, despite the fact that it is well known that oligonucleotides are not able to enter mitochondria in vivo [53]. In consequence, the obvious question is how are these transcripts targeted by ASOs? We have demonstrated that in normal human kidneys, renal cell carcinoma, mouse testis and the murine melanoma cell line B16F10, SncmtRNA and the ASncmtRNAs exit the mitochondria and are found localized in the cytoplasm and in the nucleus [42]. Consequently, our results suggest that the functional role of these molecules lies outside the organelle. Besides cell viability, ASK also drastically reduces proliferative index, anchorage-independent growth capacity, migration and invasion [52]. Taken together, our results allow us to propose that downregulation of the ASncmtRNAs constitutes an Achilles' heel of cancer cells, suggesting that the ASncmtRNAs are promising targets for cancer therapy.

In consequence, the ultimate challenge is to translate these results to an in vivo preclinical scenario with immunocompetent mice. For this purpose, we first characterized the murine noncoding mitochondrial RNAs (mncmtRNAs), which display structures similar to the human counterparts, including long double-stranded regions arising from the presence of inverted repeats. Most remarkable however is the identical expression pattern of these transcripts in both species. The mASncmtRNAs, expressed in normal proliferating cells, are downregulated in mouse tumor cells. ASK with ASO targeted to the mASncmtRNAs induces apoptotic cell death of the highly aggressive and metastatic murine melanoma cell line B16F10 *in vitro*, concomitantly with survivin downregulation [54].

We assessed the efficacy of the ASO treatment in vivo, using a B16F10 syngeneic model in C57BL6/J, where we applied a therapeutic approach similar to the clinical practice guidelines of melanoma: surgical resection of the lesion followed by systemic administration of ASO targeted to mASncmtRNAs (1560S). Remarkably, there was no visible sign of lung or liver metastasis at 120 days since the beginning of treatment with ASO, although one cannot discard the possibility of micro-metastasis [54]. In tail vein injection lung colonization assay, ASO treatment significantly reduced the number of metastatic nodules in the lungs, as well as their size [54]. Similar results were obtained in this model with a lentiviral delivery approach of therapeutic sequences. Transduction with lentiviral constructs targeted to the ASncmtRNAs induced apoptosis in murine B16F10 and human A375 melanoma cells in vitro and significantly retarded B16F10 primary tumor growth in vivo. ASK treatment drastically reduced the number of lung metastatic foci in a tail vein injection assay, compared to controls [55]. These results provide additional proof-of-concept for knockdown of ncmtRNAs for cancer therapy and altogether, our results suggest that ASncmtRNAs could be potent targets for melanoma therapy.

In the RenCa cell line, corresponding to murine renal adenocarcinoma, we showed that ASK in vitro induces apoptosis mediated by downregulation of survivin, Bcl-2 and BclxL, the latter 2 members of another family of anti-apoptotic factors [56]. ASK also induces detrimental effects on metastatic potential, such as downregulation of N-cadherin, P-cadherin and MMP9, further strengthening the potential of this strategy for renal cell carcinoma (RCC) therapy. Remarkably, our in vivo studies in a subcutaneous syngeneic model of RenCa cells in Balb/C mice show complete reversal of tumor growth [57]. Moreover, in an orthotopic assay of murine RCC induced by injection of RenCa cells into the subcapsular region of the kidney showed that all the control mice contained tumors of different size. In contrast, only one mouse treated with the therapeutic ASO exhibited a small tumor. Histological analysis of each lung showed that control mice contained several and large metastatic nodules. In contrast, only two lungs of mice treated with therapeutical ASO contained metastatic nodules, which were significantly fewer and smaller. Finally, direct metastasis assessment by tail vein injection of RenCa cells also showed a drastic reduction in lung metastatic nodules [57].

These pre-clinical results with the RenCa and B16F10 murine models establish proof-of-concept that the ASncmtRNAs constitute a potent and selective target to develop a treatment for different types of cancer and positions this approach as an attractive strategy ready for clinical testing.

In this respect, the USA Food and Drug Administration (FDA) approved an oligonucleotide directed to the human ASncmtRNAs Andes-1537) as IND for a Phase I Clinical Trial. This study, currently under way and close to completion at UCSF, California, USA, is a first-in-human, open-label, dose escalation and expansion, 2-part study to determine the safety, tolerability, and maximum tolerated dose of Andes-1537 for Injection in patients with advanced unresectable solid tumors that are refractory to standard therapy or for which no standard therapy is available (NCT02508441). The result of this trial will be very important in order to continue with the next phase to assess the antitumoral efficacy of this therapy in human cancer patients.

3. Conclusions

Downregulation of the ASncmtRNAs has been assessed in several tumor tissues, such as bladder, prostate, kidney, ovary, cervix and breast, among others [58]. The role of these transcripts in cell proliferation and tumorigenesis is not fully understood at present. However, downregulation of the ASncmtRNAs while maintaining the expression of SncmtRNA represents a universal characteristic of tumor cells. The strong inhibition of tumor growth, induction of apoptosis and even tumor remission after knockdown of these RNAs *in vivo* is an impressive phenomenon that constitutes a unique opportunity for the development of a targeted therapy against several types of cancer. Moreover, the fact that antisense therapy does not cause side effects constitutes an attribute not observed in other kinds of therapies and opens the door to the evaluation of this approach in different kinds of solid tumors.

The mechanism by which interference of these RNAs generates cell death, apoptosis and delay in metastasis is beyond the scope of this review. However, our preliminary evidence indicates that the double strand region of the antisense RNAs is a seed for generation of miRNAs, which could target mRNAs of several proteins involved in cell cycle control, cell survival, invasion and metastasis. Therefore, knockdown of these RNAs generates a pleiotropic effect that affects simultaneously several important pathways necessary throughout the whole tumorigenic process.

Mitochondrial long noncoding RNAs are novel actors in cancer metabolism and understanding the roles they fulfill in tumor cell biology will make it possible to select in the future novel targets for the development of new therapies that could be effective and of low toxicity for patients. Our target described here meets these two requirements and at present is being evaluated in a Phase I protocol soon to finish. Those results will give the necessary data to continue with the next phase and to evaluate more in depth the efficacy of our therapy.

Acknowledgements

This work was supported by Grants FONDEF D10E1090, CCTE-PFB16 Program from CONICYT, Chile and FONDECYT 1140345.

Conflict of interest

The authors declare no conflict of interest.

Nomenclature

ASO	antisense oligonucleotide
HFK	human foreskin keratinocytes
mtDNA	mitochondrial DNA

lncmtRNA	long noncoding mitochondrial ribonucleic acid
ncRNA	noncoding ribonucleic acid
SncmtRNA	sense noncoding mitochondrial ribonucleic acid
ASncmtRNA	antisense noncoding mitochondrial ribonucleic acid

Author details

Jaime Villegas Olavarria[1,2]*, Verónica A. Burzio[1,2], Vincenzo Borgna[1,3], Lorena Lobos-Gonzalez[4], Mariela Araya[2], Francisca Guevara[1], Claudio Villota[1,5] and Luis O. Burzio[1,2]

*Address all correspondence to: jvillegas@bioschile.cl

1 Facultad de Ciencias Biológicas, Universidad Andrés Bello, Chile

2 Andes Biotechnologies SpA – Fundación Ciencia para la Vida, Chile

3 Facultad de Medicina, Universidad de Santiago, Chile

4 Centro de Medicina Regenerativa, Facultad de Medicina, Clínica Alemana Universidad del Desarrollo, Chile

5 Departamento de Ciencias Químicas y Biológicas, Facultad de Salud, Universidad Bernardo O'Higgins, Santiago, Chile

References

[1] Lopez J, Tait S. Mitochondrial apoptosis: Killing cancer using the enemy within. British Journal of Cancer. 2015;**112**:957-962. DOI: 10.1038/bjc.2015.85

[2] Giampazolias E, Tait S. Mitochondria and the hallmarks of cancer. The FEBS Journal. 2016;**283**:803-814. DOI: 10.1111/febs.13603

[3] Manfredi A, Rovere-Querini P. The mitochondrion–a Trojan horse that kicks off inflammation? The New England Journal of Medicine. 2010;**362**:2132-2134. DOI: 10.1056/NEJMcibr1003521

[4] Ishikawa K, Takenaga K, Akimoto M, Koshikawa N, Yamaguchi A, Imanishi H, Nakada K, Honma Y, Hayashi J. ROS-generating mitochondrial DNA mutations can regulate tumor cell metastasis. Science. 2008;**320**:661-664. DOI: 10.1126/science.1156906

[5] Porporato P, Payen V, Perez-Escuredo J, De Saedeleer C, Danhier P, Copetti T, Dhup S, Tardy M, Vazeille T, Bouzin C, Feron O, Michiels C, Gallez B, Sonveaux P. A mitochondrial switch promotes tumor metastasis. Cell Reports. 2014;**8**:754-766. DOI: 10.1016/j.celrep.2014.06.043

[6] Seligmann H. Chimeric mitochondrial peptides from contiguous regular and swinger RNA. Computational and Structural Biotechnology Journal. 2016;**14**:283-297. DOI: 10.1016/j.csbj.2016.06.005

[7] Seligmann H. Swinger RNAs with sharp switches between regular transcription and transcription systematically exchanging ribonucleotides: Case studies. Bio Systems. 2015; **135**:1-8. DOI: 10.1016/j.biosystems.2015.07.003

[8] Seligmann H. Codon expansion and systematic transcriptional deletions produce tetra-, pentacoded mitochondrial peptides. Journal of Theoretical Biology. 2015;**38**:154-165. DOI: 10.1016/j.jtbi.2015.09.030

[9] Seligmann H. Systematically frameshifting by deletion of every 4th or 4th and 5th nucleotides during mitochondrial transcription: RNA self-hybridization regulates delRNA expression. Bio Systems. 2016;**142**:43-51. DOI: 10.1016/j.biosystems.2016.03.00

[10] Seligmann H. Undetected antisense tRNAs in mitochondrial genomes? Biology Direct. 2010;**5**:39. DOI: 10.1186/1745-6150-5-39

[11] Seligmann H. Pathogenic mutations in antisense mitochondrial tRNAs. Journal of Theoretical Biology. 2011;**269**:287-296. DOI: 10.1016/j.jtbi.2010.11.007

[12] Vendramin R, Marine JC, Leucci E. Non-coding RNAs: The dark side of nuclear-mitochondrial communication. The EMBO Journal. 2017;**36**:1123-1133. DOI: 10.15252/embj.201695546

[13] Anderson S, Bankier A, Barrell B, de Bruijn M, Coulson A, Drouin J, Eperon I, Nierlich D, Roe B, Sanger F, Schreier P, Smith A, Staden R, Young G. Sequence and organization of the human mitochondrial genome. Nature. 1981;**290**:457-465. DOI: 10.1038/290457a0

[14] O'Brien T. Evolution of a protein-rich mitochondrial ribosome: Implications for human genetic disease. Gene. 2002;**286**:73-79. DOI: 10.1016/S0378-1119(01)00808-3

[15] Pearce S, Rebelo-Guiomar P, D'Souza A, Powell C, Van Haute L, Minczuk M. Regulation of mammalian mitochondrial gene expression: Recent advances. Trends in Biochemical Sciences. 2017;**42**:625-639. DOI: 10.1016/j.tibs.2017.02.003

[16] Ojala D, Montoya J, Attardi G. tRNA punctuation model of RNA processing in human mitochondria. Nature. 1981;**290**:470-474. DOI: 10.1038/290470a0

[17] Dakubo G. Enigmatic biomolecules from the mitochondrial genome. Biological Systems: Open Access. 2015;**4**:137. DOI: 10.4172/2329-6577.1000137

[18] Holzmann J, Frank P, Loffler E, Bennett KL, Gerner C, Rossmanith W. RNase P without RNA: Identification and functional reconstitution of the human mitochondrial tRNA processing enzyme. Cell. 2008;**135**:462-474. DOI: 10.1016/j.cell.2008.09.013

[19] Lopez Sanchez M, Mercer T, Davies S, Shearwood A-M, Nygård K, Richman T, Mattick J, Rackham O, Filipovska A. RNA processing in human mitochondria. Cell Cycle. 2011;**10**: 1-13. DOI: 10.4161/cc.10.17.17060

[20] Nagaike T, Suzuki T, Katoh T, Ueda T. Human mitochondrial mRNAs are stabilized with polyadenylation regulated by mitochondria-specific poly(a) polymerase and polynucleotide phosphorylase. The Journal of Biological Chemistry. 2005;**280**:19721-19727. DOI: 10.1074/jbc.M500804200

[21] Calvo S, Clauser K, Mootha V. MitoCarta2.0: An updated inventory of mammalian mitochondrial proteins. Nucleic Acids Research. 2016;**44**:D1251-D1257. DOI: 10.1093/nar/gkv1003

[22] Smith A, Robinson A. MitoMiner v3.1, an update on the mitochondrial proteomics database. Nucleic Acids Research. 2016;**44**:D1258-D12561. DOI: 10.1093/nar/gkv1001

[23] Kim K, Noh J, Abdelmohsen K, Gorospe M. Mitochondrial noncoding RNA transport. BMB Reports. 2017;**50**:164-174. DOI: 10.5483/BMBRep.2017.50.4.013

[24] Sripada L, Tomar D, Prajapati P, Singh R, Singh AK, Singh R. Systematic analysis of small RNAs associated with human mitochondria by deep sequencing: Detailed analysis of mitochondrial associated miRNA. PLoS One. 2012;**7**:e44873. DOI: 10.1371/journal.pone.0044873

[25] Zhang L, Jiang S, Liu M. MicroRNA regulation and analytical methods in cancer cell metabolism. Cellular and Molecular Life Sciences. 2017;**74**:2929-2941. DOI: 10.1007/s00294-017-0744-1

[26] Richler C, Soreq H, Wahrman J. X-inactivation in mammalian testis is correlated with inactive X-specific transcription. Nature Genetics. 1992;**2**:192-195. DOI: 10.1038/ng1192-192

[27] Barakat T, Gribnau J. X chromosome inactivation in the cycle of life. Development. 2012;**139**:2085-2089. DOI: 10.1242/dev.069328

[28] Rinn J, Kertesz M, Wang J, Squazzo S, Xu X, Brugmann S, Goodnough L, Helms J, Farnham P, Segal E, Chang H. Functional demarcation of active and silent chromatin domains in human HOX loci by noncoding RNAs. Cell. 2007;**129**:1311-1323. DOI: 10.1016/j.cell.2007.05.022

[29] Hu W, Alvarez-Dominguez J, Lodish H. Regulation of mammalian cell differentiation by long non-coding RNAs. EMBO Reports. 2012;**13**:971-983. DOI: 10.1038/embor.2012.145

[30] Yang Y, Chen L, Gu J, Zhang H, Yuan J, Lian Q, Lv G, Wang S, Wu Y, Yang YT, Wang D, Liu Y, Tang J, Luo G, Li Y, Hu L, Sun X, Wang D, Guo M, Xi Q, Xi J, Wang H, Zhang M, Lu Z. Recurrently deregulated lncRNAs in hepatocellular carcinoma. Nature Communications. 2017;**8**:e14421. DOI: 10.1038/ncomms14421

[31] Hanahan D, Weinberg R. Hallmarks of cancer: The next generation. Cell. 2011;**144**:646-674. DOI: 10.1016/j.cell.2011.02.013

[32] Huarte M. The emerging role of lncRNAs in cancer. Nature Medicine. 2015;**21**:1253-1261. DOI: 10.1038/nm.3981

[33] Rackham O, Shearwood A-M, Mercer T, Davies S, Mattick J, Filipovska A. Long noncoding RNA are generated from the mitochondrial genome and regulated by nuclear-encoded proteins. RNA. 2011;**17**:2058-2093. DOI: 10.1261/rna.029405.111

[34] Kumarswamy R, Bauters C, Volkmann I, Maury F, Fetisch J, Holzmann A, Lemesle G, de Groote P, Pinet F, Thum T. Circulating long noncoding RNA, LIPCAR, predicts survival

in patients with heart failure. Circulation Research. 2014;**114**:1569-1575. DOI: 10.1161/CIRCRESAHA.114.303915

[35] Villegas J, Zarraga AM, Muller I, Montecinos L, Werner E, Brito M, Meneses AM, Burzio LO. A novel chimeric mitochondrial RNA localized in the nucleus of mouse sperm. DNA and Cell Biology. 2000;**19**:579-588. DOI: 10.1089/104454900439809

[36] Villegas J, Araya P, Bustos-Obregon E, Burzio LO. Localization of the 16S mitochondrial rRNA in the nucleus of mammalian spermatogenic cells. Molecular Human Reproduction. 2002;**8**:977-983. DOI: 10.1093/molehr/8.11.977

[37] Kobayashi S, Amikura R, Okada M. Presence of mitochondrial large ribosomal RNA outside mitochondria in germ plasm of Drosophila melanogaster. Science. 1993;**260**:1521-1524. DOI: 10.1126/science.7684857

[38] Kobayashi S, Amikura R, Mukai M. Localization of mitochondrial large ribosomal RNA in germ plasm of Xenopus embryos. Current Biology. 1998;**8**:1117-1120. DOI: 10.1016/S0960-9822(98)70466-X

[39] Iida T, Kobayashi S. Essential role of mitochondrially encoded large rRNA for germ-line formation in drosophila embryos. Proceedings of the National Academy of Sciences of the United States of America. 1998;**95**:11274-11278. DOI: 10.1073/pnas.95.19.11274

[40] Villegas J, Burzio V, Villota C, Landerer E, Martinez R, Santander M, Martinez R, Pinto R, Vera MI, Boccardo E, Villa LL, Burzio LO. Expression of a novel non-coding mitochondrial RNA in human proliferating cells. Nucleic Acids Research. 2007;**35**:7336-7347. DOI: 10.1093/nar/gkm863

[41] Burzio VA, Villota C, Villegas J, Landerer E, Boccardo E, Villa LL, Martinez R, Lopez C, Gaete F, Toro V, Rodriguez X, Burzio LO. Expression of a family of noncoding mitochondrial RNAs distinguishes normal from cancer cells. Proceedings of the National Academy of Sciences. 2009;**106**:9430-9434. DOI: 10.1073/pnas.0903086106

[42] Landerer E, Villegas E, Burzio VA, Oliveira L, Villota C, Lopez C, Restovic F, Martinez R, Castillo O, Burzio LO. Nuclear localization of the mitochondrial ncRNAs in normal and cancer cells. Cellular Oncology. 2011;**34**:297-305. DOI: 10.1007/s13402-011- 0018-8

[43] Villota C, Campos A, Vidaurre S, Oliveira-Cruz L, Boccardo E, Burzio VA, Varas M, Villegas J, Villa LL, Valenzuela PD, Socías M, Roberts S, Burzio LO. Expression of mitochondrial non-coding RNAs (ncRNAs) is modulated by high risk human papillomavirus (HPV) oncogenes. The Journal of Biological Chemistry. 2012;**287**:21303-21315. DOI: 10.1074/jbc.M111.326694

[44] Lewis B, Burge C, Barte, D. Conserved seed pairing, often flanked by adenosines, indicates that thousands of human genes are microRNA target. Cell. 2005;**120**:15-20. DOI: http://dx.doi.org/10.1016/j.cell.2004.12.035

[45] Bischof O, Nacerddine K, Dejean A. Human papillomavirus oncoprotein E7 targets the promyelocytic leukemia protein and circumvents cellular senescence via the Rb and p53 tumor suppressor pathways. Molecular and Cellular Biology. 2005;**25**:1013-1024. DOI: 10.1128/MCB.25.3.1013-1024.2005

[46] Siegel R, Ma J, Zou Z, Jemal A. Cancer statistics, 2014. CA: a Cancer Journal for Clinicians. 2014;**64**:9-29. DOI: 10.3322/caac.21208

[47] Tierney B, Westin SN, Schlumbrecht MP, Ramirez P. Early cervical neoplasia: Advances in screening and treatment modalities. Clinical Advances in Hematology & Oncology. 2010;**8**:547-555

[48] Villegas J, Dadlani K, Avila R, Villota C, Burzio V, Lopez C, Socias M, Zapata L, Burzio LO. The mitochondrial antisense ncRNAs are down-regulated in early cervical carcinoma. Journal of Cancer Science and Therapy. 2013;**S7**:004. DOI: 10.4172/1948-5956.S7-004

[49] Dadlani K, Lopez C, Gabler F, Roa JC, Villota C, Lina-Villa L, Boccardo E, Bustamante E, Burzio V, Burzio LO, Villegas J. Assessment of the expression of long noncoding mitochondrial RNAs (lncmtRNAs) during cervical cancer progression and cervical carcinoma. Journal of Cancer Science and Therapy. 2016;**8**:038-045. DOI: 10.4172/1948-5956.1000386

[50] Van Tilborg A, Bangma C, Zwarthoff E. Bladder cancer biomarkers and their role in surveillance and screening. International Journal of Urology. 2009;**16**:23-30. DOI: 10.1111/j.1442-2042.2008.02174.x

[51] Rivas A, Burzio V, Landerer E, Borgna V, Gatica S, Ávila R, López C, Villota C, de la Fuente R, Echenique J, Burzio LO, Villegas J. Determination of the differential expression of mitochondrial long non-coding RNAs as a noninvasive diagnosis of bladder cancer. BMC Urology 2012;**12**:37. DOI: 10.1186/1471-2490-12-37

[52] Vidaurre S, Fitzpatrick C, Burzio V, Briones M, Villota C, Villegas J, Echenique J, Oliveira-Cruz L, Araya M, Borgna V, Socías T, Lopez C, Avila R, Burzio LO. Down-regulation of the antisense mitochondrial non-coding RNAs (ncRNAs) is a unique vulnerability of cancer cells and a potential target for cancer therapy. The Journal of Biological Chemistry. 2014;**289**:27182-27198. DOI: 10.1074/jbc.M114.558841

[53] Ross M, Filipovska A, Smith R, Gait M, Murphy M. Cell-penetrating peptides do not cross mitochondrial membranes even when conjugated to a lipophilic cation: Evidence against direct passage through phospholipid bilayers. The Biochemical Journal. 2004;**383**:457-468. DOI: 10.1042/BJ20041095

[54] Lobos-González L, Silva V, Araya M, Restovic F, Echenique J, Oliveira-Cruz L, Fitzpatrick C, Briones M, Villegas J, Villota C, Vidaurre S, Borgna V, Socias M, Valenzuela S, Lopez C, Socias T, Varas M, Díaz J, Burzio LO, Burzio V. Targeting antisense mitochondrial ncRNAs inhibits murine melanoma tumor growth and metastasis through reduction in survival and invasion factors. Oncotarget. 2016;**7**:58331-58350. DOI: 10.18632/oncotarget.11110

[55] Varas-Godoy M, Lladser A, Farfan N, Villota C, Villegas J, Tapia JC, Burzio LO, Burzio VA, Valenzuela PDT. In vivo knockdown of antisense non-coding mitochondrial RNAs by a lentiviral-encoded shRNA inhibits melanoma tumor growth and lung colonization. Pigment Cell & Melanoma Research. 2018;(1):64-72. DOI: 10.1111/pcmr.12615

[56] Besbes S, Mirshahi M, Pocard M, Billard C. New dimension in therapeutic targeting of BCL-2 family proteins. Oncotarget. 2015;**6**:12862-12871. DOI: 10.18632/oncotarget.3868

[57] Borgna V, Villegas J, Burzio V, Belmar S, Araya M, Jeldes E, Lobos-González L, Silva V, Villota C, Oliveira-Cruz L, Lopez C, Socias T, Castillo O, Burzio LO. Mitochondrial ASncmtRNA-1 and ASncmtRNA-2 as potent targets to inhibit tumor growth and metastasis in the RenCa murine renal adenocarcinoma model. Oncotarget. 2017;**8**:43692-43708. DOI: 10.18632/oncotarget.18460

[58] Borgna V, Lobos-González L, Burzio V, Araya M, Avila R, Jeldes E, Silva V, Briones M, Socias T, Guevara F, López C, Villota C, Bustamante E, Bendek M, Fitzpatrick C, Burzio LO, Villegas J. Non-coding mitochondrial RNAs (ncmtRNAs) in gynecological and urinary malignancies: Universal targets for development of and efficient therapy? In: Watanabe HS, editor. Horizons in Cancer Research. Vol. 65. New York: Nova Science Publisher, Inc; 2017. pp. 91-117

Chapter 10

Mitochondrial DNA Variations in Tumors: Drivers or Passengers?

Edoardo Errichiello and Tiziana Venesio

Additional information is available at the end of the chapter

http://dx.doi.org/10.5772/intechopen.75188

Abstract

Mitochondrial DNA alterations, including point mutations, deletions, inversions and copy number variations, have been widely reported in many age-related degenerative diseases and tumors. However, numerous studies investigating their pathogenic role in cancer have provided inconsistent evidence. Furthermore, biological impacts of mitochondrial DNA variants vary tremendously, depending on the proportion of mutant DNA molecules carried by the neoplastic cells (the so-called heteroplasmy). The recent discovery of inter-genomic crosstalk between nucleus and mitochondria has reinforced the role of mitochondrial DNA variants in perturbing this essential signaling pathway and thus indirectly targeting nuclear genes involved in tumorigenic and invasive phenotype. Therefore, mitochondrial dysfunction is currently considered a crucial hallmark of carcinogenesis as well as a promising target for anticancer therapy. This chapter describes the role of different types of mitochondrial DNA alterations by mainly considering the paradigmatic model of colorectal carcinogenesis and, in particular, it revisits the issue of whether mitochondrial mutations are causative cancer drivers or simply genuine passenger events. The advent of high-throughput next-generation sequencing techniques, as well as the development of genetic and pharmaceutical interventions for the treatment of mitochondrial dysfunction in cancer, are also discussed.

Keywords: mitochondrial DNA variants, heteroplasmy, nuclear-mitochondrial crosstalk, oxidative stress, mtDNA copy number alterations, D-loop, cancer therapy, mitogenomics

1. Introduction

Mitochondria are highly dynamic organelles whose biogenesis and functions are tightly regulated by the nucleus through a constant bidirectional crosstalk. Indeed, only about 1%

of mitochondrial proteins are encoded by mitochondrial DNA (mtDNA), with all the others encoded by the nuclear genome, including proteins involved in mtDNA replication and transcription [1].

The human mtDNA is a small circular double-stranded DNA molecule of approximately 16.6 kb that encodes for 2 ribosomal RNAs (12S and 16S), 22 transfer RNAs required for protein synthesis and 13 essential protein subunits of the oxidative phosphorylation system (OXPHOS) (**Figure 1**) [2]. The electron transport chain, the primary metabolic pathway which generates energy in the form of ATP, is composed of five protein complexes (I–V) localized in the inner membrane of mitochondria, including complex II that is exclusively coded by the nuclear genome. This system includes seven subunits of respiratory enzyme complex I, one subunit of complex III, three subunits of complex IV and two subunits of complex V. As mentioned before, all other mitochondrial proteins, including those involved in mtDNA replication, transcription and translation, are encoded by nuclear genes and are targeted to the mitochondrion by specific transport systems. The discovery of over 2000 mitochondrial small non-coding RNAs (mitosRNAs), playing a pivotal role in the control of normal mitochondrial gene expression, revealed an underestimated level of mitochondrial functional complexity [3]. Furthermore, studies on antisense anti-termination tRNAs and delRNAs shed new light on novel mechanisms expanding the coding potential of mitogenome [4, 5].

Byproducts of the electron transport chain (ETC) constantly generate reactive oxygen species (ROS) that may severely damage the mitochondrial DNA. If not efficiently repaired, the accumulation of oxidative lesions in the mtDNA molecules lead to gradual mitochondrial dysfunction, which is reflected in changes in the number, morphology and functioning of mitochondria, as observed in cancer cells [6].

mtDNA is more susceptible to mutations than nuclear DNA, due to the lack of histones and chromatin protective structures, paucity of introns, less efficient mtDNA repair mechanisms and a higher exposure to deleterious ROS generated during ATP synthesis within the mitochondrial compartment [7].

Although low levels of intracellular ROS normally regulate cellular signaling and are essential for normal cell survival and proliferation, aberrant ROS production is frequently observed in neoplastic cells. In the mitochondrial free radical theory of aging accumulation of damaging mtDNA mutations, impairment of oxidative phosphorylation as well as an imbalance in the expression of antioxidant enzymes results in exponential overproduction of ROS. This elicited condition forms a "vicious cycle" that is the basis of a wide range of pathologies, termed as "free radical diseases" such as cancer, neurodegeneration, atherosclerosis, diabetes mellitus and chronic inflammation [8]. Importantly, besides the obvious induction of oxidative nucleotide damage to mtDNA, ROS promotes tumorigenesis through several other mechanisms, including stabilization of hypoxia-inducible factor (HIF)-α, increased calcium flux, inactivation of key phosphatases, such as Pten and PP2A, and activation of both the NRF2 and NF-κB transcription factors [9–11].

Since the Warburg theory of cancer postulated in 1956 [12], mitochondrial dysfunction has been regarded as a hallmark of cancer progression and as a promising target for anticancer t herapies [13, 14]. For instance, enhancing complex I activity has been demonstrated to inhibit tumorigenicityandmetastasisofbreastcancercells[15].Morerecently,mitochondrialdysfunction

http://dx.doi.org/10.5772/intechopen.75188

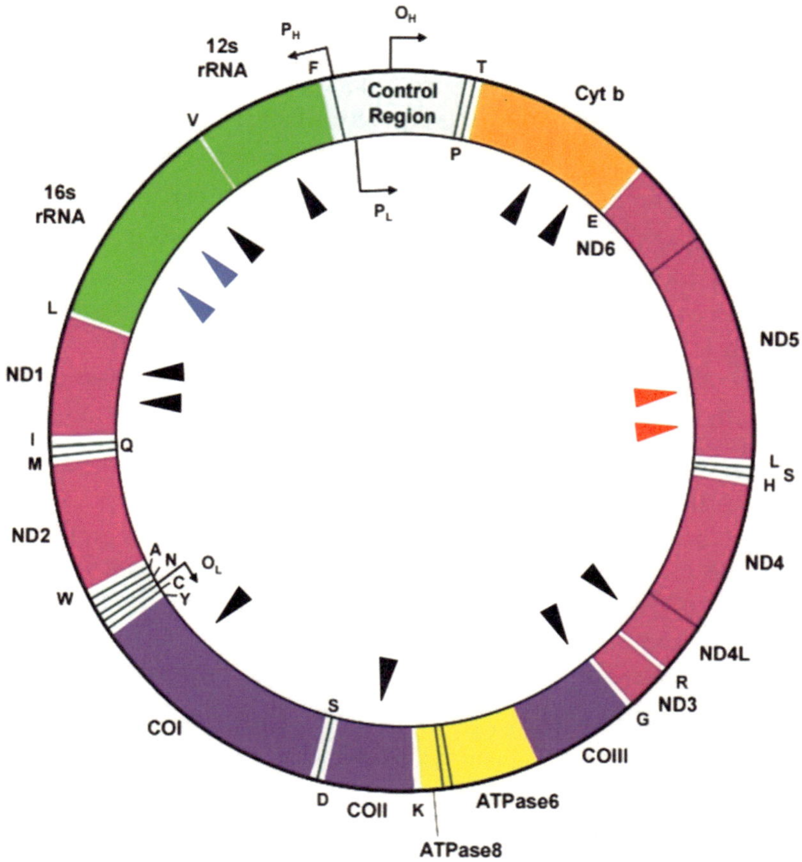

Figure 1. Map of the human mitochondrial DNA and distribution of somatic variants in colorectal cancer. mtDNA somatic mutations are mainly represented by homoplasmic alterations (black arrowheads), although rarer heteroplasmic substitutions (blue arrowheads) have been detected in the MT-RNR2 (16S) region or mixed homoplasmic/heteroplasmic variants (red arrowheads) in the MT-ND5 locus.

has also been associated with a crucial step for tumorigenesis, that is, epithelial-to-mesenchymal transition (EMT), enabling cancer dissemination and metastatic spread [16]. Importantly, mtDNA alterations may also disrupt the inter-genomic crosstalk between nucleus and mitochondrion and is associated with increased oxidative stress, ROS and cytosolic calcium accumulation, reduction of cell ATP levels and an imbalance in the NADH/NAD+ ratio. Moreover, ROS-induced oxidative stress may also affect the expression of nuclear genes involved in tumorigenic and invasive phenotypes, as it has been shown in colorectal cancer cells [17].

2. mtDNA alterations: a focus on colorectal carcinogenesis

2.1. Somatic mtDNA variants

Cancer is caused by the accumulation of multiple genetic alterations, such as point mutations, copy number variations (CNVs), inversions and epigenetic modifications [18]. This multi-step process has been depicted in detail for colorectal cancer, which represents an ideal paradigm of tumorigenesis. In 1990, Fearon and Vogelstein [19] postulated a multi-step model of colorectal carcinogenesis, the long established "adenoma-carcinoma sequence", in which the inactivation of the APC tumor-suppressor gene occurs first in normal colonic epithelial cells, followed by activating mutations in the KRAS gene and subsequent additional alterations in other tumor-suppressor genes, such as TP53 and TGF-β pathway genes.

Accumulating evidence emphasizes the functional role of mtDNA abnormalities in mitochondrial dysfunction and colorectal carcinogenesis. In a whole-genome comparative study of five different tumors, it has been demonstrated that the frequencies of deleterious non-synonymous somatic variants vary tremendously across tumor types, with the higher frequency (63%) in colorectal adenocarcinomas [20]. The vast majority of these mtDNA variants were represented by G > A and C > T transitions, the typical molecular fingerprint due to oxidative stress in mtDNA [21].

Thus far, mtDNA variants have been found to affect different regions with an essential role in mitochondrial protein synthesis machinery and oxidative phosphorylation (**Figure 1**) [22–24]. Importantly, it has been shown that mtDNA mutations may generate unprocessed transcripts by precluding RNA processing that impair mitochondrial biogenesis and energy maintenance [25, 26]. It is noteworthy to mention that mtDNA variants not only affect genes directly involved in the ETC, but also genes related to mitochondrial metabolism, such as tRNA genes, in which pathogenic mutations are 6.5 times more frequent than in other mitochondrial loci [27, 28].

MUTHY-associated polyposis (MAP) patients carry a significant increase of non-synonymous changes in conserved amino acid residues of the MT-CO_2 gene, particularly the hotspot m.7763G > A transition [29]. Nevertheless, there is no compelling evidence in the literature propending for a single common coding-region mtDNA variant or haplogroup that may strongly influence the risk of developing a colorectal adenocarcinoma. Alternatively, it is likely that mtDNA alterations influencing colorectal cancer risk may be in the form of heteroplasmic low frequency variants, possibly restricted to specific subsets of patients with colorectal cancer [30]. Curiously, it has been demonstrated that mutations disrupting the respiratory complex I in pituitary adenomas are somatic modifiers of tumorigenesis associated with less aggressive and genome-stable oncocytic lesions [31].

It is commonly believed that mtDNA variants arise due to positive selection of those "driver" variants conferring clonal growth advantage. Accordingly, we observed that likely non-pathogenic mtDNA variants ("passengers") reverted to the wild-type homoplasmic status during tumor progression in colorectal cancer patients [29]. On the contrary, the mtDNA variants that are positively selected during tumor progression might be considered the most tolerable alterations for neoplastic cells. However, a deleterious impact of mtDNA passenger variants on cancer progression may not be completely excluded, as it has been previously evidenced in nuclear DNA passenger alterations [32].

2.2. Mitochondrial DNA heteroplasmy

Mitochondrial DNA heteroplasmy has been involved in a large spectrum of human diseases. Beside classical mitochondrial diseases, such as mitochondrial myopathy, myoclonic epilepsy with ragged red fibers, and mitochondrial encephalomyopathy, lactic acidosis, and stroke-like episodes (MELAS), mitochondrial heteroplasmy also plays a pivotal role in complex disorders, including type 2 diabetes mellitus, late-onset neurodegenerative diseases and cancer [30].

mtDNA variants are maternally-inherited or arise as *de novo* somatic mutations in a fraction (heteroplasmic) or all (homoplasmic) mitochondrial genomes within each cell containing hundreds of copies of mtDNA molecules. Over time, the proportion of the mutant mtDNA within the cell may vary and drift toward predominantly mutant or wild-type form to achieve homoplasmy. Accordingly, the biological impact of a mtDNA variant may fluctuate, depending on the proportion of mutant mtDNA molecules carried by the neoplastic cell. Moreover, the level of heteroplasmy increases significantly with age and may vary between tissues and ethnic groups [33, 34]. By using high-throughput sequencing technology, Guo et al. [35] showed that very low heteroplasmy variants, down to almost 0.1%, are generally inherited from the mother, thus implying their likely neutral effect, and that this inheritance begins to decrease at about 0.5%. Accordingly, it has been demonstrated that high heteroplasmic mtDNA mutation loads, generally above 80%, are required to trigger substantial dysfunctions in the oxidative phosphorylation process. For instance, the m.3571insC mutation in the MTND1 gene of respiratory complex I is commonly detected in oncocytic tumors, in which it causes a severe mitochondrial dysfunction when mutant load is above 83% [36]. Importantly, this mitochondrial threshold effect strictly regulates the balance between tumor growth and suppression [37]. Interestingly, low-level mitochondrial heteroplasmies are commonly found in healthy individuals, and the advent of next-generation sequencing (NGS) technologies revealed that 25–65% of the general population harbor at least one heteroplasmic variant across the entire mitochondrial genome [38, 39]. By studying human colorectal cancer cell lines, Polyak et al. [40] showed that the vast majority of mutations were ROS-related homoplasmic transitions, indicating that mtDNA molecules could rapidly become homogeneous under high clonal selection conditions. Nevertheless, several other *in vivo* studies demonstrated that mtDNA heteroplasmy is far more common in colorectal neoplasms [41–43]. As occasionally observed in the case of revertant mosaicism, a naturally occurring phenomenon involving spontaneous correction of a pathogenic mutation in a somatic cell, heteroplasmic somatic variants may also naturally revert to wild-type homoplasmy [44, 45].

2.3. mtDNA copy number alterations

Epidemiological studies have indicated significant association of leukocyte mtDNA copy number with risk of several malignancies, including glioma, colorectal and breast tumors, and its use has been proposed as a potential biomarker to select patients who benefit from adjuvant chemotherapy [46–50]. A reduced mtDNA content has also been correlated with lymph node metastasis and lower survival rates in patients with colorectal cancer [51].

In the past years, it has been demonstrated that mtDNA depletion leads to tumorigenesis by inducing changes in the redox status, membrane potential, ATP levels, gene expression, nucleotide pools, and increased chromosomal instability (e.g. translocations) [52, 53]. However, other findings reported a gain of mtDNA copy number, thus suggesting that mtDNA replication could be increased to compensate for detrimental metabolic effects caused by mtDNA variations and/or oxidative stress [54]. These conflicting data may be partly explained by the non-homogeneous timing of blood DNA analyses for mtDNA copy number determination. Interestingly, depletion of mtDNA results in significant changes in methylation patterns of a number of nuclear-encoded genes, and these epigenetic modifications are reversed by the restoration of mtDNA content [55].

The molecular mechanism altering mtDNA copy number is still under investigation. In a study of 65 colorectal cancers, it has been suggested that hypomethylation of specific sites on CpG islands of the D-loop promoter may be involved in the regulation of mtDNA copy numbers [56]. Moreover, it has been reported that polymorphisms within the nuclear-encoded polymerase gamma gene (POLG), which codifies for a key component of the mitochondrial genome maintenance machinery, may lead to a decrease in mtDNA content and mitochondrial dysfunction [57]. Curiously, a homozygous polymorphic insertion (AluYb8MUTYH) in the 15th intron of the MUTYH base excision repair gene has been associated with a significant reduction of the type 1 MUTYH protein that localizes to mitochondria as well as lowered mtDNA content in age-related diseases [58]. Since biallelic mutations of MUTYH are associated with the MAP syndrome, it might be speculated that homozygous or compound heterozygous MUTYH variants may correlate with the mtDNA content in colorectal cancer [30].

2.4. D-loop and mitochondrial instability

The non-coding D-loop region contains essential transcription and replication elements and is formed by two hypervariable regions, namely HV-I (nt. 16,024–16,383) and HV-II (nt. 57–333) [59]. The latter includes the D310 sequence, a polycytidine repeat (nt. 303–309), which is essential for mtDNA replication in virtue of the H-strand replication origin. Replication of the leading strand initiates at the origin of H-strand synthesis and proceeds unidirectionally, displacing the parental H-strand as single-stranded DNA [60]. The D-loop is a well-known hotspot for somatic mutations in many types of cancer, with a mutation rate 100- to 200-fold higher than nuclear DNA. This finding may be partly explained by considering the direct relationship between mutational frequency and single-strandedness during mitochondrial replication [61].

mtDNA variants in the D-loop region have been repeatedly associated with risk and survival rates in cancer patients and, thus, they have been proposed as valuable prognostic markers. However, it has been argued that most of these studies could be biased due to artifacts related to genotyping errors or inadequate experimental design [62]. Mitochondrial microsatellite instability (mtMSI), that is a change in length in the repetitive sequences of the D-loop segment between normal and tumor tissues, has been described as a frequent molecular event in different cancers, but its prognostic value is still debated [63]. The variation of the homopolymeric tract length mainly arises through replication slippage of mitochondrial DNA polymerase and, importantly, this process may affect mtDNA replication and transcription. Intriguingly, the oxidative damage to mitochondrial polymerase γ may also contribute to the alteration in the length of the polycytidine repeat by impacting on mtDNA replication [64].

Instability of the D-loop hypervariable region-II (HV-II) has been associated with variants specifically grouped inside the MT-CO_2 gene in MAP patients, thus suggesting that genome instability might contribute to drive non-random accumulation of MT-CO_2 variants in the early stages of MAP colorectal tumorigenesis [29]. Therefore, D-loop mutations probably do not directly drive carcinogenesis but are more likely an epiphenomenon, used as a universal clonal marker ("molecular clock") to estimate the relative mitotic history of tumors [65, 66].

3. Mitochondrial-nuclear crosstalk

Tight coordination between the nucleus and mitochondria is required for proper mitochondrial functioning and includes both anterograde (nucleus to mitochondria) and retrograde (mitochondria to nucleus) signals. This crosstalk is critical for the maintenance of cellular homeostasis, and accumulated mtDNA variants may perturb this subtle pathway [67]. It has been demonstrated that somatically acquired mitochondrial-nuclear genome fusion sequences are present in human cancer cells [68]. Although most of the genes encoding proteins of the OXPHOS machinery are transcribed in the nucleus (anterograde signaling), mitochondria may also exert retrograde regulatory control over the nucleus in terms of nuclear gene expression modulation [69]. This phenomenon suggests a strong association between nuclear and mitochondrial DNA alterations in driving tumor development and progression. Variants in nuclear-encoded mitochondrial genes, such as fumarate hydratase, iso-citrate dehydrogenase and succinate dehydrogenase) have been associated with a wide variety of human cancers, such as paragangliomas, uterine leiomyomas, renal carcinomas, breast cancers, gastrointestinal stromal cancers, leukemia, prostate cancer, glioblastomas and colorectal carcinomas [70–78]. Furthermore, it has been demonstrated that mtDNA changes and MAPK pathway alterations synergize to drive colorectal malignant transformation [79].

In a study on colorectal adenoma and adenocarcinoma samples, an increased number of mutations in nuclear genes encoding proteins involved in critical mitochondrial processes, such as fusion, fission and localization were found [80]. It has also been suggested that mtDNA depletion may disrupt crucial nuclear processes, leading to centrosome amplification and mitotic spindle multipolarity, both participating in cancer cell transformation [81, 82]. mtDNA variants have the potential to induce molecular signals through the mitochondrial-nuclear crosstalk mechanism, thereby promoting nuclear compensation in response to mitochondrial malfunction [67]. Interestingly, some typical nuclear transcription factors, such as the tumor-suppressor p53 and estrogen receptor (ER), are localized within mitochondria, where they exert various transcription-independent functions [83]. By using transmitochondrial cybrid systems ("cybrids"), Kaipparettu et al. [69] elegantly demonstrated that mitochondria derived from the non-transformed breast epithelial cell line MCF10A reverse the tumorigenic properties of osteosarcoma metastatic cells (e.g. cell proliferation and viability under hypoxic conditions, anchorage-independent cell growth, resistance to anticancer drugs) by suppressing several oncogenic pathways involving HER2, SRC, RAS and TP53; on the other hand, some of the tumor-suppressor genes including VHL, PTEN and RB1 were overexpressed in cytoplasmic hybrids (cybrids) with non-cancerous mitochondria.

Other studies suggested that mitochondrial dysfunction may induce epigenetic modifications within the nuclear genome, such as aberrant methylation patterns in CpG-rich regions [84, 85]. These epigenetic alterations, including DNA and chromatin modifications and signaling through small RNAs, may contribute to the maintenance of mitochondria-mediated oncogenic transformation. However, the mitochondrial signals that potentially might trigger these epigenetic changes in the nucleus remain still largely unknown [30].

ROS-induced mitochondrial deregulation has been reported to trigger a survival response by inducing the nuclear factor NF-κB pathway and stimulating the synthesis of anti-apoptotic molecules (such as Bcl-xL/Bcl-2), which in turn promote cell survival and proliferation [86].

Moreover, oxidative stress may also affect the expression of nuclear genes involved in tumorigenic and invasive phenotypes [87]. Altogether these findings suggest that targeting the retrograde signaling could be a successful therapeutic strategy for cancer.

4. Targeting mitochondria for cancer therapy

Numerous studies suggested that mtDNA alterations may contribute to chemotherapy resistance and affect radiotherapy outcome. For instance, Guerra et al. [88] showed that mutations in the NADH dehydrogenase subunit 4 (MT-ND4) lead to acquired chemoresistance during treatment with paclitaxel carboplatin.

In the last few years, spindle transfer, a promising emerging strategy aimed at generating clinical germline gene therapy against inherited mitochondrial disorders, has supported the idea of a possible gene therapy approach for the editing of somatic mtDNA alterations [89]. Ideally, repairing the mutated mtDNA sequence would also restore the normal mitochondrial function and likely induce tumor regression. Taylor et al. [90] proposed a strategy that aimed to specifically block the replication of the mutant mtDNA by peptide nucleic acid (PNA), thereby allowing the selective propagation of the wild-type DNA. Moreover, mitochondrial dysfunction might also be restored by stimulating the mitophagy process in order to eliminate the deleterious mtDNA variants [91]. Targeting DNA repair enzymes to mitochondria may be a suitable strategy to correct mtDNA mutations. For instance, cell transfection with an expression vector containing the gene coding the DNA repair enzyme human 8-oxoguanine DNA glycosylase/apurinic lyase (hOGG1) has been used to reduce free fatty acids (FFAs)-induced mtDNA damage [92]. Furthermore, overexpression of hOGG1 in mitochondria has been shown to attenuate breast cancer progression and metastasis in transgenic mice [93]. Although hOGG1 has been the most frequently employed enzyme to enhance mtDNA repair, alternative strategies targeting other proteins transferred to mitochondria, such as endonuclease III (EndoIII) and endonuclease VIII (EndoVIII), have been proposed in the last years [94–96]. Other therapeutic approaches for patients carrying mtDNA mutations are based on allotopic gene expression, as preliminary demonstrated in different mitochondrial disorders [97], and targeted restriction endonucleases. In this regard, SmaI and PstI have been used as a powerful tool for treatment of mitochondrial dysfunction, resulting in the elimination of the mutant mtDNA and restoration of normal mitochondrial functionality [98]. In the last decade, many other approaches and compounds targeting dysfunctional mitochondria have been experienced, such as signal peptides. Lipophilic cations, cell-penetrating peptides and nanoparticles. A promising approach is based on the reprogramming of energy metabolism in colorectal cancer cells, through specific mitochondria-targeting agents, such as the second-generation rosamine analogs that target complex II and ATP synthase activities of the mitochondrial oxidative phosphorylation pathway [99]. More recently, it has been argued that mitochondria of tumor-initiating cells (TICs), which play a prominent role in cancer initiation, metastasis and resistance to therapy, may be targeted by mitocan vitamin E succinate in a complex II-dependent manner [100]. Another original approach has been developed to trigger cell death signaling pathways in colorectal cancer cells [101], such as ROS-dependent apoptosis and autophagy [102]. The recent improvement of high-throughput drug-screening platforms allowed the identification of novel non-toxic mitochondrial inhibitors, as in the case of diphenyleneiodonium chloride (DPI), a strong inhibitor of mitochondrial complex I and II flavin-containing enzymes, which effectively depletes cancer stem-like cells (CSCs), one of the main drivers of poor clinical outcome in a wide variety of tumor types and especially in advanced disease states [103]. Interestingly, mitochondrial inhibition with VLX600 has also been proposed in combination with imatinib in the treatment of drug-resistant gastrointestinal stromal tumors (GISTs) [104].

Recently, morphological and ultrastructural changes in the mitochondrial cristae structure (cristae remodeling), for example, through the optic atrophy 1 (OPA1) pathway, represent an important step in apoptosis and autophagy, and a potential target for future pharmacological modulation in cancer [105].

Chromosomal translocations generating in-frame oncogenic gene fusions also represent successful examples of targeted cancer therapies, and recently it has been shown that the FGFR3-TACC3 (F3–T3) gene fusion—initially discovered in human glioblastoma and then reported in many other cancers—promotes oxidative phosphorylation, mitochondrial biogenesis and tumor growth [106–108].

5. Ultra-sensitive next-generation sequencing techniques and mitogenomics

Whole mitochondrial genome analysis by high-throughput next-generation sequencing (NGS) techniques enables the detection of low-level heteroplasmic mtDNA variants and completely revolutionized mitogenomics in the last few years [109]. This approach has been extensively applied to different mitochondrial disorders to carefully investigate the transmission dynamics of low-level maternal germline mtDNA variants across generations [110–112]. In a comparative analysis, it has been demonstrated that Sanger sequencing is valid for quantification of heteroplasmies with more than 10% of cells/mitochondria carrying the mutation, whereas NGS is capable of reliably detecting and quantifying heteroplasmic variants down to the 1% level [113]. Recently, a massive parallel sequencing (MPS) protocol reliably quantified low frequency, large mtDNA deletions in single cells with a lower detection limit of 0.5% [114]. mtDNA NGS has been also suggested as a useful quality check of pluripotent stem cells for drug discovery and regenerative medicine purposes [115].

Conventionally, DNA variants detected in a tumor sample but not in the germline counterpart (such as peripheral blood, buccal swab or saliva) are scored as somatic (likely pathogenic) mtDNA variants, otherwise they are considered as germinal variants (likely polymorphic/benign). High-throughput NGS approaches may unveil low-level germinal heteroplasmies having a tumoral tissue counterpart with higher heteroplasmy simply because of increased cell replication rate or random genetic drift phenomena and, therefore, without any deleterious oncogenic effect. The ultra-sensitive detection rate of NGS methods may be used to monitor even subtle shifts in the heteroplasmy levels of the tumor during time and potentially correlate them with tumor evolution [116]. Moreover, the possibility to easily analyze the circulating cell-free mtDNA isolated from plasma/serum ("liquid biopsy") or urine [117–119], may allow non-invasive serial sampling from the same patient.

6. Conclusions

In the last decades, evidence on the contribution of mtDNA variants to tumorigenesis has incredibly grown. Therefore, mitochondria are actually considered one of the most promising targets for novel anticancer therapies. Accordingly, mtDNA variants can be regarded as useful tumor biomarkers for clinical practice, whereas the tight communication between nuclear and mitochondrial genomes sheds new light on the molecular and functional mechanisms underlying the onset and progression of complex human diseases, such as cancer and neurodegenerative diseases.

Conflict of interest

The authors declare no conflicts of interest. This article does not contain any studies with human participants performed by the authors.

Author details

Edoardo Errichiello[1]* and Tiziana Venesio[2]

*Address all correspondence to: edoardo.errichiello@unipv.it

1 Department of Molecular Medicine, University of Pavia, Pavia, Italy

2 Unit of Pathology, Candiolo Cancer Institute-FPO, IRCCS, Candiolo, Italy

References

[1] Bogenhagen DF. Mitochondrial DNA nucleoid structure. Biochimica et Biophysica Acta. 2012;**1819**(9-10):914-920. DOI: 10.1016/j.bbagrm.2011.11.005

[2] Taylor RW, Turnbull DM. Mitochondrial DNA mutations in human disease. Nature Reviews. Genetics. 2005;**6**(5):389-402. DOI: 10.1038/nrg1606

[3] Ro S, Ma HY, Park C, Ortogero N, Song R, Hennig GW, Zheng H, Lin YM, Moro L, Hsieh JT, Yan W. The mitochondrial genome encodes abundant small noncoding RNAs. Cell Research. 2013;**23**(6):759-774. DOI: 10.1038/cr.2013.37

[4] Seligmann H. Two genetic codes, one genome: Frameshifted primate mitochondrial genes code for additional proteins in presence of antisense antitermination tRNAs. Bio Systems. 2011;**105**(3):271-285. DOI: 10.1016/j.biosystems.2011.05.010

[5] Seligmann H. Codon expansion and systematic transcriptional deletions produce tetra-, pentacoded mitochondrial peptides. Journal of Theoretical Biology. 2015;**387**:154-165. DOI: 10.1016/j.jtbi.2015.09.030

[6] Gottfried E, Kreutz M, Mackensen A. Tumor metabolism as modulator of immune response and tumor progression. Seminars in Cancer Biology. 2012;**22**(4):335-341. DOI: 10.1016/j.semcancer.2012.02.009

[7] Druzhyna NM, Wilson GL, LeDoux SP. Mitochondrial DNA repair in aging and disease. Mechanisms of Ageing and Development. 2008;**129**(7-8):383-390. DOI: 10.1016/j.mad.2008.03.002

[8] Georgieva E, Ivanova D, Zhelev Z, Bakalova R, Gulubova M, Aoki I. Mitochondrial dysfunction and redox imbalance as a diagnostic marker of "free radical diseases". Anticancer Research. 2017;**37**(10):5373-5381. DOI: 10.21873/anticanres.11963

[9] Calvani M, Comito G, Giannoni E, Chiarugi P. Time-dependent stabilization of hypoxia inducible factor-1α by different intracellular sources of reactive oxygen species. PLoS One. 2012;**7**(10):e38388. DOI: 10.1371/journal.pone.0038388

[10] Gebremedhin D, Terashvili M, Wickramasekera N, Zhang DX, Rau N, Miura H, Harder DR. Redox signaling via oxidative inactivation of PTEN modulates pressure-dependent myogenic tone in rat middle cerebral arteries. PLoS One. 2013;**8**(7):e68498. DOI: 10.1371/journal.pone.0068498

[11] Nakahata S, Morishita K. PP2A inactivation by ROS accumulation. Blood. 2014;**124**(14):2163-2165. DOI: 10.1182/blood-2014-08-594093

[12] Warburg O. On the origin of cancer cells. Science. 1956;**123**:309-314

[13] Sharma LK, Fang H, Liu J, Vartak R, Deng J, Bai Y. Mitochondrial respiratory complex I dysfunction promotes tumorigenesis through ROS alteration and AKT activation. Human Molecular Genetics. 2011;**20**(23):4605-4616. DOI: 10.1093/hmg/ddr395

[14] Woo DK, Green PD, Santos JH, D'Souza AD, Walther Z, Martin WD, Christian BE, Chandel NS, Shadel GS. Mitochondrial genome instability and ROS enhance intestinal tumorigenesis in APC(min/+) mice. The American Journal of Pathology. 2012;**180**(1):24-31. DOI: 10.1016/j.ajpath.2011.10.003

[15] Santidrian AF, Matsuno-Yagi A, Ritland M, Seo BB, LeBoeuf SE, Gay LJ, Yagi T, Felding-Habermann B. Mitochondrial complex I activity and NAD+/NADH balance regulate breast cancer progression. The Journal of Clinical Investigation. 2013;**123**(3):1068-1081. DOI: 10.1172/JCI64264

[16] Guerra F, Guaragnella N, Arbini AA, Bucci C, Giannattasio S, Moro L. Mitochondrial dysfunction: A novel potential driver of epithelial-to-mesenchymal transition in cancer. Frontiers in Oncology. 2017;**7**:295. DOI: 10.3389/fonc.2017.00295

[17] Webb E, Broderick P, Chandler I, Lubbe S, Penegar S, Tomlinson IP, Houlston RS. Comprehensive analysis of common mitochondrial DNA variants and colorectal cancer risk. British Journal of Cancer. 2008;**99**(12):2088-2093. DOI: 10.1038/sj.bjc.6604805

[18] Wang C, Zhao S, Du Y, Guo Z. Single nucleotide polymorphisms in the D-loop region of mitochondrial DNA is associated with colorectal cancer outcome. Mitochondrial DNA. Part A, DNA Mapping, Sequencing, and Analysis. 2016;**27**(6):4361-4363. DOI: 10.3109/19401736.2015.1089502

[19] Fearon ER, Vogelstein B. A genetic model for colorectal tumorigenesis. Cell. 1990;**61**(5):759-767

[20] Larman TC, DePalma SR, Hadjipanayis AG, Cancer Genome Atlas Research Network, Protopopov A, Zhang J, Gabriel SB, Chin L, Seidman CE, Kucherlapati R, Seidman

JG. Spectrum of somatic mitochondrial mutations in five cancers. Proceedings of the National Academy of Sciences of the United States of America. 2012;**109**(35):14087-14091. DOI: 10.1073/pnas.1211502109

[21] Kamiya H, Ueda T, Ohgi T, Matsukage A, Kasai H. Misincorporation of dAMP opposite 2-hydroxyadenine, an oxidative form of adenine. Nucleic Acids Research. 1995;**23**(5):761-766

[22] Abu-Amero KK, Alzahrani AS, Zou M, Shi Y. High frequency of somatic mitochondrial DNA mutations in human thyroid carcinomas and complex I respiratory defect in thyroid cancer cell lines. Oncogene. 2005;**24**(8):1455-1460. DOI: 10.1038/sj.onc.1208292

[23] Greaves LC, Preston SL, Tadrous PJ, Taylor RW, Barron MJ, Oukrif D, Leedham SJ, Deheragoda M, Sasieni P, Novelli MR, Jankowski JA, Turnbull DM, Wright NA, McDonald SA. Mitochondrial DNA mutations are established in human colonic stem cells, and mutated clones expand by crypt fission. Proceedings of the National Academy of Sciences of the United States of America. 2006;**103**(3):714-719. DOI: 10.1073/pnas.0505903103

[24] Kassem AM, El-Guendy N, Tantawy M, Abdelhady H, El-Ghor A, Abdel Wahab AH. Mutational hotspots in the mitochondrial D-loop region of cancerous and precancerous colorectal lesions in Egyptian patients. DNA and Cell Biology. 2011;**30**(11):899-906. DOI: 10.1089/dna.2010.1186

[25] Rackham O, Busch JD, Matic S, Siira SJ, Kuznetsova I, Atanassov I, Ermer JA, Shearwood AM, Richman TR, Stewart JB, Mourier A, Milenkovic D, Larsson NG, Filipovska A. Hierarchical RNA processing is required for mitochondrial ribosome assembly. Cell Reports. 2016;**16**(7):1874-1890. DOI: 10.1016/j.celrep.2016.07.031

[26] Kuznetsova I, Siira SJ, Shearwood AJ, Ermer JA, Filipovska A, Rackham O. Simultaneous processing and degradation of mitochondrial RNAs revealed by circularized RNA sequencing. Nucleic Acids Research. 2017;**45**(9):5487-5500. DOI: 10.1093/nar/gkx104

[27] Mohammed F, Rezaee Khorasany AR, Mosaieby E, Houshmand M. Mitochondrial A12308G alteration in tRNA(Leu(CUN)) in colorectal cancer samples. Diagnostic Pathology. 2015;**10**:115. DOI: 10.1186/s13000-015-0337-6

[28] Seligmann H. Pathogenic mutations in antisense mitochondrial tRNAs. Journal of Theoretical Biology. 2011;**269**(1):287-296. DOI: 10.1016/j.jtbi.2010.11.007

[29] Errichiello E, Balsamo A, M1 C, Venesio T. Mitochondrial variants in MT-CO2 and D-loop instability are involved in MUTYH-associated polyposis. Journal of Molecular Medicine (Berlin). 2015;**93**(11):1271-1281. DOI: 10.1007/s00109-015-1312-0

[30] Errichiello E, Venesio T. Mitochondrial DNA variants in colorectal carcinogenesis: Drivers or passengers? Journal of Cancer Research and Clinical Oncology. 2017;**143**(10):1905-1914. DOI: 10.1007/s00432-017-2418-2

[31] Kurelac I, MacKay A, Lambros MB, Di Cesare E, Cenacchi G, Ceccarelli C, Morra I, Melcarne A, Morandi L, Calabrese FM, Attimonelli M, Tallini G, Reis-Filho JS, Gasparre G. Somatic complex I disruptive mitochondrial DNA mutations are modifiers of

tumorigenesis that correlate with low genomic instability in pituitary adenomas. Human Molecular Genetics. 2013;**22**(2):226-238. DOI: 10.1093/hmg/dds422

[32] McFarland CD, Korolev KS, Kryukov GV, Sunyaev SR, Mirny LA. Impact of deleterious passenger mutations on cancer progression. Proceedings of the National Academy of Sciences of the United States of America. 2013;**110**(8):2910-2915. DOI: 10.1073/pnas.1213968110

[33] Sondheimer N, Glatz CE, Tirone JE, Deardorff MA, Krieger AM, Hakonarson H. Neutral mitochondrial heteroplasmy and the influence of aging. Human Molecular Genetics. 2011;**20**(8):1653-1659. DOI: 10.1093/hmg/ddr043

[34] Ramos A, Santos C, Mateiu L, Gonzalez Mdel M, Alvarez L, Azevedo L, Amorim A, Aluja MP. Frequency and pattern of heteroplasmy in the complete human mitochondrial genome. PLoS One. 2013;**8**(10):e74636. DOI: 10.1371/journal.pone.0074636

[35] Guo Y, Li CI, Sheng Q, Winther JF, Cai Q, Boice JD, Shyr Y. Very low-level heteroplasmy mtDNA variations are inherited in humans. Journal of Genetics and Genomics. 2013;**40**(12):607-615. DOI: 10.1016/j.jgg.2013.10.003

[36] Musicco C, Cormio A, Calvaruso MA, Iommarini L, Gasparre G, Porcelli AM, Timperio AM, Zolla L, Gadaleta MN. Analysis of the mitochondrial proteome of cybrid cells harbouring a truncative mitochondrial DNA mutation in respiratory complex I. Molecular BioSystems. 2014;**10**(6):1313-1319. DOI: 10.1039/c3mb70542k

[37] Gasparre G, Porcelli AM, Lenaz G, Romeo G. Relevance of mitochondrial genetics and metabolism in cancer development. Cold Spring Harbor Perspectives in Biology. 2013;**5**(2). DOI: 10.1101/cshperspect.a011411

[38] Sosa MX, Sivakumar IK, Maragh S, Veeramachaneni V, Hariharan R, Parulekar M, Fredrikson KM, Harkins TT, Lin J, Feldman AB, Tata P, Ehret GB, Chakravarti A. Next-generation sequencing of human mitochondrial reference genomes uncovers high heteroplasmy frequency. PLoS Computational Biology. 2012;**8**(10):e1002737. DOI: 10.1371/journal.pcbi.1002737

[39] Ye K, Lu J, Ma F, Keinan A, Gu Z. Extensive pathogenicity of mitochondrial heteroplasmy in healthy human individuals. Proceedings of the National Academy of Sciences of the United States of America. 2014;**111**(29):10654-10659. DOI: 10.1073/pnas.1403521111

[40] Polyak K, Li Y, Zhu H, Lengauer C, Willson JK, Markowitz SD, Trush MA, Kinzler KW, Vogelstein B. Somatic mutations of the mitochondrial genome in human colorectal tumours. Nature Genetics. 1998;**20**(3):291-293. DOI: 10.1038/3108

[41] Chatterjee A, Mambo E, Sidransky D. Mitochondrial DNA mutations in human cancer. Oncogene. 2006;**25**:4663-4674. DOI: 10.1038/sj.onc.1209604

[42] He Y, Wu J, Dressman DC, Iacobuzio-Donahue C, Markowitz SD, Velculescu VE, Diaz LA Jr, Kinzler KW, Vogelstein B, Papadopoulos N. Heteroplasmic mitochondrial DNA mutations in normal and tumour cells. Nature. 2010;**464**(7288):610-614. DOI: 10.1038/nature08802

[43] Mehrabi S, Akwe JA, Adams G Jr, Grizzle W, Yao X, Aikhionbare FO. Analysis of mtDNA sequence variants in colorectal adenomatous polyps. Diagnostic Pathology 2010;**5**:66. DOI:10.1186/1746-1596-5-66

[44] JE1 L-C, McGrath JA, Uitto J. Revertant mosaicism in skin: Natural gene therapy. Trends in Molecular Medicine. 2011;**17**(3):140-148. DOI: 10.1016/j.molmed.2010.11.003

[45] Errichiello E, Berrino E, Panero M, Sapino A, Venesio T. Frequent Homoplasmic Wild-Type Reversion of Cytochrome b Variants in MUTYH-Associated Polyposis. Conference "Mitochondrial Medicine: Developing New Treatments for Mitochondrial Disease". Hinxton, Cambridge, UK: Wellcome Genome Canpus Conference Center; 4-6 May 2016. P28

[46] Thyagarajan B, Wang R, Barcelo H, Koh WP, Yuan JM. Mitochondrial copy number is associated with colorectal cancer risk. Cancer Epidemiology, Biomarkers & Prevention. 2012;**21**(9):1574-1581. DOI: 10.1158/1055-9965.EPI-12-0138-T

[47] Huang B, Gao YT, Shu XO, Wen W, Yang G, Li G, Courtney R, Ji BT, Li HL, Purdue MP, Zheng W, Cai Q. Association of leukocyte mitochondrial DNA copy number with colorectal cancer risk: Results from the Shanghai Women's health study. Cancer Epidemiology, Biomarkers & Prevention. 2014;**23**(11):2357-2365. DOI: 10.1158/1055-9965.EPI-14-0297

[48] Hofmann JN, Hosgood HD 3rd, Liu CS, Chow WH, Shuch B, Cheng WL, Lin TT, Moore LE, Lan Q, Rothman N, Purdue MP. A nested case-control study of leukocyte mitochondrial DNA copy number and renal cell carcinoma in the prostate, lung, colorectal and ovarian cancer screening trial. Carcinogenesis. 2014;**35**(5):1028-1031. DOI:10.1093/carcin/bgt495

[49] Chen Y, Zhang J, Huang X, Zhang J, Zhou X, Hu J, Li G, He S, Xing J. High leukocyte mitochondrial DNA content contributes to poor prognosis in glioma patients through its immunosuppressive effect. British Journal of Cancer. 2015;**113**(1):99-106. DOI: 10.1038/bjc.2015.184

[50] Jiang H, Zhao H, Xu H, Hu L, Wang W, Wei Y, Wang Y, Peng X, Zhou F. Peripheral blood mitochondrial DNA content, A10398G polymorphism, and risk of breast cancer in a Han Chinese population. Cancer Science. 2014;**105**(6):639-645. DOI: 10.1111/cas.12412

[51] Cui H, Huang P, Wang Z, Zhang Y, Zhang Z, Xu W, Wang X, Han Y, Guo X. Association of decreased mitochondrial DNA content with the progression of colorectal cancer. BMC Cancer. 2013;**13**:110. DOI:10.1186/1471-2407-13-110

[52] Delsite R, Kachhap S, Anbazhagan R, Gabrielson E, Singh KK. Nuclear genes involved in mitochondria-to-nucleus communication in breast cancer cells. Molecular Cancer. 2002;**1**:6

[53] Desler C, Munch-Petersen B, Stevnsner T, Matsui S, Kulawiec M, Singh KK, Rasmussen LJ. Mitochondria as determinant of nucleotide pools and chromosomal stability. Mutation Research. 2007;**625**(1-2):112-124. DOI: 10.1016/j.mrfmmm.2007.06.002

[54] Feng S, Xiong L, Ji Z, Cheng W, Yang H. Correlation between increased copy number of mitochondrial DNA and clinicopathological stage in colorectal cancer. Oncology Letters. 2011;**2**(5):899-903. DOI: 10.3892/ol.2011.322

[55] Smiraglia DJ, Kulawiec M, Bistulfi GL, Gupta SG, Singh KK. A novel role for mitochondria in regulating epigenetic modification in the nucleus. Cancer Biology & Therapy. 2008;**7**(8):1182-1190

[56] Gao J, Wen S, Zhou H, Feng S. De-methylation of displacement loop of mitochondrial DNA is associated with increased mitochondrial copy number and nicotinamide adenine dinucleotide subunit 2 expression in colorectal cancer. Molecular Medicine Reports. 2015;**12**(5):7033-7038. DOI: 10.3892/mmr.2015.4256

[57] Linkowska K, Jawień A, Marszałek A, Malyarchuk BA, Tońska K, Bartnik E, Skonieczna K, Grzybowski T. Mitochondrial DNA polymerase γ mutations and their implications in mtDNA alterations in colorectal Cancer. Annals of Human Genetics. 2015;**79**:320-328. DOI: 10.1111/ahg.12111

[58] Guo W, Zheng B, Cai Z, Xu L, Guo D, Cao L, Wang Y. The polymorphic AluYb8 insertion in the MUTYH gene is associated with reduced type 1 protein expression and reduced mitochondrial DNA content. PLoS One. 2013;**8**(8):e70718. DOI: 10.1371/journal.pone.0070718

[59] Tipirisetti NR, Govatati S, Pullari P, Malempati S, Thupurani MK, Perugu S, Guruvaiah P, Rao KL, Digumarti RR, Nallanchakravarthula V, Bhanoori M, Satti V. Mitochondrial control region alterations and breast cancer risk: A study in south Indian population. PLoS One. 2014;**9**(1):e85363. DOI: 10.1371/journal.pone.0085363

[60] Brown TA, Cecconi C, Tkachuk AN, Bustamante C, Clayton DA. Replication of mitochondrial DNA occurs by strand displacement with alternative light-strand origins, not via a strand-coupled mechanism. Genes & Development. 2005;**19**(20):2466-2476. DOI: 10.1101/gad.1352105

[61] Seligmann H. Coding constraints modulate chemically spontaneous mutational replication gradients in mitochondrial genomes. Current Genomics. 2012;**13**(1):37-54. DOI: 10.2174/138920212799034802

[62] Salas A, García-Magariños M, Logan I, Bandelt HJ. The saga of the many studies wrongly associating mitochondrial DNA with breast cancer. BMC Cancer. 2014;**14**:659. DOI: 10.1186/1471-2407-14-659

[63] Venderbosch S, van Vliet S, Craenmehr MH, Simmer F, de Haan AF, Punt CJ, Koopman M, Nagtegaal ID. Mitochondrial microsatellite instability in patients with metastatic colorectal cancer. Virchows Archiv. 2015;**466**(5):495-502. DOI:10.1007/s00428-015-1733-8

[64] Graziewicz MA, Day BJ, Copeland WC. The mitochondrial DNA polymerase as a target of oxidative damage. Nucleic Acids Research. 2002;**30**(13):2817-2824

[65] Máximo V, Soares P, Lima J, Cameselle-Teijeiro J, Sobrinho-Simões M. Mitochondrial DNA somatic mutations (point mutations and large deletions) and mitochondrial DNA variants in human thyroid pathology a study with emphasis on Hürthle cell tumors. The American Journal of Pathology. 2002;**160**(5):1857-1865. DOI: 10.1016/S0002-9440(10)61132-7

[66] Schwartz S Jr, Alazzouzi H, Perucho M. Mutational dynamics in human tumors confirm the neutral intrinsic instability of the mitochondrial D-loop poly-cytidine repeat. Genes, Chromosomes & Cancer. 2006;**45**(8):770-780. DOI:10.1002/gcc.20340

[67] Horan MP, Cooper DN. The emergence of the mitochondrial genome as a partial regulator of nuclear function is providing new insights into the genetic mechanisms underlying age-related complex disease. Human Genetics. 2014;**133**(4):435-458. DOI: 10.1007/s00439-013-1402-4

[68] Ju YS, Tubio JM, Mifsud W, Fu B, Davies HR, Ramakrishna M, et al. Frequent somatic transfer of mitochondrial DNA into the nuclear genome of human cancer cells. Genome Research. 2015;**25**(6):814-824. DOI: 10.1101/gr.190470.115

[69] Kaipparettu BA, Ma Y, Park JH, Lee TL, Zhang Y, Yotnda P, Creighton CJ, Chan WY, Wong LJ. Crosstalk from non-cancerous mitochondria can inhibit tumor properties of metastatic cells by suppressing oncogenic pathways. PLoS One. 2013;**8**(5):e61747. DOI: 10.1371/journal.pone.0061747

[70] Dwight T, Mann K, Benn DE, Robinson BG, McKelvie P, Gill AJ, Winship I, Clifton-Bligh RJ. Familial SDHA mutation associated with pituitary adenoma and pheochromocytoma/paraganglioma. The Journal of Clinical Endocrinology and Metabolism. 2013;**98**(6):E1103-E1108. DOI: 10.1210/jc.2013-1400

[71] Lehtonen R, Kiuru M, Vanharanta S, Sjöberg J, Aaltonen LM, Aittomäki K, et al. Biallelic inactivation of fumarate hydratase (FH) occurs in nonsyndromic uterine leiomyomas but is rare in other tumors. The American Journal of Pathology. 2004;**164**(1):17-22. DOI: 10.1016/S0002-9440(10)63091-X

[72] Ricketts C, Woodward ER, Killick P, Morris MR, Astuti D, Latif F, Maher ER. Germline SDHB mutations and familial renal cell carcinoma. Journal of the National Cancer Institute. 2008;**100**(17):1260-1262. DOI: 10.1093/jnci/djn254

[73] Janeway KA, Kim SY, Lodish M, Nosé V, Rustin P, Gaal J, et al. Defects in succinate dehydrogenase in gastrointestinal stromal tumors lacking KIT and PDGFRA mutations. Proceedings of the National Academy of Sciences of the United States of America. 2011;**108**(1):314-318. DOI: 10.1073/pnas.1009199108

[74] Simões RV, Serganova IS, Kruchevsky N, Leftin A, Shestov AA, Thaler HT, Sukenick G, Locasale JW, Blasberg RG, Koutcher JA, Ackerstaff E. Metabolic plasticity of metastatic breast cancer cells: Adaptation to changes in the microenvironment. Neoplasia. 2015;**17**(8):671-684. DOI: 10.1016/j.neo.2015.08.005

[75] Paschka P, Schlenk RF, Gaidzik VI, Habdank M, Krönke J, Bullinger L, et al. IDH1 and IDH2 mutations are frequent genetic alterations in acute myeloid leukemia and confer adverse prognosis in cytogenetically normal acute myeloid leukemia with NPM1 mutation without FLT3 internal tandem duplication. Journal of Clinical Oncology. 2010;**28**(22):3636-3643. DOI: 10.1200/JCO.2010.28.3762

[76] Parsons DW, Jones S, Zhang X, Lin JC, Leary RJ, Angenendt P, et al. An integrated genomic analysis of human glioblastoma multiforme. Science. 2008;**321**(5897):1807-1812. DOI: 10.1126/science.1164382

[77] Taylor BS, Schultz N, Hieronymus H, Gopalan A, Xiao Y, Carver BS, et al. Integrative genomic profiling of human prostate cancer. Cancer Cell. 2010;**18**(1):11-22. DOI: 10.1016/j.ccr.2010.05.026

[78] Li WL, Xiao MS, Zhang DF, Yu D, Yang RX, Li XY, Yao YG. Mutation and expression analysis of the IDH1, IDH2, DNMT3A, and MYD88 genes in colorectal cancer. Gene. 2014;**546**(2):263-270. DOI: 10.1016/j.gene.2014.05.070

[79] Venesio T, Balsamo A, Errichiello E, Ranzani GN, Risio M. Oxidative DNA damage drives carcinogenesis in MUTYH-associated-polyposis by specific mutations of mitochondrial and MAPK genes. Modern Pathology. 2013;**26**(10):1371-1381. DOI: 10.1038/modpathol.2013.66

[80] de Araujo LF, Fonseca AS, Muys BR, Plaça JR, Bueno RB, Lorenzi JC, Santos AR, Molfetta GA, Zanette DL, Souza JE, Valente V, Silva WA Jr. Mitochondrial genome instability in colorectal adenoma and adenocarcinoma. Tumour Biology 2015;**36**(11):8869-8879. DOI:10.1007/s13277-015-3640-7

[81] Donthamsetty S, Brahmbhatt M, Pannu V, Rida PC, Ramarathinam S, Ogden A, Cheng A, Singh KK, Aneja R. Mitochondrial genome regulates mitotic fidelity by maintaining centrosomal homeostasis. Cell Cycle. 2014;**13**(13):2056-2063. DOI: 10.4161/cc.29061

[82] Saunders W. Centrosomal amplification and spindle multipolarity in cancer cells. Seminars in Cancer Biology. 2005;**15**(1):25-32. DOI: 10.1016/j.semcancer.2004.09.003

[83] Wickramasekera NT, Das GM. Tumor suppressor p53 and estrogen receptors in nuclear-mitochondrial communication. Mitochondrion. 2014;**16**:26-37. DOI: 10.1016/j.mito.2013.10.002

[84] Bellizzi D, D'Aquila P, Giordano M, Montesanto A, Passarino G. Global DNA methylation levels are modulated by mitochondrial DNA variants. Epigenomics. 2012;**4**(1):17-27. DOI: 10.2217/epi.11.109

[85] Minocherhomji S, Tollefsbol TO, Singh KK. Mitochondrial regulation of epigenetics and its role in human diseases. Epigenetics. 2012;**7**(4):326-334. DOI: 10.4161/epi.19547

[86] Formentini L, Sánchez-Aragó M, Sánchez-Cenizo L, Cuezva JM. The mitochondrial ATPase inhibitory factor 1 triggers a ROS-mediated retrograde prosurvival and proliferative response. Molecular Cell. 2012;**45**(6):731-742. DOI: 10.1016/j.molcel.2012.01.008

[87] Kang KA, Zhang R, Kim GY, Bae SC, Hyun JW. Epigenetic changes induced by oxidative stress in colorectal cancer cells: Methylation of tumor suppressor RUNX3. Tumour Biology. 2012;**33**(2):403-412. DOI: 10.1007/s13277-012-0322-6

[88] Guerra F, Perrone AM, Kurelac I, Santini D, Ceccarelli C, Cricca M, Zamagni C, De Iaco P, Gasparre G. Mitochondrial DNA mutation in serous ovarian cancer: Implications

for mitochondria-coded genes in chemoresistance. Journal of Clinical Oncology. 2012;**30**(36):e373-e378. DOI: 10.1200/JCO.2012.43.5933

[89] Tachibana M, Amato P, Sparman M, Woodward J, Sanchis DM, Ma H, et al. Towards germline gene therapy of inherited mitochondrial diseases. Nature. 2013;**493**(7434):627-631. DOI: 10.1038/nature11647

[90] Taylor RW, Chinnery PF, Turnbull DM, Lightowlers RN. Selective inhibition of mutant human mitochondrial DNA replication in vitro by peptide nucleic acids. Nature Genetics. 1997;**15**(2):212-215. DOI: 10.1038/ng0297-212

[91] van Gisbergen MW, Voets AM, Starmans MH, de Coo IF, Yadak R, Hoffmann RF, Boutros PC, Smeets HJ, Dubois L, Lambin P. How do changes in the mtDNA and mitochondrial dysfunction influence cancer and cancer therapy? Challenges, opportunities and models. Mutation Research, Reviews in Mutation Research 2015;**764**:16-30. DOI:10.1016/j.mrrev.2015.01.001

[92] Hashizume M, Mouner M, Chouteau JM, Gorodnya OM, Ruchko MV, Potter BJ, Wilson GL, Gillespie MN, Parker JC. Mitochondrial-targeted DNA repair enzyme 8-oxoguanine DNA glycosylase 1 protects against ventilator-induced lung injury in intact mice. American Journal of Physiology. Lung Cellular and Molecular Physiology. 2013;**304**(4):L287-L297. DOI: 10.1152/ajplung.00071.2012

[93] Yuzefovych LV, Kahn AG, Schuler MA, Eide L, Arora R, Wilson GL, Tan M, Rachek LI. Mitochondrial DNA repair through OGG1 activity attenuates breast Cancer progression and metastasis. Cancer Research. 2016;**76**(1):30-34. DOI: 10.1158/0008-5472.CAN-15-0692

[94] Rachek LI, Grishko VI, Alexeyev MF, Pastukh VV, LeDoux SP, Wilson GL. Endonuclease III and endonuclease VIII conditionally targeted into mitochondria enhance mitochondrial DNA repair and cell survival following oxidative stress. Nucleic Acids Research. 2004;**32**(10):3240-3247. DOI: 10.1093/nar/gkh648

[95] Gebb SA, Decoux A, Waggoner A, Wilson GL, Gillespie MN. Mitochondrial DNA damage mediates hyperoxic dysmorphogenesis in rat fetal lung explants. Neonatology. 2013;**103**(2):91-97. DOI: 10.1159/000342632

[96] Yang XM, Cui L, White J, Kuck J, Ruchko MV, Wilson GL, Alexeyev M, Gillespie MN, Downey JM, Cohen MV. Mitochondrially targeted endonuclease III has a powerful anti-infarct effect in an in vivo rat model of myocardial ischemia/reperfusion. Basic Research in Cardiology. 2015;**110**(2):3. DOI: 10.1007/s00395-014-0459-0

[97] Manfredi G, Fu J, Ojaimi J, Sadlock JE, Kwong JQ, Guy J, Schon EA. Rescue of a deficiency in ATP synthesis by transfer of MTATP6, a mitochondrial DNA-encoded gene, to the nucleus. Nature Genetics. 2002;**30**(4):394-399. DOI: 10.1038/ng851

[98] Tanaka M, Borgeld HJ, Zhang J, Muramatsu S, Gong JS, Yoneda M, et al. Gene therapy for mitochondrial disease by delivering restriction endonuclease SmaI into mitochondria. Journal of Biomedical Science. 2002;**9**(6 Pt 1):534-541. DOI: 64726

[99] Lim SH, Wu L, Kiew LV, Chung LY, Burgess K, Lee HB. Rosamines targeting the cancer oxidative phosphorylation pathway. PLoS One. 2014;**9**(3):e82934. DOI: 10.1371/journal.pone.0082934

[100] Yan B, Stantic M, Zobalova R, Bezawork-Geleta A, Stapelberg M, Stursa J, Prokopova K, Dong L, Neuzil J. Mitochondrially targeted vitamin E succinate efficiently kills breast tumour-initiating cells in a complex II-dependent manner. BMC Cancer. 2015;**15**:401. DOI: 10.1186/s12885-015-1394-7

[101] Koehler BC, Jäger D, Schulze-Bergkamen H. Targeting cell death signaling in colorectal cancer: Current strategies and future perspectives. World Journal of Gastroenterology. 2014;**20**(8):1923-1934. DOI: 10.3748/wjg.v20.i8.1923

[102] Wilson TR, McEwan M, McLaughlin K, Le Clorennec C, Allen WL, Fennell DA, Johnston PG, Longley DB. Combined inhibition of FLIP and XIAP induces Bax-independent apoptosis in type II cancer cells. Oncogene. 2009;**28**(1):63-72. DOI: 10.1038/onc.2008.366

[103] Ozsvari B, Bonuccelli G, Sanchez-Alvarez R, Foster R, Sotgia F, Lisanti MP. Targeting flavin-containing enzymes eliminates cancer stem cells (CSCs), by inhibiting mitochondrial respiration: Vitamin B2 (riboflavin) in cancer therapy. Aging (Albany NY). 2017;**9**(12):2610-2628. DOI: 10.18632/aging.101351

[104] Vitiello GA, Medina BD, Zeng S, Bowler TG, Zhang JQ, Loo JK, Param NJ, Liu M, Moral JA, Zhao JN, Rossi F, Antonescu CR, Balachandran VP, Cross JR, DeMatteo RP. Mitochondrial inhibition augments the efficacy of imatinib by resetting the metabolic phenotype of gastrointestinal stromal tumor. Clinical Cancer Research. 2018;**24**(4): 972-984. DOI:10.1158/1078-0432.CCR-17-2697

[105] Burke PJ. Mitochondria, bioenergetics and apoptosis in cancer. Trends in Cancer. 2017;**3**(12):857-870. DOI: 10.1016/j.trecan.2017.10.006

[106] Costa R, Carneiro BA, Taxter T, Tavora FA, Kalyan A, Pai SA, Chae YK, Giles FJ. FGFR3-TACC3 fusion in solid tumors: Mini review. Oncotarget. 2016;**7**(34):55924-55938. DOI: 10.18632/oncotarget.10482

[107] Lasorella A, Sanson M, Iavarone A. FGFR-TACC gene fusions in human glioma. Neuro-Oncology. 2017;**19**(4):475-483. DOI: 10.1093/neuonc/now240

[108] Frattini V, Pagnotta SM, Tala FJJ, Russo MV, Lee SB, et al. A metabolic function of FGFR3-TACC3 gene fusions in cancer. Nature. 2018;**553**(7687):222-227. DOI: 10.1038/nature25171

[109] Briscoe AG, Hopkins KP, Waeschenbach A. High-throughput sequencing of complete mitochondrial genomes. Methods in Molecular Biology. 2016;**1452**:45-64. DOI: 10.1007/978-1-4939-3774-5_3

[110] Li M, Schönberg A, Schaefer M, Schroeder R, Nasidze I, Stoneking M. Detecting heteroplasmy from high-throughput sequencing of complete human mitochondrial DNA genomes. American Journal of Human Genetics. 2010;**87**(2):237-249. DOI: 10.1016/j.ajhg.2010.07.014

[111] Goto H, Dickins B, Afgan E, Paul IM, Taylor J, Makova KD, Nekrutenko A. Dynamics of mitochondrial heteroplasmy in three families investigated via a repeatable re-sequencing study. Genome Biology. 2011;**12**(6):R59. DOI: 10.1186/gb-2011-12-6-r59

[112] Dames S, Chou LS, Xiao Y, Wayman T, Stocks J, Singleton M, Eilbeck K, Mao R. The development of next-generation sequencing assays for the mitochondrial genome and 108 nuclear genes associated with mitochondrial disorders. The Journal of Molecular Diagnostics. 2013;**15**(4):526-534. DOI: 10.1016/j.jmoldx.2013.03.005

[113] Kloss-Brandstätter A, Weissensteiner H, Erhart G, Schäfer G, Forer L, Schönherr S, et al. Validation of next-generation sequencing of entire mitochondrial genomes and the diversity of mitochondrial DNA mutations in oral squamous cell carcinoma. PLoS One. 2015;**10**(8):e0135643. DOI: 10.1371/journal.pone.0135643

[114] Zambelli F, Vancampenhout K, Daneels D, Brown D, Mertens J, Van Dooren S, Caljon B, Gianaroli L, Sermon K, Voet T, Seneca S, Spits C. Accurate and comprehensive analysis of single nucleotide variants and large deletions of the human mitochondrial genome in DNA and single cells. European Journal of Human Genetics. 2017;**25**(11):1229-1236. DOI: 10.1038/ejhg.2017.129

[115] Perales-Clemente E, Cook AN, Evans JM, Roellinger S, Secreto F, Emmanuele V, Oglesbee D, Mootha VK, Hirano M, Schon EA, A1 T, Nelson TJ. Natural underlying mtDNA heteroplasmy as a potential source of intra-person hiPSC variability. The EMBO Journal. 2016;**35**(18):1979-1990. DOI: 10.15252/embj.201694892

[116] Pagani IS, Kok CH, Saunders VA, Van der Hoek MB, Heatley SL, Schwarer AP, Hahn CN, Hughes TP, White DL, Ross DM. A method for next-generation sequencing of paired diagnostic and remission samples to detect mitochondrial DNA mutations associated with Leukemia. The Journal of Molecular Diagnostics. 2017;**19**(5):711-721. DOI: 10.1016/j.jmoldx.2017.05.009

[117] Yu M. Circulating cell-free mitochondrial DNA as a novel cancer biomarker: Opportunities and challenges. Mitochondrial DNA. 2012;**23**(5):329-332. DOI: 10.3109/19401736.2012.696625

[118] Lu H, Busch J, Jung M, Rabenhorst S, Ralla B, Kilic E, Mergemeier S, Budach N, Fendler A, Jung K. Diagnostic and prognostic potential of circulating cell-free genomic and mitochondrial DNA fragments in clear cell renal cell carcinoma patients. Clinica Chimica Acta. 2016;**452**:109-119. DOI: 10.1016/j.cca.2015.11.009

[119] He WS, Bishop KS. The potential use of cell-free-circulating-tumor DNA as a biomarker for prostate cancer. Expert Review of Molecular Diagnostics. 2016;**16**(8):839-852. DOI: 10.1080/14737159.2016.1197121